TREATING IMPULSIVE, ADDICTIVE, AND SELF-DESTRUCTIVE BEHAVIORS

Treating Impulsive, Addictive, and Self-Destructive Behaviors

Mindfulness and Modification Therapy

Peggilee Wupperman

Foreword by Robert L. Leahy

THE GUILFORD PRESS

New York   London

The author has checked with sources believed to be reliable in her efforts to provide information that is complete and generally in accord with the standards of practice that are accepted at the time of publication. However, in view of the possibility of human error or changes in behavioral, mental health, or medical sciences, neither the author, nor the editor and publisher, nor any other party who has been involved in the preparation or publication of this work warrants that the information contained herein is in every respect accurate or complete, and they are not responsible for any errors or omissions or the results obtained from the use of such information. Readers are encouraged to confirm the information contained in this book with other sources.

Library of Congress Cataloging-in-Publication Data

Names: Wupperman, Peggilee, author.
Title: Treating impulsive, addictive, and self-destructive behaviors : mindfulness and modification
    therapy / Peggilee Wupperman ; foreword by Robert L. Leahy.
Description: New York : The Guilford Press, [2019] | Includes bibliographical references and index.
Identifiers: LCCN 2018061356| ISBN 9781462538836 (paperback) | ISBN 9781462538843 (hardcover)
Subjects: LCSH: Self-destructive behavior—Treatment. | Mindfulness-based cognitive therapy. |
    BISAC: PSYCHOLOGY / Psychopathology / Post-Traumatic Stress Disorder (PTSD). | MEDICAL /
    Psychiatry / General. | SOCIAL SCIENCE / Social Work.
Classification: LCC RC569.5.S45 W87 2019 | DDC 616.85/8200835—dc23
LC record available at *https://lccn.loc.gov/2018061356*

To my mom, dad, and aunt

About the Author

Peggilee Wupperman, PhD, is Associate Professor of Psychology at John Jay College of the City University of New York. She is also Assistant Clinical Professor at the Yale School of Medicine. Dr. Wupperman is invested in improving the understanding and treatment of individuals with dysregulated emotions and behaviors. With this aim, she has conducted basic and applied research related to mindfulness and modification therapy for more than a decade. Her publications have focused on behavior dysregulation, mindfulness, emotion regulation, emotion processing, and personality disorders. Dr. Wupperman regularly teaches classes and workshops for mental health professionals and trainees. She sees clients through the American Institute for Cognitive Therapy and through various clinical trials.

Foreword

Any clinician working in the real world of clients struggling with difficulties knows that emotion dysregulation is the key impediment to getting better. Whether it is the client with substance abuse problems, eating disorders, borderline personality, posttraumatic stress disorder, problematic behavioral habits, or even couple issues, the inability to cope with difficult emotions is a fundamental issue. If the client remains dysregulated, no amount of insight, no amount of compassion, and no structured treatment plan will get very far. The experienced clinician knows this; after going down dark alleys that lead nowhere, the clinician comes to understand that clients will stand still in an existential malaise if they cannot cope with the difficult, often overwhelming, emotions that keep them from moving forward.

Some readers will already be familiar with the castle metaphor in psychotherapy. The image is one of trying to reach the castle that is in the distance. Each step along the way may bring us closer to our destination. It is in the castle that we want to be. Along the way there are detours, ruts, chasms into which we fall, and difficult obstacles. But we keep moving toward the castle. Therapy with clients with dysregulation issues is like this journey toward the castle, except that we are on the journey with them. Sometimes we also fall down along the way.

Peggilee Wupperman's singularly insightful book is the guide along this journey. This is a book I wish I had had when I was first learning how to do therapy. It is a book that even now I have benefited from reading. It is a book any clinician, with any orientation, can find valuable. Each chapter identifies what is going on in clients' minds, the obstacles and demons that are perplexing them, and how a gifted, wise, sensitive, and experienced therapist can help along this journey. Wupperman seems to have climbed inside the head of the clients and is able to see what they see. This is a unique gift—one that she is generous to share with us. I must say that many clinical books read like they are written in a formulaic way, burdened by the dry academic jargon that makes one feel that there are no real people in the room. Wupperman's book reads like you are looking over the shoulder of someone who has walked and traveled and even stumbled along this precarious but important journey.

Her integration of mindfulness, motivational interviewing, emotion regulation strategies, and just simply excellent wisdom in working with clients is unique, in my view. While presenting ideas about clarifying values and identifying goals, Wupperman anticipates exactly the kinds of objections the client will have. She makes sense of these objections, and with empathy, compassion, and a gentle and wise nudge, she directs us in helping the client to overcome resistance to change. And while providing metaphors, insights, and detailed examples of dialogues, she also reveals the thoughts, feelings, and inevitable mistakes that we as therapists will make. This is not to criticize—no, it is to humanize the process. After all, we are human, aren't we? Let's not forget that.

I found myself fascinated with how the very techniques and concepts of mindfulness and modification therapy (MMT) are relevant to helping the therapist with his or her countertransference as well. (Is *countertransference* a word with which we, in cognitive-behavioral therapy, can cope? Yes.) If you work with dysregulated clients, you may become dysregulated yourself, or you may sit there with your patronizing diagnostic labels dismissing the client as "borderline." We all have our ways of coping; we all have defenses. But what is so refreshing and enlightening about Wupperman's book is that reading it, you know that she understands you—the therapist—and she has ideas, techniques, and insights that will help you overcome yourself. Sometimes we as therapists can be one of the obstacles in the room. Sometimes we need to get out of the way.

Each chapter in this wonderful book is filled with structured approaches, forms for clients, examples of questions that might arise, and the answers that will put them to rest. Each chapter is an example of how we can do better therapy with clients who struggle with what seems insurmountable. The metaphors throughout give a sense of richness to the journey that clients are on and soften the message for those who may feel like they are in a cauldron, falling into a chasm, or spinning in their chairs. Judgments and labels that clients use are often a reflection of the messages that they have gotten all their lives about their emotions and how they cope. Wupperman reminds us of how problematic coping makes sense, how it "works" at the moment, and how one can change this without debating, coercing, humiliating, controlling, or dismissing clients.

There is wisdom in these pages. I found myself thinking, "I wish I had said that," when I read some of these dialogues. I was comforted to see that I am not the only therapist with irrational and unhelpful thoughts—and I was especially grateful that this gifted clinician gave me the insight to change those thoughts and feelings and the permission to be imperfect.

If we see the castle in the distance as we travel along the landscape with each client, we will find that this excellent book will keep us moving forward. And, someday, if we are lucky, we will reach the castle.

ROBERT L. LEAHY, PhD
Director, American Institute for Cognitive Therapy
Clinical Professor of Psychology,
Department of Psychiatry,
Weill Cornell Medical College

Acknowledgments

I am extremely grateful to have had the chance to interact with a variety of caring, talented, and inspirational individuals while developing mindfulness and modification therapy (MMT).

Tremendous thanks go out to Robert Leahy and Richard Rogers, without whose guidance and support this book literally would not exist.

Warm thanks are also offered to the additional experts who contributed to MMT either directly or by providing mentoring in research or treatment development: G. Alan Marlatt, Bruce Rounsaville, Matthias Berking, Seth Axelrod, Sarah Bowen, Deborah Haller, Craig S. Neumann, Marsha Linehan, and Duane Fehon—as well as everyone at the Yale Psychotherapy Development Center, the American Institute for Cognitive Therapy, and the Psychology Department at John Jay College. Big thanks also go out to The Guilford Press, especially Senior Editor Jim Nageotte, for believing in MMT and providing invaluable editorial guidance. Thanks also to Senior Assistant Editor Jane Keislar, for expertly managing the editing process, and to Senior Production Editor Anna Nelson for skillfully managing the production process.

I extend gratitude to the professionals who worked to develop and evaluate the treatments that influenced MMT, which include motivational interviewing, dialectical behavior therapy, mindfulness-based relapse prevention, acceptance and commitment therapy, cognitive-behavioral therapy, and mentalization-based psychotherapy. (I won't list individual names, as I'm afraid I'll accidentally forget to include someone.)

I also offer heartfelt thanks to all the wonderful MMT project managers, research assistants, and research therapists whose contributions have been invaluable (and who will always be considered part of the MMT family): Faith Unachukwa, Briana Ryan, Michal Yehezkel Tirado, Mia Gintoft Cohen, Jennifer Varley, Jessica Dong, Ashley Spada, Emily Edwards, Eugenia Garcia Dubus, Nicole Mulvihill-Rivera, Rakhel Shapiro, Martin Viola, Qian Li, Monique DiNapoli, Amanda Reed, Amy Cunningham, Kathryn James, Melissa Fickling, Which One, Jacqueline Douglas, Jenny "Em" Mitchell, Nancy Burns, and Cameron Pugach. (Additional shout-out to Cameron and Nancy for their extensive input and their tireless proofreading of this entire book.)

For providing funding of MMT studies and related research, I thank the Donaghue Medical Research Foundation, the Research Foundation of the City University of New York, the Professional Staff Congress at CUNY, the John Jay Office for the Advancement of Research, and the National Institute on Drug Abuse.

I want to thank my family and other loved ones for their support, humor, and patience during this oh-so-long process. You know who you are, and you are cherished beyond words.

Finally, I am grateful to the therapy clients who move and inspire me on a regular basis. Deepest gratitude, respect, and affection go out to the clients who have allowed me into their lives over the years. I am honored and awed to have had the chance to work with you.

Contents

PART I

A Transdiagnostic Treatment for Dysregulated Behavior

Dysregulated behaviors are behaviors that provide relief and often pleasure, but that lead to negative consequences over time (e.g., Mezzich et al., 1997; Wupperman et al., 2015). By the time clients attend treatment for dysregulated behavior, they have likely suffered substantial negative consequences across several areas of their lives. Despite these consequences, clients often report that they feel utterly unable to resist their urges to engage in the dysregulated behavior. As a result, clients often enter treatment feeling some combination of shame, discouragement, self-hatred, helplessness, and/or ambivalence about treatment. (See the box on p. 2 and Chapter 1 for further definition of dysregulated behavior.)

The aim of this book is to help therapists improve the lives of clients who struggle with dysregulated behavior. This book provides guidelines for conducting mindfulness and modification therapy (MMT), a transdiagnostic treatment for dysregulated behavior that can be customized to target each client's specific needs and behaviors. MMT was developed to help clients move past their suffering and move closer to lives that feel fulfilling and meaningful. MMT also addresses constructs that underlie dysregulated behavior, as well as related issues with treatment engagement and motivation.

MMT strategically integrates key principles and techniques from six treatments with evidence for treating dysregulated behavior: motivational interviewing (MI; Miller & Rollick, 2012), mindfulness-based relapse prevention (MBRP; Bowen, Chawla, & Marlatt, 2010), dialectical behavior therapy (DBT; Linehan, 1993a), acceptance and commitment therapy (ACT; Hayes, Strosahl, & Wilson, 2011), cognitive-behavioral therapy (CBT; e.g., Witkiewitz & Marlatt, 2007), and mentalization-based psychotherapy (MBP; Bateman & Fonagy, 2004). By systematically focusing these evidence-based principles and techniques on dysregulated behavior, MMT provides a cohesive protocol for implementing these components strategically and efficiently.

1

Several treatments for dysregulated behavior already exist. Why would therapists want to learn yet another intervention?

- Most therapists are busy (to say the least). Learning and mastering MMT is substantially less costly, less time-consuming, and easier than learning six separate interventions.
  - Even if therapists did become proficient at all six treatments, therapists who did not know MMT would have to spend time selecting relevant components of each treatment and integrating those components into an intervention aimed at dysregulated behavior. The alternative would be to use components of different treatments without any overall strategy or unified plan.
  - In contrast, MMT allows therapists to use key components of these empirically supported treatments in a way that is strategic and efficient.
- Many clients who present with one dysregulated behavior also struggle with a second or third. MMT is the only therapy for dysregulated behavior that provides all of the following: a transdiagnostic protocol, structured guided mindfulness practices, and the ability to treat clients who are actively engaging in dysregulated behavior when entering therapy.
- Finally, due to its targeted nature, MMT can be implemented in clinical settings that might not have the resources to implement more complex, comprehensive treatments.

How does MMT compare to existing treatments?

Chapter 1 provides further details comparing MMT to specific existing treatments—including situations in which an existing treatment might be a more optimal choice than MMT. However, regardless of how laudable a current treatment might be, no treatment works for every client. MMT provides options for improving outcome for clients (and clinics) for whom existing treatments might not be the best fit.

Dysregulated behaviors are also known as *impulsive, addictive,* or *self-destructive* behaviors. When therapists hear the term *dysregulated behavior,* they often think of substance misuse, eating-disordered behavior, nonsuicidal self-injury, or issues with anger/aggression. However, dysregulated behavior includes any behavior that a person has extreme trouble resisting despite long-term harmful consequences. Examples of behaviors that may become dysregulated include spending/shopping, gambling, sexual behavior, video gaming, Internet browsing, hand washing, pornography viewing, texting exes, checking behavior, trichotillomania, kleptomania, and napping for hours.

CHAPTER 1

Challenges of Treating Dysregulated Behavior

If you are reading this book, you are likely a mental health professional who provides therapy to clients with dysregulated behavior. You may work in a setting that specializes in treating dysregulated behavior (e.g., a clinic targeting substance misuse or disordered eating), or you may work in a general setting but realize that dysregulated behavior is a problem for many of your clients.

Regardless, you are likely invested in conducting treatment that offers your clients the best possible outcomes. Although you and I may use different phrases to describe *best possible outcomes*, I believe we would agree that a desired outcome is one in which a client (1) overcomes any dysregulated behavior that interferes with living a valued life, and (2) takes steps to move closer to a life that feels more satisfying and fulfilling.

However, clients with dysregulated behavior often have great difficulty in treatment. They often feel as though the dysregulated behavior is impossible to resist, even while being aware of the negative consequences of the behavior. Consequently, they tend to display fluctuating motivation, difficulty with treatment engagement, and high dropout rates. Even for clients who don't drop out, therapy may be hindered by problems with attendance and home practice, risky behaviors, and disappointing outcomes (McFarlane, Olmstead, & Trottier, 2008; Miller, Walters, & Bennett, 2001). Even success in treatment may be a temporary accomplishment, as relapse rates are greater than 50% across dysregulated behaviors (McFarlane et al., 2008; McLellan, Lewis, O'Brian, & Kleber, 2000; Miller et al., 2001).

As a result, therapists treating clients with dysregulated behavior are at risk for developing emotional exhaustion and doubts about their effectiveness as clinicians (Koekkoek, van Meijel, & Hutschemaekers, 2006). Over time, these therapists may often experience feelings of disengagement and judgmental attitudes toward clients (e.g., Koekkoek, Hutschemaekers, van Meijel, & Schene, 2011). In other words, therapists who treat clients with dysregulated behavior are at risk of becoming less effective in helping the very clients they have chosen to treat.

The ultimate purpose of this book is to describe MMT, an approach that will improve the chances of positive outcomes for clients with dysregulated behavior. Secondary benefits may include decreasing your own chances of burnout, while also increasing your work satisfaction and improving your effectiveness as a therapist. By systematically integrating evidence-based clinical models and interventions, MMT offers a transdiagnostic intervention for improving client motivation, engagement, and (ultimately) outcome.

> **A strong word of caution before proceeding:** Therapists are often busy, which means that you may feel the urge to skip the first chapters of this book and jump straight to the guidelines and handouts for the treatment sessions. (You would not be the first therapist to skip the how-to chapters of a treatment guide.) Please resist that urge! Chapters 2–7 provide important instructions on principles, strategies, techniques, and tracking that are essential in conducting MMT effectively. In MMT, the *way* you interact with the clients is every bit as vital as whether you assign the correct mindfulness practices or handouts. To phrase it more directly: If you only utilize the session handouts without reading Chapters 2–7, you will not be providing MMT to your clients. Instead, you will be providing a treatment without any backing or rationale. The results will likely be poor for your clients and discouraging for you. Thus, you are strongly encouraged to read Chapters 2–7 before moving to Chapter 8. (To facilitate this process, Chapters 2–7 were written to be as practical and direct as possible.)

Part I of this book presents an overview of MMT, as well as guidelines for conceptualizing and collaborating with clients. Part II describes five basic MMT strategies for improving motivation, engagement, and treatment outcome. These strategies are core components that are meant to be integrated throughout every MMT session. Finally, Part III contains guidelines for conducting MMT sessions, along with handouts and therapist sheets for each session topic.

Throughout the clinical chapters, handouts and therapist sheets are labeled as *H* or *TS* (respectively), followed by the letter of the relevant session and a number signifying the order in the session. For example, *H-C1* is the first handout in Session C; *TS-F3* is the third therapist sheet in Session F; and *TS-SF1* is the first therapist sheet in a semi-flex session

WHAT *Is* DYSREGULATED BEHAVIOR?

As mentioned in the Introduction to Part I, the "dysregulated" behaviors that MMT targets are those that provide short-term relief or pleasure, but that cause harm over time (e.g., Mezzich et al., 1997). Individuals who routinely engage in dysregulated behavior tend to have extreme difficulty inhibiting the behavior, even when they know it is causing harm and even when they make sincere efforts to abstain or resist. Although these behaviors are often called *impulsive*, *addictive*, or *self-destructive* behaviors, none of these terms provide accurate descriptions of all dysregulated behaviors (e.g., Raymond et al., 1999; Wupperman et al., 2012). First, some dysregulated behaviors occur after hours of rumination and planning, so they are not consistent with the definition of *impulsive*. (A former smoker may receive a negative work review in the morning and spend the rest of the day planning how she will buy cigarettes on the way home.) Second, many behaviors do not fit the standard model of addictions. (Someone may routinely react to stress by punching walls or starting fights, but few would say that the person was *addicted* to aggressive behavior.) Third, the term *self-destructive* is problematic in that it is judgmental and also implies intent—as though the person's motive for the behavior is solely to damage or destroy her- or himself. However, most dysregulated behavior is aimed at regulating affect or decreasing urges (e.g., Goodman, 2008)—as opposed to damaging oneself. (Although damage to self and others may be one of the eventual consequences of dysregulated behavior, such damage is rarely the purpose of the behavior. Even nonsuicidal self-injury is often primarily an attempt to regulate affect or urges; Klonsky, 2007; Nixon, Cloutier, & Aggarwal, 2002). Thus, since *impulsive, addictive,* and *self-destructive* are often not accurate adjectives, this book uses the umbrella term *dysregulated behavior* (e.g., Selby et al., 2010; Wupperman et al., 2015).

> MMT has been conducted with many clients who reported current suicidal ideation and/or histories of suicide attempts; however, very few MMT clients have reported *active* suicidal urges. Although those clients progressed satisfactorily, the data are limited. Considering the severity of potential consequences, the limited amount of data, and the substantial evidence supporting DBT and other evidence-based treatments for suicidality, it is recommended that any clients seeking treatment for suicidality enter a therapy with evidence for treating this specific population.

Conventional treatments for dysregulated behavior can often be stymied because these behaviors rarely occur alone. Instead, therapists are often confronted with an array of dysregulated behaviors. For example, a client who abuses alcohol or drugs has an increased likelihood of binge eating, aggression, gambling, compulsive sex, self-injury, and smoking (e.g., Bulik, Sullivan, Cotter, & Joyce, 1997; Goodman, 2008; Klonsky & Muehlenkamp, 2007; Petry, Stinson, & Grant, 2005). From another perspective, a client who engages in binge eating has an increased probability of alcohol/drug abuse, compulsive sex, compulsive spending, self-injury, and problematic anger (e.g., Allen, Byrne, Oddy, & Crosby, 2013; Goodman, 2008; Krug et al., 2008; Vansteelandt et al., 2013).

As a further challenge, clients treated for one dysregulated behavior often segue to a "replacement" behavior once the first is addressed. For example, a person may quit drinking but begin smoking; the person may then quit smoking but begin overeating (e.g., Manley & Boland, 1983). What's more, dysregulated behaviors may even interfere with therapy itself. *Therapy-interfering behavior* is any behavior that impedes treatment engagement or outcome, such as difficulty attending sessions or problems completing home practice assignments.

As a result of the above, therapists often feel they are treating a moving target. They may become overwhelmed and uncertain when facing multiple target behaviors, transitions from one dysregulated behavior to another, and/or an array of therapy-interfering behaviors.

WHY MMT?

Therapists treating clients with dysregulated behavior need (1) a transdiagnostic treatment that includes (2) a systematic integration of therapy components with evidence for treating dysregulated behaviors. This treatment should be able to target multiple dysregulated behaviors, while also allowing customization for each client's specific behavior(s).

An Integrated Intervention Specifically Designed to Target Behavior Dysregulation

To address this need, MMT was designed by integrating key strategies and principles from six evidence-based treatments: motivational interviewing (MI), mindfulness-based relapse prevention (MBRP), dialectical behavior therapy (DBT), acceptance and commitment therapy (ACT), cognitive-behavioral therapy (CBT), and mentalization-based psychotherapy (MBP). Strategies and procedures from each of these treatments were identified, systematically integrated, and targeted toward the aim of decreasing dysregulated behavior.

MMT is a threefold intervention. It consists of explicit evidence-based methods for addressing (1) multiple dysregulated behaviors, (2) "replacement" dysregulated behaviors, and (3) broad constructs that underlie and contribute to this spectrum of behaviors. MMT also specifically targets the related clinical issues of low motivation, problems with engagement, and frequent dropout, as well as high relapse rates.

MMT is a partially manualized treatment that includes general session templates, guidelines, and principles, while also allowing the therapist to customize the treatment to fit each client's specific needs and behaviors. In implementing MMT, clinical judgment and skills are not just important; they are essential. As a therapist, you will have substantial opportunity to creatively tailor the treatment within the general MMT framework. The ultimate goals of MMT are to help each client move past dysregulated behavior and begin to move toward a life that feels more satisfying and fulfilling.

Mindfulness in the Treatment of Dysregulated Behavior

Dysregulated behaviors are commonly conceptualized as attempts to avoid or regulate negative affect and urges (Baker, Piper, McCarthy, Majeskie, & Fiore, 2004; Cooper, Frone, Russell, & Mudar, 1995; Williams, Fennell, Barnhofer, Crane, & Silverton, 2015; Witkiewitz & Bowen, 2010). In this conceptualization, negative affect can include emotions such as sadness, anxiety, or boredom, but it can also include *dissatisfaction* with the current state of being. For example, a person may think she should feel happier than she does after receiving a promotion, so she uses drugs to feel happier. Or a person may want to feel confident around friends, so he drinks to seem more confident. In both cases, the individuals did not necessarily feel *unhappy* or *unconfident* initially; instead they just didn't feel *as* happy or *as* confident as they thought they *should* feel. They were dissatisfied with what they were experiencing.

However, despite research supporting dysregulated behaviors as efforts to avoid or change negative affect and urges, the negative affect and urges may not be the primary drivers of the behaviors. After all, we all experience negative affect on a fairly regular basis, but we do not all routinely engage in harmful dysregulated behaviors. Instead, a primary problem that often underlies such behaviors is *the perceived inability to experience and tolerate* (and thus adaptively cope with) the negative affect and urges. In other words, the problem may be difficulties with mindfulness.

Mindfulness involves being aware of, attentive to, and accepting of the present moment, without feeling the need to avoid or suppress one's experiences (Kabat-Zinn, 1982). Consistently, mindfulness is negatively related to a wide variety of dysregulated behaviors (Borders, Earleywine, & Jajodia, 2010; Lavender, Jardin, & Anderson, 2009; Lundh, Karim, & Quilisch, 2007; Spinella, Martino, & Ferri, 2013; Wupperman, Fickling, Klemanski, Berking, & Whitman,

2013). Mindfulness is also associated with enhancements in neural pathways related to self-regulation (e.g., Holzel et al., 2011; Witkiewitz, Lustyk, & Bowen, 2013).

The mindfulness practices in MMT were designed to address a central construct underlying dysregulated behaviors. By integrating mindfulness with other empirically supported methods, MMT helps clients process and habituate to negative emotions and urges, thus reducing the perceived need to avoid the emotions or to act on the urges (Wupperman et al., 2012, 2015). MMT's mindfulness practices are also designed to help clients (1) become aware of conditioned reactions, and (2) tolerate their affect long enough to choose adaptive strategies for regulating emotions and behaviors—instead of responding automatically with habitual reactions (e.g., Berking & Whitely, 2014; Bowen et al., 2014; Witkiewitz et al., 2013; Wupperman, Neumann, & Axelrod, 2008). In addition, mindfulness is integrated with techniques designed to decrease interpersonal conflict and increase awareness of positive emotions (e.g., Wupperman et al., 2015)—which may also reduce the perceived need to engage in dysregulated behaviors.

Of course, mindfulness is not a magic cure for dysregulated behavior. (*Considering some of the recent hype about mindfulness, this point cannot be stressed enough.*) Clients who struggle with dysregulated behavior tend to have problems coping in a variety of areas and require more than just mindfulness to be treated effectively. Mindfulness practice also does not immediately address the difficulties with therapy alliance, motivation, homework completion, retention, and communication often experienced by such clients. Thus, although a mindfulness component may be beneficial in treating dysregulated behavior, it is not sufficient on its own. Instead, MMT strategically integrates mindfulness with other evidence-based components for addressing dysregulated behavior.

MMT: An Integrated Intervention for Behavior Dysregulation

Despite growing research supporting the potential utility of mindfulness in treatment for behavior dysregulation (e.g., Bowen et al., 2014; de Souza et al., 2015; Fix & Fix, 2013; Godfrey, Gallo, & Afari, 2015), there is still a need for a transdiagnostic treatment that can target a variety of dysregulated behaviors, including treatment-interfering behaviors. Conventional mindfulness interventions have shown great promise for treating specific areas of dysregulation (e.g., mindfulness-based eating awareness training; Kristeller, 2015) and/or targeting relapse prevention in clients no longer actively engaging in the behavior (e.g., MBRP for addictive behaviors; Bowen et al., 2010). In contrast, although MMT draws on core elements of conventional mindfulness treatments, it was designed to be transdiagnostic and to focus on individuals who are actively engaging in dysregulated behavior(s) at intake. For example, MMT (1) targets general behavior dysregulation, while also tailoring sessions and practices for specific behaviors; (2) stresses the therapy relationship; (3) includes methods for addressing motivational issues; and (4) includes methods for targeting problems with attendance and homework completion. MMT can also be customized for each client's overall goals and values, and when compared to most mindfulness-based treatments, MMT contains a greater range of skills (including mindful emotion regulation and communication skills that are specifically relevant to dysregulated behavior).

Accordingly, conventional mindfulness treatments may be more beneficial for (1) settings in which a more didactic style is needed; (2) situations in which a brief, concentrated treatment is appropriate; (3) larger groups; and/or (4) situations in which clients have already stopped the behavior but need relapse prevention skills. In contrast, MMT may be more beneficial for clients who (1) are currently engaging in the dysregulated behavior, (2) need a more individualized approach, (3) have trouble with treatment engagement, and/or (4) have multiple dysregulated behaviors (and/or the potential for multiple behaviors).

MMT also incorporates key principles and techniques of DBT and ACT (a balance of acceptance and change, as well as a focus on long-term values); however, MMT is also distinct from these treatments. MMT is a focused treatment specifically aimed at reducing dysregulated behaviors that interfere with clients' lives. All sessions and exercises involve mindfulness, and the brief added focus on mindful emotion regulation and communication is aimed primarily at decreasing dysregulated behaviors and relapse. Further, MMT includes formal, audio-guided mindfulness practices (as opposed to informal practices in DBT and ACT), a simpler range of skills and processes, and more structured home assignments.

In contrast, DBT and ACT are both comprehensive treatments. DBT was developed to alleviate suicidal behaviors and other symptoms related to borderline personality disorder. Although DBT has been adapted to target additional dysregulated behaviors (Dimeff & Koerner, 2007), these adaptations are largely comprehensive treatments that include individual therapy, group therapy, between-session coaching calls, and therapists' consultation groups. Further, DBT skills training spends equal time on mindfulness, distress tolerance, emotion regulation, and interpersonal skills. ACT is also a comprehensive treatment that has been used to treat full diagnoses or spectrums of dysfunction. It involves six interconnected therapeutic processes (the hexaflex) and is based on a theory of the relation of language to acquired stimuli.

Thus, DBT or ACT may be the clear choices when a therapist's primary goal is to provide comprehensive treatment for suicidal behaviors, borderline personality disorder, or the disorders targeted in ACT treatment manuals (e.g., anxiety, depression, chronic pain, etc.). In contrast, MMT may offer advantages when targeting dysregulated behavior is a primary goal. MMT focuses on core interventions specifically designed to target dysregulated behavior. Compared to DBT and ACT, these core interventions can be less costly, less time-consuming, and more accessible for therapists to learn and gain expertise. Treatment implementation can also be more time and cost efficient, and MMT's less complex skills were designed to be simpler for clients to learn and master. (For further information comparing MMT to mindfulness-based treatments, DBT, and ACT, see Wupperman et al., 2012, 2015.)

> This book is written for mental health professionals, regardless of whether they describe themselves as psychologists, therapists, counselors, clinicians, social workers, psychiatrists, or any other mental-health-related label. Although this book uses the term *therapist*, feel free to mentally substitute the label with which you identify, and feel free to mentally substitute *counseling* for *therapy* if that term feels more relevant to you.

BASIC DESCRIPTION OF MMT

MMT helps clients (1) clarify life values and (2) develop the capability to experience the moment—including negative emotions, thoughts, and urges—without engaging in dysregulated behaviors. MMT also targets risk factors for dysregulated behavior, such as difficulty living according to personal values, lack of pleasurable/fulfilling life experiences, difficulty with basic regulation of emotions, and problems with relationships/lack of social support.

The primary evidence for MMT is the simple fact that it systematically integrates relevant components from evidence-supported interventions for dysregulated behavior. MMT thus allows therapists to implement evidence-based principles and techniques in a cohesive protocol that is strategic, efficient, and focused.

In addition, preliminary studies of MMT's systematic integration have been conducted in four small trials and in multiple case studies. Results have shown significant decreases in a range of dysregulated behaviors. Trials have focused on (1) women court-referred for alcohol abuse and aggression (Wupperman et al., 2012), (2) adults self-referred for drug/alcohol problems and anger issues (Wupperman et al., 2015), (3) community and college adults self-referred for binge eating and depressive symptoms (Wupperman, Burns, Edwards, Pugach, & Spada, 2019a), and (4) adults with mild psychotic and/or manic features who were self-referred for opioid addiction (Wupperman, Burns, Pugach, & Edwards, 2019b). All effect sizes were large, and retention rates were consistently greater than 80%. In addition, clinical case studies of MMT for men and women of varied socioeconomic backgrounds have shown decreases in combinations of trichotillomania, smoking, bulimic episodes, compulsive checking behavior, shopping/spending, alcohol abuse, anger outbursts, computer gaming, general avoidant behaviors, and obsessively texting romantic interests (Wupperman, Burns, Spada, Pugach, & Shapiro, 2018). Thus, although the studies have been small and have not yet included a randomized controlled trial, these results—combined with MMT's integration of empirically supported methods—provide a promising evidence base. Additionally, larger trials are also scheduled.

Finally, clients in all studies tended to rate MMT as highly helpful (average ratings of 8.67–9.62 on a scale of 1–10) and reported more than 80% confidence that they would continue practicing at least some of the skills after treatment ended.

Although MMT has most often been conducted in weekly individual sessions, the frequency and format of sessions can be customized based on needs of clients and clinics. Initial sessions focus on building rapport, enhancing motivation, identifying the client's values, and improving the client's ability to mindfully experience neutral stimuli (e.g., physical sensations) without reacting to them reflexively. In later sessions, clients visualize upsetting situations and purposely experience the resulting emotions, thoughts, and urges without engaging in habitual reactions.

Ensuing sessions continue to include these elements, while also targeting issues relevant to individuals with dysregulated behaviors, including (1) mindful regulation of emotions; (2) mindful communication, understanding of others, and refusal skills; and (3) integration and generalization. After the first five sessions, therapists are encouraged to modify the order of session topics to best meet the needs of the client.

Mindfulness and related skills are taught and practiced in every session; in addition, home assignments include:

- Guided audio practices (6–15 minutes; 5 times weekly),
- Daily informal practice (average 2–3 minutes),
- Daily Log of emotions, urges, and dysregulated behaviors, and
- Further assignments that broaden daily practices.

Daily Logs and other assignments are reviewed at the beginning of each session. If necessary, the therapist nonjudgmentally helps the client recognize antecedents to lapse(s), recommit to treatment goals, and rehearse future coping. Along with the focus on mindfulness and skills training, MMT also includes a strong focus on the therapeutic relationship, with active reflection and affirmation throughout treatment.

SUGGESTED SESSION STRUCTURE: BRIEF OUTLINE

The following suggested structure applies to the second session and forward. The timelines can be somewhat flexible to allow you to modify sessions based on the client's needs.

- First 20 minutes: Greet the client and review the previous week.
  - Listen to the client's experiences and concerns; show the client that you are interested in him or her as a human being.
  - Review and discuss the Daily Log and home practice.
  - Address any issues with home practice and/or target behavior.
- Next 20–25 minutes: Introduce and discuss the current session topic.
  - Customize your explanation to fit the client's needs, values, and concerns.
  - Conduct relevant mindfulness/experiential exercise.
  - Discuss the client's understanding of and reactions to the topic.
  - Assign the home practice for the upcoming week.
- Last 5 minutes: Conduct any additional planning for the upcoming week and wrap up the session.

This book is written to be practice-focused and selectively manualized. It offers a framework for treatment, while also providing guidance on how you can tailor MMT to fit the needs of your clients and settings. In other words, MMT is not a cookie-cutter therapy. Your clinical skills and expertise are not just important; they are essential.

Depending on need, MMT can be:

1. Delivered on its own for clients who primarily need help decreasing dysregulated behavior,
2. Delivered as a "first step" treatment to decrease dysregulated (and treatment-interfering) behaviors prior to further treatment (e.g., for trauma), or
3. Integrated with treatments for disorders comorbid with dysregulated behavior (e.g., social anxiety), which might decrease co-occurring and future dysregulated behaviors.

Upcoming chapters guide you in selecting and implementing MMT components in order to customize the treatment for the specific dysregulated behavior(s), values, and needs of each client. You will also be instructed on delivering MMT in individual or group sessions.

This book provides:

1. Several hypothetical case examples and vignettes, as well as examples of dialogues from therapy sessions that cover common experiences (e.g., what to say when a client doesn't complete home practice).
2. Weekly therapist guidelines and client handouts/worksheets. The handouts/worksheets are also available on the publisher's website to download and print (see the box at the end of the table of contents). Since MMT is transdiagnostic, the handouts/worksheets use the term *target behavior* for the dysregulated behaviors. You are encouraged to download and customize the documents to fit each client's specific behavior.
3. Audios for all guided mindfulness practices, with instructions on sharing the files with your clients (see the box at the end of the table of contents).

Important note: If you are a mental health professional, you are probably pressed for time, so you may feel tempted to skim through this book as fast as possible. *Please remember that it is crucial for you to read Chapters 2–7 (on the basic MMT strategies and general guidelines) before moving to the detailed session descriptions that begin in Chapter 8.* (Thank you for your patience in reading these reminders.)

Chapter Summary

- Dysregulated behaviors provide short-term relief or pleasure, but lead to negative consequences over time. Persons who routinely engage in dysregulated behavior tend to have extreme difficulty resisting the behavior, even when they know it is causing harm.

- MMT is a transdiagnostic therapy that integrates evidence-supported methods for addressing (1) multiple dysregulated behaviors, (2) "replacement" dysregulated behaviors, and (3) broad constructs that underlie and contribute to this spectrum of behaviors. MMT also specifically targets the related clinical issues of low motivation, problems with engagement, and frequent dropout, as well as high relapse rates.

- The overriding purpose of MMT is to help each client (1) take steps toward a life that feels more satisfying and fulfilling, and (2) overcome any dysregulated behavior that interferes with moving toward such a life.

CHAPTER 2

Conceptualization and Professional Stance

Consistent with most treatments for dysregulated behaviors (Bowen et al., 2010; Linehan, 1993a; Miller & Rollnick, 2012), MMT stresses the need for a nonjudgmental and empathic conceptualization of clients. Therapists communicate this nonjudgmental empathy to clients while also working to help them make changes to move toward lives that fit their values.

If you have chosen to work with clients who engage in dysregulated behavior, you are likely a caring and empathic individual. However, clients with dysregulated behavior can be difficult to treat. I say this not to imply that the clients themselves are inherently difficult or flawed in any way. Clients with dysregulated behavior tend to react in the same ways many people would react if they had the same combination of biology and history: with a conditioned use of dysregulated behavior as a way to cope. However, these reactions sometimes have the potential to impede the therapy process unless therapists are mindful of their own responses to such reactions.

For example, many clients with dysregulated behavior arrive to treatment with expectations that can interfere with therapeutic rapport. These clients often have long histories of being judged and criticized—by family, authority figures, and even therapists. Many have been told (repeatedly) that they are selfish, weak, lazy, and/or characterologically flawed because they continue to engage in the behavior despite costs to self and others. They often expect you to have similar judgments about them, to the extent that they may initially perceive you to be judging even when you are not doing so—and they may react accordingly. Thus, building rapport can be especially challenging.

In addition, many skilled and compassionate therapists sometimes have trouble with their own reactions when treating clients with dysregulated behavior. The obvious example is a therapist's personal countertransference when a client exhibits a dysregulated behavior similar to that of an important person in the therapist's life. In these instances, you may experience frustrations and resentments similar to those that you experience toward the person in your own life.

Moreover, most therapists experience positive emotions when they feel they are successful in building rapport and helping a client make progress. We care about our clients' well-being, and we tend to feel more positively about our *own* skills as therapists when clients are "doing well." In contrast, when clients are *not* making progress, therapists may question their own skills (even when such questioning isn't warranted). Questioning along these lines can feel uncomfortable and discouraging—especially when a therapist has invested considerable emotional effort into helping a client. Instead, it is often easier to judge the client for the lack of progress (e.g., the client isn't making progress because he doesn't want to change, is selfish, isn't willing to do the work, is lazy). Once those judgments start, it can be easy to decide that the client needs to be treated with a more confrontational, critical, or dismissive style—or that the client needs to "hit rock bottom" before improving. Unfortunately, such a view is not uncommon among some therapists who treat individuals with dysregulated behavior, so blaming and labeling the client may be reinforced by other therapists.

Even extremely compassionate and empathic therapists may sometimes find themselves feeling irritated and judgmental. However, despite the large number of treatments and theories focused on various forms of dysregulated behavior, one finding has been consistent across treatments and clinical trials: Empathic, nonjudgmental communication by the therapist is one of the biggest predictors of treatment success. In contrast, a confrontational, critical, dismissive style predicts higher dropout and poorer outcomes (e.g., Miller, Benefield, & Tonigan, 1993; Moyers & Miller, 2013).

This point is so crucial that I am going to emphasize it in ***bold italics:***

Therapist expression of empathy and nonjudgmental communication predicts improved treatment outcome. A confrontational, critical, or dismissive style predicts increased dropout and less successful outcome.

Now, talking (or writing) about the importance of nonjudgmental empathy is all well and good, but the question becomes: How does a therapist remain nonjudgmental and empathic if a client routinely misses sessions (perhaps without calling), arrives late, avoids home practice, and/or engages in target behaviors that he or she knows will lead to negative consequences for him-/herself or others?

Answer: The therapist works to understand what is going on with the client. In other words, the key to maintaining an empathic stance is to conduct an accurate case conceptualization.

The following section describes the way MMT conceptualizes dysregulated behavior. This conceptualization is based on research and consistent with the biopsychosocial formulations of many established treatments. The primary difference in MMT is the way in which the therapist explains the formulation to the clients (described in Strategy 3A, pp. 51–56).

MMT's Conceptualization of Dysregulated Behavior

An empathic formulation helps the therapist and the client understand the client's behavior in a way that facilitates treatment engagement and improves chances of a successful outcome. Since dysregulated behaviors span a variety of actions and syndromes, the following conceptualization is general instead of specific. As with any psychological construct, all aspects may not apply to every client; thus, the explanation may be modified to fit particular clients and particular behaviors.

The description in the next paragraph provides an overview of a basic research-based explanation of the biopsychosocial conceptualization. Strategy 3A describes this conceptualization in the way you will explain it to clients. (The description in Strategy 3A is easier for clients to understand and remember. It is also more fun; see the "Boiling Pot Metaphor," pp. 51–56.)

According to the biopsychosocial theory, behavior dysregulation is the result of an interaction between biological, environmental, and psychological factors (e.g., Griffiths, 2005). Individuals who have a pattern of difficulty resisting dysregulated behavior(s) tend to be born with temperaments that leave them more emotionally vulnerable to such behaviors (Cheetham, Allen, Yücel, & Lubman, 2010; Eisenberg & Morris, 2002; Griffiths, 2005). These individuals are often described as having heightened emotional reactivity. In addition, some dysregulated behaviors, such as alcohol misuse, have a genetic component (Goldman, Oroszi, & Ducci, 2005). Finally, some prenatal experiences (use of drugs/alcohol by mother, poor nutrition, etc.) may also contribute to an increased vulnerability to dysregulated behaviors (Day, Helsel, Sonon, & Goldschmidt, 2013). However, persons without any known genetic predispositions or suboptimal prenatal conditions can also be born with vulnerable temperaments.

A temperamental predisposition does not mean that a person will definitely—or even probably—develop problems with dysregulated behavior. Instead, such persons have a vulnerability to developing such issues under the "right" environmental circumstances. This fact is noteworthy, because *contrary to popular expectations, the belief that dysregulated behaviors are caused by inalterable biological factors causes more stigma—not less* (e.g., Racine, Bell, Zizzo, & Green, 2015). This belief in patients also decreases their motivation to work toward change. After all, why make an effort to change something that is predetermined by biology?

Environmental risk factors for dysregulated behavior usually involve repeated adverse or invalidating childhood experiences (Gratz, 2006; Krause, Mendelson, & Lynch, 2003; Moulton, Newman, Power, Swanson, & Day, 2015). Adverse childhood experiences include those in which important others (often caretakers) fail to provide acknowledgment and empathy in response to the child's emotions and in response to the child herself. These experiences can leave the child doubting and judging her emotional reactions as wrong or bad. Examples include:

- Physical abuse, sexual abuse, emotional abuse, or neglect.
- Being raised by family members who:
  - have less reactive temperaments and thus might misunderstand and criticize the child's strong emotional reactions (leaving the child to believe that something about his or her emotions are wrong), or
  - lack the ability to adaptively tolerate and regulate their own emotions, and thereby model invalidation and dysregulated behavior to the child.
- Adverse experiences entirely outside of the home, such as mistreatment by another caretaker; victimization by bullying or sexual assault; "routine" mistreatment related to racism, sexism, homophobia, xenophobia, or other forms of bigotry (see the box on p. 15); routine exclusion by other school children (leaving the child to feel like she must be unlikable or "wrong" since she does not fit in), etc.

Repeated adverse experiences are emotionally painful for anyone. In individuals with emotionally reactive temperaments, such experiences are even more painful. Eventually, the pain begins to feel unbearable. As a consequence, the individuals often begin fearing and avoiding any situation with even the potential of evoking distressing or even uncomfortable emotions. Unfortunately, avoidance of emotions tends to cause the emotions to persist and become more intense over time (e.g., Hayes, Beevers, Feldman, Laurenceau, & Perlman, 2005), which can eventually lead the emotions to seem even more intolerable (and even more crucial to avoid). In situations when these individuals *cannot* avoid negative emotions (which happens regularly for most people), they may feel compelled to react with dysregulated behaviors aimed at quickly "turning off" the dreaded emotions. These behaviors work all too well in providing relief and decreasing negative emotions in the short term—which only reinforces the behaviors, rendering them more likely to occur again. Over time, the dysregulated behaviors may become automatic reactions to any sign of possible discomfort.

> Research shows that differential treatment based on race, culture, gender, sexual orientation, and other forms of diversity is a given, even when not obvious or intentional (e.g., Koch, D'Mello, & Sackett, 2015; Milkman, Akinola, & Chugh, 2015; Saucier, Miller, & Doucet, 2005; Tenenbaum & Ruck, 2007). Although overt acts of bigotry can be conceptualized more obviously as adverse experiences, therapists are also encouraged to be aware of more subtle forms of differential treatment that can also affect clients' experiences.

In addition to instigating dysregulated behaviors, adverse childhood experiences can also contribute to the maintenance of these behaviors. Adverse childhood experiences usually do not reinforce adaptive behaviors—but *do* reinforce maladaptive behaviors, such as:

- Dysregulated behaviors aimed at "turning off" negative emotions that seem intolerable. (As described above, the dysregulated behaviors can often mute painful emotions.)
- Extreme reactions that occur in desperation when individuals feel that they need help or that nobody understands how distressed they are.
  - Extreme reactions may include anger outbursts, threatening to harm self or others, crying in response to situations that may not seem to warrant such a reaction, or any reactions that may seem more intense than justified by the situation.
  - Such reactions may sometimes be the only behaviors that motivate dismissive or invalidating others to offer help, so the person becomes conditioned to such reactions as the only way to receive help when he feels helpless or despairing.
  - Extreme reactions may also be the only reactions that lead dismissive or invalidating others to acknowledge the person's suffering, so the person becomes conditioned to such reactions as an effort to communicate pain and distress.

When drinking, binge eating, indulging in compulsive sex, or other dysregulated behaviors are the main methods a person knows for coping with emotions that seem intolerable, these behaviors will often become conditioned responses to *any* emotional discomfort. Similarly, when extreme reactions are the only actions that result in validation or help from others, these reactions may be reinforced to the point that they occur automatically without conscious intention.

THE THERAPIST'S STANCE TOWARD CLIENTS WITH DYSREGULATED BEHAVIOR

MMT views dysregulated behavior and extreme responses not as overreactions, provocations, or manipulations, but instead as *understandable responses to long-established intrapsychic and environmental reinforcers.*

> You are human (or, at least, so I assume), so you will definitely find yourself feeling judgmental about clients at times. You might also feel resistant about letting go of those judgments. Especially if you were trained to treat dysregulated behavior with a confrontational style of treatment, you might believe the client *needs* to be judged and harshly confronted. Such a reaction is natural. However, please remember that providing nonjudgmental communication is *not* the same as coddling or enabling clients. Providing empathy and nonjudgmental communication *is* the way to be most effective in helping clients change. You will still work to help clients change—even while expressing empathy about the difficulty/ambivalence/pain in doing so.
>
> If you find yourself feeling resistant when reading the preceding paragraph, please know that you are probably not alone. It might help to ask yourself the following questions:
>
> - What is your purpose in doing this work?
>   - Is your purpose to discipline or chastise clients whose behavior you do not like?
>   - Or is it to provide the kind of treatment that is most likely to lead clients to overcome their dysregulated behavior?
>
> If you chose the latter option, then I urge you to work to provide nonjudgmental, empathic communication to clients. I also understand that it can be very difficult to do so. Feeling resistance or struggling with this concept does not mean you are not a good therapist or a kind person. It just means that you might have to work a little harder to let go of previously learned methods of dealing with clients.
>
> (P.S. See how I just encouraged you to change while also communicating nonjudgmental empathy?)

Even when therapists understand how clients became caught in the spiral of dysregulated behavior, they may become frustrated when clients continue to have difficulty stopping the behavior while receiving treatment. Again, the trick is to continue working to help the client move toward change while also doing your best to remain compassionate and nonjudgmental. More strategies for moving toward change are included in ensuing chapters. However, nonjudgmental empathy by the therapist is required before any significant change is possible.

The following reminders are provided to help clarify your understanding of how clients can find dysregulated behavior seemingly impossible to resist. This understanding is essential not just for you to be able to provide effective treatment, but also for you to help the clients understand their own difficulties with stopping the behavior. Whether they admit it to you or not, many clients are more frustrated with themselves than you can ever be with them.

- People who struggle with dysregulated behavior tend to have one primary way of coping with pain: dysregulated behavior (which I call the *target behavior*). Pain can include a variety of emotions: sadness, anxiety, loneliness, emptiness, guilt, shame, stress, self-doubt, anger, jealousy, hopelessness, fear, boredom (often a secondary emotion covering emptiness or meaninglessness), etc.

- The target behavior eases the pain and provides a release—at least for the short term.
    - Often it is the only thing that provides a release, so it is the only thing that seems to "work."
    - Over time, any pain or discomfort automatically leads to intense urges to engage in the target behavior (see "MMT's Conceptualization of Dysregulated Behavior" above).
    - The target behavior can become such a conditioned response to a variety of situations that even the situations themselves can trigger urges—even when painful emotions are not initially present. (For example, if a person becomes conditioned to drinking whenever he watches TV, he may have strong urges to drink whenever he watches TV, even if he is not experiencing any negative emotions.) However, these urges can feel so intense that attempts to resist the urges can also lead to pain and discomfort.
- Human beings are wired to try to stop the experience of pain.
    - If a person knows one primary method of stopping pain, she will likely have extreme difficulty giving up that method—even if it causes long-term harm.
    - Along with decreasing pain, the target behavior may also decrease shyness, increase self-perception of having social skills and being liked, increase feelings of belonging, and increase feelings of pleasure and comfort. Thus, giving up the target behavior can also lead to feelings of grief, a sense of isolation, and a loss of pleasure (i.e., more pain).
- However, the target behavior *increases* pain over time.
    - The more one avoids emotions, the more frightening, intolerable, and intense the emotions become. Thus, the perceived need to engage in behaviors to "turn off" the distressing emotions continues to increase over time.
    - Therein lies the dark irony: The target behavior may temporarily decrease uncomfortable emotions—but it harms the ability to tolerate future uncomfortable emotions.
    - What's more, environmental consequences of target behavior often also lead to more pain (e.g., problems with relationships, problems with work or school, and negative health consequences).
    - Some target behaviors (e.g., drug or alcohol use, binge eating) also lead to biological changes that make stopping the behavior even more difficult.
- Eventually, the target behavior becomes such a central form of coping with life that even a short period without the behavior can lead to severe urges that feel overwhelming and excruciating.
- If a human being is in enough pain, he will do whatever it takes to get out of that pain.
- Little by little, the behavior can begin to feel like one of the most essential things in the person's life—regardless of how much that person cares about anything or anyone else. Clients often are in this stage by the time they seek treatment. Is it any wonder they may have trouble stopping the behavior?

Here is another tool to remember when you start to feel judgmental about a client. Ask yourself, "Have *I* ever done something that was beneficial in the short term, but that I knew would have negative consequences in the long term?" Have you ever eaten a second donut at lunch, even though you knew you would feel guilty and sluggish the rest of the afternoon? Have you ever hit "snooze" one more time, even though you knew you might be late for work and incur the boss's reaction? Have you ever stayed up an extra hour (or two or three) surfing the Internet, even though you knew you would feel tired the next day? Have you ever skipped a workout, even though you knew you would regret it later? Have you ever binge-watched a TV show, even though you knew you would be stressed the next day because you put off that project or the cleaning you had planned to do?

We all do things that feel pleasant or relieve stress in the short term but that we regret in the long term. (If you do not, then you should write your own book to share your secret with the rest of us.) Staying up too late or eating too much at a meal may not have comparable negative consequences as routinely binge eating, gambling, or other dysregulated behaviors. But you also may not have had the same combination of temperament and adverse environment as your clients. Or if you have, then perhaps you also had some protective factors that helped keep you from being pulled as deeply into the spiral of dysregulation. Regardless, recognizing those behaviors in yourself can help you empathize with what your clients may experience when they do things that attenuate stress in the short term but increase suffering later.

The importance of introspection when working with these clients cannot be stressed enough. I have known therapists who have openly judged and criticized clients for continuing to get drunk despite negative consequences, even though those therapists continued to eat sweets despite being diabetic. I have known a therapist who threw up his hands in disgust when a client engaged in self-injury despite knowing the negative consequences, even though the therapist routinely took cigarette breaks throughout the day (with the rationale that he needed to smoke to relieve the stress of working with such "difficult" clients).

Whenever you find yourself thinking, "How could she have engaged in that target behavior when she *knew* it would hurt her in the long run?" just remind yourself of the workouts you have missed, the extra donuts you have eaten, or the times you procrastinated on that project you kept telling yourself you would start.

Remember: *It is OK to sometimes feel frustrated with a client—as long as you can continue to feel nonjudgmental compassion and empathy at the same time.*

Finally, this section would not be complete without talking about a word that I urge you to expunge from your vocabulary (at least when talking about clients). That word is *manipulating*. Unfortunately, the word *manipulating* (or *manipulative*) has become a fairly standard label for any client who behaves in ways a therapist does not like. Even kind-hearted, well-meaning therapists can easily find themselves using the word when they feel irritated with a client, especially after hearing other therapists use the word to describe *their* clients. (A cousin to the word *manipulative* is *provocative*, which also usually means that the client engaged in behavior the therapist did not like.)

Before interpreting the client's behavior as manipulative, ask yourself two questions:

1. Is it an accurate way to describe the client's behavior?
2. Is it an effective way to describe the client's behavior?

Is it accurate? Is the client really manipulating?

The word *manipulating* implies that the client is controlling your behavior through unfair, insidious, and unscrupulous tactics (*Merriam-Webster Online*, n.d.). If you say the client is manipulating you, this would imply that the client is so functional and powerful that she can *plan and implement* a strategy to actually control others—including a trained therapist! (And if you label a client as manipulative [which implies a stable trait], that would mean the client was functional and powerful enough to plan and implement strategies to control people on a regular basis!) Even more notably, calling a client *manipulative* describes her behavior in a way that sounds like she is purposely doing something that is much more unfair and unscrupulous than what most people do. Let's put aside the problem with judgments for a moment and just focus on whether the label is accurate.

Therapists sometimes call clients *manipulative* when they behave in ways the therapist interprets as "overdramatic" attempts to gain the therapist's sympathy or attention. Other times the label is used when clients become angry at one person and talk about the anger to another person. For both of these types of behaviors, I urge you to remember the MMT's conceptualization of clients. Clients with dysregulated behavior tend to feel emotions more strongly than others do, and they are often conditioned to display their emotions in ways that may seem exaggerated or dramatic, without any conscious intention of doing so. Considering the client's biosocial history, such behavior is natural—not manipulative.

However, the instances when therapists are most likely to describe the client's behavior as *manipulative* are when the client is caught lying. Often the lies involve the client's contention that he did not engage in dysregulated behavior when he actually did. Sometimes the lies involve reasons for missing a session or skipping home practice that the therapist knows to be false. Sometimes the lies even involve the client's exaggeration or fabrication of qualities about himself or incidents in his life that he thinks will seem interesting to the therapist. Basically, the lies can be divided into two types: (1) fabrications to keep from getting into trouble and/or disappointing you, or (2) fabrications to increase the chance you will care about him and/or find him interesting.

When finding yourself wanting to judge such falsehoods as manipulations, ask yourself the following:

> "Have I ever stretched the truth to keep someone from being irritated at me and/or to keep from getting into trouble?"
>
> "Have I ever insinuated that the reason I did not return an email was that I had no free time the last few days, when actually I just forgot or did not feel like taking the time to reply?"
>
> "Have I ever responded to someone's request to make plans by saying I was booked that evening, when I was actually free but did not feel like socializing?"
>
> "When I was a student, did I ever tell the professor that I missed class because I wasn't feeling well, when really I just wanted to take extra time to study or rest?"

If you answered "yes" to any of these questions, do you think of yourself as an unscrupulous manipulator? If not, then why is it OK for you (or your friends) to make excuses to stay in someone's positive regard—but not OK when the client does so, often with much higher stakes?

As for the client potentially exaggerating or even inventing qualities or circumstances that might seem likable or noteworthy, consider these self-reflective questions: Did you ever have a crush on someone and insinuate that you liked that person's favorite band or sports team a little more than you actually did? Did you ever apply for a job and exaggerate your experience a little—or perhaps modify the description of your experience to better fit what you knew the company wanted?

Most people stretch the truth at one time or another, but most people are not immediately labeled as manipulators when they do so. Again, a little introspection can be essential in maintaining empathy.

The second point to consider before labeling a client as manipulative is, Is it effective?

In short: *No,* it is not effective. Nonjudgmental communication is essential for effective treatment. Empathy is a predictor of positive treatment outcome. By labeling a client as manipulative, you are increasing the chance that you will judge and even dislike the client, and you are decreasing the chance that you will be able to provide effective treatment. Thus, if you find yourself wanting to label a client as manipulative, to yourself or others, do your best to reread this section and think of the questions above. Do your best to let go of judgment, and resist using this label when describing any of your clients.

> Clients who express anger are often also described as *splitting.* Although splitting is a psychodynamic term that was not originally meant to be judgmental, it is usually used in a judgmental way that is dismissive to the client. ("The client complained that the doctor didn't listen to her, but she was probably just splitting.") Therefore, *splitting* is also a term not used in MMT. Instead, you are encouraged to work to understand the client's reactions, which will help you to be more effective in treatment.

ASSESSMENT

The purpose of MMT is to move clients closer to lives that feel more valuable and fulfilling. Consequently, a thorough assessment of the client's values and goals is critical (to say the least). Instructions on eliciting clients' values and goals appear in Strategy 2 (on p. 46) and in the description of the intake session (on pp. 102–108). For now, just keep in mind that the client's values and goals are vital in conceptualizing the client and tailoring the treatment to fit his or her individual needs.

Regarding dysregulated behavior, the amount, extent, and consequences of the target dysregulated behavior are assessed in the intake session(s) prior to conducting MMT. Therapists are encouraged to use empirically validated assessments of the client's particular dysregulated behavior(s) if possible. MMT is a transdiagnostic treatment that can be customized to target a variety of dysregulated behaviors. Since dysregulated behaviors can include any behavior a person routinely has trouble resisting despite negative consequences, this book does not have room to provide (nor do you have time to read) details about every empirically supported assessment for every possible dysregulated behavior. However, it is worthwhile to take time to research and access validated measures for assessing the extent and consequences of the specific dysregulated behaviors with which your clients present.

Recommendations for conducting an unstructured assessment of the target behavior are provided in Chapter 7, which also includes broad guidelines for the overall intake session(s). Ongoing assessment of the behavior will occur through the client's use of the Daily Log, which is assigned every week and reviewed by the therapist at the beginning of each session.

Finally, assessing the function of dysregulated behavior is achieved by conducting a functional analysis, which is described in Chapter 6. Understanding the function of a client's dysregulated behavior is essential to treatment. However, the instructions for conducting a functional analysis are presented after the basic MMT strategies (Chapters 3–5) because the strategies describe methods of interacting with clients that are necessary for an effective functional analysis. The strategies also provide unstructured methods of understanding factors that reinforce dysregulated behaviors.

CHAPTER SUMMARY

- When conducting MMT, an empathic conceptualization of the client and her or his behavior is not just important; it is essential for successful treatment. An empathic conceptualization helps the therapist and the client understand the client's behavior in a way that facilitates treatment engagement and improves chances of a successful outcome.

- According to the biopsychosocial theory, behavior dysregulation is the result of an interaction among biological, environmental, and psychological factors.

- When conceptualizing a client, work to identify his or her values and goals, as well as the extent and function of the behavior(s) you are targeting.

- If you notice that you're having trouble remaining empathic and nonjudgmental toward a client, please refer back to this chapter to help yourself realign your attitude.

PART II

FIVE BASIC MMT STRATEGIES

MMT is grounded in five basic strategies to optimize motivation, cooperation, and outcome. These strategies are essential for effective treatment delivery. Part II (1) provides descriptions of these strategies and their primary components, (2) explains how to implement these strategies in session, and (3) offers examples of relevant therapy vignettes. The five basic strategies are presented in the following box. In addition, the primary components of each strategy are listed in boxes toward the beginning of each strategy's description. Part III of this book provides the guidelines for conducting each MMT session, with the expectation that the five basic strategies will be integrated into every component of every session.

FIVE BASIC MMT STRATEGIES

1. Maintain a strong focus on the therapeutic relationship by providing active, nonjudgmental reflection, validation, and affirmation.
2. Maintain a strong focus on client values (and how the target behavior interferes with a life consistent with those values).
3. Maintain a strong focus on helping the client understand self, behavior, and treatment.
4. Provide lots of structure and home practice (to foster habit).
5. Actively shape client behaviors, with a heavy use of validation, fostering the relationship, and supporting client values.

CHAPTER 3

Strategy 1

Strong Focus on the Therapeutic Relationship

The importance of the therapeutic relationship cannot be stressed enough. A strong therapeutic relationship is crucial for building motivation in clients who may feel ambivalent or hopeless about giving up the dysregulated behavior (and ambivalent or even resentful about attending therapy).

A. Use nonjudgmental communication to provide active reflection, validation, and affirmation.
   - Find the kernel of truth.
   - Focus on emotions whenever possible.
   - Also ask open-ended questions (but sparingly).

B. Communicate respect and positive regard whenever possible—and you have to mean it!

C. Don't argue with clients.

D. When you do (gently) push clients, explain why you are doing so and communicate caring.

E. Reflect and validate what the client brings, but sometimes (maybe often) place a little extra focus on the . . . negative.

Along with building motivation, a strong therapeutic relationship can help:

- Personalize the treatment to fit the client's values and goals.
- Reinforce treatment cooperation.
- Model the ability to mindfully experience, tolerate, and express emotions.
- Provide a corrective experience for processing emotional reactions within an empathic relationship.
- Foster basic mentalization (increased understanding of mental states of self and others).
- Help the client feel valued as a human being, which—sadly enough—is an experience that some clients may have felt rarely if ever (e.g., Castonguay & Hill, 2012; Moyers, Miller, & Hendrickson, 2005; Wolfe, Kay-Lambkin, Bowman, & Childs, 2013).

The importance of the therapy relationship is also supported by MMT trials: When clients were given end-of-treatment surveys that asked which aspects of treatment they found most helpful, more than 70% wrote answers that included the therapeutic relationship. (Common answers included "getting to talk to someone who understands me" and "talking to someone who doesn't judge me.") The surveys also provided another response that highlights the importance of the relationship: When clients were asked what they thought about treatment when they first started attending, approximately 10% reported little-to-no confidence that the treatment would work. Many of these clients said that they continued attending sessions and doing the home practice during this time at least partially because they liked talking with their therapist. Only later did they more fully believe that they could be helped by the treatment (e.g., Wupperman et al., 2018).

Sometimes clients who have recently stopped engaging in their target behavior will say to their therapist, "I'm not sure if I'm giving up this behavior *for me*. I may be doing it to please you. Is that a problem?" The answer: It's not a problem at all! It is fine if the client initially stops the behavior (or attends session or completes home practice) in order to please the therapist. (It is also fine if the client stops the behavior based on an ultimatum from a loved one or as part of a court referral.) Regardless of the reason the client initially complies with treatment, the critical elements are that the client:

- Learns to experience and tolerate uncomfortable emotions and urges without feeling compelled to engage in the target behavior.
- Learns adaptive ways of coping with emotions and moving toward a valued life.
- Understands that the dysregulated behavior interferes with living a life that fits the client's values (and with feeling like the kind of person the client wants to be).

Once clients master these three concepts and gain the ability to live without feeling controlled by the target behavior, they tend to naturally want to continue working toward regulating the behavior—regardless of how ambivalent they originally felt. The difficult part can be getting the client to the point of understanding and mastering these concepts. Getting clients to that point is one of the areas in which the therapeutic relationship is key.

Of course, talking about the importance of a strong therapeutic relationship is one thing. Actually building and maintaining such a relationship is another. *Remember:* Many of these clients have long histories of being openly judged and demeaned for their target behavior, including by previous therapists. Consequently, they may automatically assume that *you* are judging them (or will judge them if they cannot immediately succeed at stopping the behavior).

- Thus, it is understandable that some clients have difficulty trusting a therapist or showing any vulnerability.
- It also makes sense that some clients may feel defensive or initially appear defiant and resentful.

However, although building a strong relationship can be difficult, it is not impossible. The following tips can help.

STRATEGY 1A: Use nonjudgmental communication to provide active reflection, validation, and affirmation.

Important: Providing nonjudgmental communication does not mean that you will stop working for change. Providing nonjudgmental communication does *mean that you will provide the most effective method for helping the client change.* When conducting MMT, you are encouraged to actively listen for opportunities to offer nonjudgmental reflections, validations, and affirmations throughout each session.

Reflections involve rephrasing, paraphrasing, or focusing on underlying emotions. The use of reflections builds rapport by communicating that you are listening attentively and are interested in what the client just said (Miller & Rollnick, 2012). Reflections should be a frequent response throughout all sessions—especially when working to build motivation, reviewing the client's week and home practice, and discussing the difficulties of stopping the dysregulated behavior. Reflections should also be incorporated into the portion of each session that focuses on new skills. Examples of reflections include:

- *You had a busy day!*
- *He finally noticed all the work you've been doing.*
- *You're wondering if this process will be worth the effort.*
- *It sounds like the thought of living without your target behavior feels scary.*
- *You seem sad when you talk about that.*
- *How exciting!*

Along with building rapport, reflections also encourage a client to continue talking about the topic that is reflected, so reflections can be used to direct the session without subjecting the client to a barrage of questions.

CLIENT: I woke up yesterday, and all of a sudden I thought about how nice it would be to just spend the day engaging in the dysregulated behavior. I didn't do it—but I really wanted to.

THERAPIST: You felt some really strong urges.

CLIENT: Yes. And I was surprised, because I've been feeling so good and haven't had urges that strong in a while.

THERAPIST: That must have felt pretty scary.

CLIENT: It did. I started worrying that I was getting worse again.

THERAPIST: That does sound scary! And upsetting.

CLIENT: It was upsetting! I know you keep saying that it's normal for urges to come and go and that I'd probably feel them again, but I guess I thought that I was past that. (*Shakes head.*)

THERAPIST: It's natural to feel that way. [Validation] And it can be discouraging to work so hard and feel like you're finally past all the struggles—and then find out that you've still got some struggling ahead.

CLIENT: I didn't think I'd have to struggle with urges like that anymore. I want to be past all this!

THERAPIST: Of course you do! (*Pause*) But even though you were having urges—and feeling scared and discouraged—you didn't actually engage in the behavior.

CLIENT: Right. I just made myself keep busy. I went to the park and ran for a while, and then I sat at a coffee shop and played games on my smartphone.

THERAPIST: Good for you! I'm impressed. [Affirmation] That couldn't have been easy. How did you get yourself to go to the park instead of acting on the urge?

Notice how the therapist originally focused on emotions as she encouraged the client to talk about the experience of urges—which then prompted the client to further explore his emotions. When the therapist eventually reflected the client's response to the urges ("But . . . you didn't actually engage in the behavior"), the client changed focus to report how he kept from engaging in the behavior. The reflections by the therapist directed the focus of the session, while also likely seeming more natural than a series of questions ("What did you feel when you had the urges?"; "What was that like for you?"; "How did you keep from engaging in the behavior?").

Of course, questions can sometimes be necessary and effective. The therapist eventually segued to an open-ended question to encourage the client to talk about ways in which he coped. (Knowledge of effective coping strategies may be useful for the therapist in the future. In addition, such knowledge helps the client reexperience adaptive behavior—which the therapist can affirm, thus building efficacy.) However, the question about coping was likely more effective after a series of reflections than it would have been after four or five questions had already been asked.

Along with communicating interest and directing the session, reflections can also help clients experience, understand, and adaptively express emotions. *Remember:* Unpleasant emotions are often cues for dysregulated behavior, and one goal of treatment is helping clients learn how to experience and tolerate emotions. Thus, reflections that focus on emotions can help clients process and habituate to negative emotions in a setting that feels "safe" and nonjudgmental. Such reflections can also model the fact that negative emotions do not have to be scary or harmful.

Finally, reflections can also be double-sided. For example, the first "side" may reflect what the client just said (including talk that may include potential obstacles to change), and the second "side" may reflect previous client statements or actions that are related to adaptive change. (In MI, these sides are called *sustain talk* vs. *change talk*; Miller & Rollnick, 2012.) The client tends to continue talking about the topic the therapist covers last, so be sure to end with the topic you'd like the client to continue discussing.

> *Seems like you feel sad whenever you think about not going out to drink with your friends—which is understandable. I also know you've said you were sick of the way your life was going when you were drinking and would do anything not to go back to that life.*

> *Your urges were so intense that they felt almost unbearable—yet you were still able to get through the entire weekend without binge eating.*

*So, since you've stopped smoking, you've had more trouble concentrating and felt a little
more anxious. You've also noticed that you've had more energy to play sports with your
kids and you've felt like a better father.*

As shown in these examples, the *change* side can include talk about confidence, hope,
intentions, or actions related to change. In addition, discussing the client's unhappiness with
aspects of his former or current life (if still engaging in the dysregulated behavior) can also be
relevant to change, as the client's dissatisfaction can be a motivator for action.

Double-sided reflections can consist of just one or two sentences (as in the preceding examples above), or they can include a pause between the two sides—with several reflections on the
first side before moving to the *change* side. This allows the client to process thoughts and emotions related to difficulties, while also demonstrating that the therapist understands the extent
of those difficulties. In other words, it shows that the therapist understands how much the client
is struggling and perhaps suffering—which is often necessary before the client can trust the
therapist when the therapist expresses confidence that the client can change.

Warning: *Moving away from difficulties too quickly can backfire!* Sometimes the client
might need to feel her difficulties have been heard and understood before she can even consider
the possibility of change. Thus, moving toward change too quickly can risk the client's feeling
as though she needs to work harder to convince the therapist how difficult change would be.
By spending time on the difficulty before moving toward change, the therapist decreases the
chance that the client will feel defensive or unheard when the therapist moves the talk toward
change.

What happens if the therapist moves to the change side and the client continues to talk
about obstacles to change, perhaps even more strongly than before? No need to worry; it happens to the best of therapists. When the client continues to talk about obstacles in response
to your attempts to move forward, the client is just communicating that he is not ready to talk
about change at the moment. You can then move back to reflecting the obstacles for a few sentences or even several minutes (or sometimes even most of a session). Clients are not robots, and
sometimes they don't process emotions in the timeframe we might think they should. Eventually, you can use another double-sided reflection to move back toward change (possibly toning
down the level of positivity on the change side)—and/or you can utilize one of the other MMT
strategies. (Additional information about responding to ambivalence and building motivation
can be found throughout the five basic strategies, as well as in Chapter 6.)

Validation involves communicating that the person's emotions, thoughts, and/or behaviors
are understandable considering the circumstances. (These circumstances may include the client's experience[s] in the session, the client's current situation[s] outside the session, and/or the
client's childhood history.) Like reflection, validation builds rapport and motivation, while also
fostering habituation to emotions. Validation also helps clients understand their own reactions,
which in turn makes those reactions seem less scary, less shameful, and more tolerable. Validation can focus on the entire emotion/thought/behavior or on an aspect of an emotion/thought/
behavior. For example:

- *I understand how that would be scary for you.*
- *It makes sense that you would feel sad after your friend moved away.*

- *It's natural to feel anxious before a job interview. Most people would feel anxious.*
- *Of course you're having trouble concentrating! You had only 3 hours of sleep last night, and it's natural to have trouble concentrating after not getting enough sleep.*
- *Urges are normal. They don't mean you're getting worse. I know they can feel excruciating, and I'm sorry you have to feel them—but they're just a normal part of the process of getting past the target behavior.*
- *I completely get how you'd be angry by that. I'd feel angry, too.*
- *When a person is in a lot of pain, it's understandable that she or he would want to do whatever it takes to stop feeling the pain. At some point, you learned that the target behavior helped turn off the pain—at least for the short term.*
- *So it's natural that you have strong urges to engage in the behavior whenever you feel sad or scared. It doesn't mean that there's something wrong with you. [Optional:] But the trouble is that the behavior causes more pain in the long term—so we need to work to find other ways to deal with the pain.*

Of note is that validation has a lot of overlap with reflection. For example, the therapist's response of "how frustrating" could be seen as a reflection (reflecting underlying emotion) or a validation (validating that the client's frustration is understandable). The purpose of listing reflection and validation separately is to provide as much nuance and as many examples as possible. It does not really matter whether you mentally label a response as a validation or reflection. In other words, it is essential that you use reflection/validation in session; it is *not* essential (or effective) for you to get caught up in trying to find the "correct" label.

Affirmation involves reinforcing or expressing respect or appreciation. Affirmations can build rapport, self-efficacy, and motivation. When you affirm a behavior, that behavior often increases in frequency or intensity, so be sure to affirm behavior you'd like to increase. For example, providing an affirmation after a client shares emotions has the potential to increase the likelihood the client will share emotions in the future. Examples of affirmations include:

- *Thank you for being honest with me. I know it was difficult, and I appreciate that.*
- *I'm proud of you.*
- *I can tell you care a lot about your daughter; I respect that.*
- *You've been putting a lot of effort into this, and I want you to know that I see that.*
- *It took a lot of courage to come here and open up about your struggles.*
- *That's very insightful.*

The main point to remember about affirmations (and reflections and validations as well) is that they must be genuine. You *must* mean what you say. Therapists in MMT trainings sometimes ask whether affirmations might be viewed by clients as being overly positive, fake, or condescending. The answer is almost always "no"—as long as the therapist is genuine and realistic when providing affirmations. The keys to providing effective affirmations are:

- Be genuine. If you don't mean it, don't say it. However, there are ways to help you be more aware of *why* a client's behavior deserves affirmation (and therefore to be genuine in providing affirmation that you otherwise may not have considered). For more information, see the upcoming box, "How to Be Genuine in Reflecting, Validating, and Affirming," on pages 32–33.
- Make sure the intensity of the affirmation fits the situation. Otherwise, the client might think you are inauthentic or condescending.
  - Appropriate affirmations to a client who refrained from target behavior for a week include:
    - *I'm happy for you!*
    - *Great job!*
    - *You've made a lot of progress.*
    - *That's impressive.*
    - *I know you worked really hard for this.*
  - Responses that may be perceived as condescending or overly positive:
    - *That's utterly amazing!*
    - *You can do anything you set your mind to!*
- Be vigilant in looking for client behaviors to affirm. It is much easier to notice behavior that is potentially harmful than to notice behavior that is adaptive. Affirmations will eventually come naturally to you, but in the beginning, you might have to work hard to notice affirmation-worthy behavior.

When affirming client behavior, be sure to communicate that you will continue to think highly of the client even if she isn't always perfect. Otherwise, a client may be afraid of disappointing you if she has a lapse or doesn't understand the home practice, with the result that the client may have trouble attending session or being forthcoming if she thinks her recent behavior may change the way you feel about her.

> *Great job going a second week without any aggressive behavior. I'm proud of you!* (Pause) *I do want you to know that I wouldn't think less of you if you ever did have a lapse. Of course, I'd rather you* not *have a lapse, because I know that your anger outbursts get in the way of the kind of life you want. But I wouldn't think less of you or be disappointed in you. I'd just think that we would need to work together to get you back on track.*

Finally, as a client continues to make progress, therapists sometimes get so caught up in providing affirmations and reflecting positive emotions that they forget that the client probably still feels substantial negative emotions and struggles with urges at times. Consequently, clients will sometimes feel like they would disappoint their therapists if they bring up these emotions and struggles—so instead they try to hide them. ***Be sure to communicate your awareness of continued difficulty even when providing affirmations.***

> *You've made a lot of progress. I know you're not where you want to be and that it's still really difficult at times, but I'm impressed with the work you've done so far.*

How to Be Genuine in Reflecting, Validating, and Affirming

Genuineness is essential when interacting with clients. The key is to be mindful of situations from the client's perspective, and to find the kernel of truth in the emotions, thoughts, and/or behaviors.

Reflections are the easiest, as you can just rephrase what the client said and/or guess at underlying emotions.

Validations become easier when you view clients' actions based on their circumstances— and when you *don't take clients' actions personally.*

For example, you may initially have trouble understanding why a client continues to engage in dysregulated behavior when the behavior causes harm to him and distress to others. You might gain understanding if you learned that this client had a history of living in adverse environments and that the behavior was the only thing that helped him "turn off" emotions that felt unbearable. (See "MMT's Conceptualization of Dysregulated Behavior," Chapter 2, pp. 13–15, and Strategy 3A, Chapter 4, pp. 51–56.) With that knowledge in mind, it becomes understandable (and authentic to validate) that the client might:

- Feel sad and anxious when he thinks about never engaging in the behavior again.
- Feel ambivalent about stopping the behavior, since the behavior is the only thing that has worked at decreasing pain and discomfort.
- Have increased urges to engage in the behavior when feeling stress and other uncomfortable emotions.

Or, if you know that a client has a history of being treated as though his needs are not valuable, you will be more likely to understand why he may be angry and anxious when you had to reschedule a session with little notice.

I can understand how you'd feel irritated and anxious right now. You've had too many times when you've been treated like your needs don't matter—so it makes sense that you might be afraid I'm just one more person discounting your needs when I rescheduled at the last minute. I want to explain again that the reason I had to reschedule is that the office shut down due to a gas leak—not because I didn't think your needs were valuable. But it's OK if you have a little trouble trusting me for a while. I understand, and we can still work toward moving you closer to a life that feels more like the kind of life you want.

Affirmations can initially seem the most difficult; the solution is to be mindful of the client's circumstances and also look for behavior you would like to increase or maintain. For example, if you know a client feels anxious when making a phone call (which is more common than you may think), you will have an easier time affirming a client's call to set an appointment. ("Good for you! [Affirmation]. I know that phone calls take a lot of effort.")

Once you become accustomed to looking for adaptive behavior, you will find that many behaviors have some aspect that is adaptive. For example: A client misses two sessions without calling, engages in the target behavior several times since your last session, and then shows up to the current session 15 minutes late. You'll clearly need to talk about the maladaptive behavior; however, what can you possibly affirm or validate to increase the chance that your talk will be effective? Answer:

I'm glad to see you again. [Affirmation] I know it can be hard to come back to session after missing, so good for you for showing up. [Affirmation] Now, we do need to talk about the last couple of weeks. I want to help you move toward the point where you can get a job and start feeling good about your life again [Client goals], and I can't do that unless you're here to work with me. But you're here now [Implicit affirmation], so let's talk about what happened the last couple of weeks so you can get back on track.

Along with the benefits discussed above, reflections, validations, and affirmations can also decrease the chances that clients will feel defensive when you talk about problems (e.g., missing session) or behavior change. Genuine reflections and validations show the client that she is valuable enough for you to make the effort to see the situation from her point of view. Genuine affirmations show that you are aware of the client's adaptive behaviors even when you are prompting her to examine or change other behaviors. The crucial element is to be genuine. The following are responses that combine affirmations and reflections/validations with encouragement to change.

For a client who lapsed and engaged in the target behavior the previous week:

Thank you for being honest with me. That took courage, and I really appreciate it. [Series of affirmations] I know you're feeling discouraged [Reflection], but let's talk about what was going on around the time you decided to engage in the target behavior. I say this not to criticize or judge—but because if we can work to understand what was going on at the time, we can plan for ways to decrease the chance that it will happen again.

For a client who didn't do the home practice:

OK, so you didn't do the home practice—but you have *been coming to sessions. And that's important. I want you to know that I do see that you're making an effort. [Series of affirmations] I know that you're busy and that the home practice can feel tedious. [Reflection/ validation] The thing is that the home practice is important for moving toward the life you want and being able to stop binge eating—which keeps you stuck and leaves you feeling bad about yourself. [Reflection] Let's talk about what might be getting in the way of doing the home practice.*

For a client who has committed to treatment but not yet gone a week without at least one instance of target behavior—and who always has a reason why last week was the "last time":

Look, I respect you enough that I'm going to be straight with you. [Affirmation] I know you've said the reason you haven't gone a full week without the target behavior is because of unexpected crises that have been beyond your control. [Reflection] And I understand that you have a lot of things going on in your life that are hard to cope with. [Validation] The problem is that because you do have so much going on, I'm worried this pattern will keep repeating—that week after week will go by, and a crisis will happen every week, and 6 months from now you're still going to be stuck where you are now. And I care about you enough that I don't want that to happen. So I'd like to talk about ways you can get through the next week without any target behavior—even if a crisis happens that is beyond your control. Are you willing to work even harder than you've already worked so you can get past this roadblock?

Some therapists have asked whether using some of these techniques might be manipulating the client. Here is what keeps the techniques from being manipulative. In MMT, the therapist helps the client (1) identify how his or her life could feel more fulfilling and valuable, (2) overcome dysregulated behaviors that interfere with such a life, and (3) begin to take steps toward that life. Thus, these techniques are not used to meet some hidden agenda of the therapist; instead, they are used to help each client become more effective in *moving toward a life he/she has identified as a life that would fit his/her individual values.*

(This use of these techniques is also appropriate for clients who are attending therapy due to court referral or other outside pressures. See MMT Strategy 2, pp. 44–45, and Chapter 8 for more details.)

> This book uses the term *urges* to describe both the impulse and the desire to engage in dysregulated behavior. In some treatment areas (e.g., substance use, disordered eating), the term *urges* is used to describe impulses, and the term *craving* is used to indicate the desire to engage in the dysregulated behavior. However, since MMT is a transdiagnostic treatment, this book uses the term *urges* to describe both experiences.

STRATEGY 1B:
Communicate respect and positive regard whenever possible.

The reason this substrategy may sound like it is repeating points from the previous substrategy is that . . . it *is* repeating points from the previous substrategy. But this point is crucial enough that it is worth additional discussion.

Remember: Many of these clients arrive to therapy feeling frustrated and/or disgusted with themselves. They have often been criticized by most of the important (and not so important) people in their lives. They often feel strong shame about themselves and their behavior. Thus, they need (and deserve!) to receive respect and positive regard.

A goal for the first few sessions is to have the client leave each session feeling better about her-/himself than before the session. This goal is met not through insincere compliments or condescending praise, but through finding the qualities that deserve respect—in the client's behavior and/or in the client as a person. Again, you must be genuine to be effective.

For example, potential areas of focus for court-referred clients include the following:

- *Thanks for showing up for today's session. Some court-referred clients don't show up for their first session, so I appreciate that you're here.*
- *I appreciate your being so cooperative. I can understand how you'd feel resentful about being here, so I'm impressed that you've been so polite and nice about the whole thing. That says a lot about you.*
- *It takes a lot of courage to come here and be bombarded with questions by someone you don't even know—especially when you don't want to be here in the first place. Thank you for showing up and cooperating.*

Potential areas of focus for any clients include the following:

- *It takes courage to come to therapy and reveal personal details to someone you've just met. Many people know that they need therapy and tell themselves that they'll start therapy someday—but then never get the courage to actually start. It's a big deal that you took this step.*
- *You've been working very hard and putting a lot of effort into this process. I just want you to know that I get that.*
- *Thank you for being so open with me. I know it wasn't easy.*

It's important to note that sometimes clients feel uncomfortable about anything resembling praise. They may think you just don't know them well enough to know how flawed they are—or they may be afraid they will fail to live up to your expectations and disappoint you. Therefore, therapists are encouraged to ask clients about their reactions to any praise. A little discomfort is acceptable; in fact, therapists can even validate and process the discomfort. However, if the praise actually feels outright aversive to the client, the therapist can just scale back the intensity of future affirmations, at least for a while. However, the therapist should *not* stop the affirmations altogether.

STRATEGY 1C: Don't argue with clients.

Arguing isn't effective, and it will *decrease* the chance of the client being compliant (White & Miller, 2007). Now, sometimes arguing with a client might initially *seem* beneficial or even necessary. (The key word here is *seem*.) For example, a client might tell you that he is going to do something that you believe will be harmful (e.g., spend time with friends who will be engaging in the target behavior), or he might tell you that he will *not* do something you believe is necessary for progress (e.g., not attend therapy for 2 weeks while work is hectic). This substrategy does not mean that you should express agreement with everything a client says. Instead, it focuses on using strategies that are *effective* in communicating. Immediately disagreeing with a client's wants/needs/plans (and then continuing to argue your point when the client does not immediately change his mind) is *not* effective.

If/when you do find yourself tempted to argue with a client, or even feeling as though you and the client are on opposing sides, you need to step back mentally and reevaluate your next move. *The most effective strategy is to switch to reflection or validation for a few moments.* By taking a moment—or several moments—to reflect and validate, you can gain understanding of what the client is feeling, which will allow you to be more empathic and effective in your subsequent communication. Reflection and validation also show that:

1. You care about what the client is experiencing.
2. You are willing to listen instead of immediately jumping to the stereotypical therapist mode of trying to make the client fit what *you* think is "healthy."
3. You "get" the extent of the client's objections, hardships, and difficulties—while still believing in the client's ability to move toward a more valued life.

Once you gain greater understanding of the client's point of view, you may decide that the issue is not urgent enough to continue pressing at the moment. Or you might decide that you need to continue the discussion. Which bring us to Strategy 1D.

STRATEGY 1D: When you do (gently) push a client (or express an opinion that differs from the client's), explain why you are doing so and communicate caring.

First, pushing clients should be used sparingly—and should then be done gently and respectfully. Pushing clients who are ambivalent, unmotivated, or unconfident in their abilities—or who just have trouble being compliant—can lead to reactance and resistance. (Pushing *anyone* who feels ambivalent will usually just lead to that person's arguing *against* what you are pushing her to do. It is part of human nature.)

However, by explaining the reason(s) behind your pushing and the fact that you care, you communicate that you are doing your best to be on the same side as the client—as opposed to just being an authority figure trying to impose your own values. You also show that you value and respect the client enough to explain why you are pushing and how the behavior you are advocating can help the client—as opposed to just expecting the client to assume that you are right.

I'm a little concerned that I'm pushing you too hard to talk about your lapse last week, because I understand you don't want to talk about it. I don't want you to feel pressured—or to feel irritated at me for pressuring you. But the reason I want to talk about it is because I know how bad you feel about yourself when you engage in the target behavior—and I want to do whatever I can to help you stop feeling that way. By working to understand what happened when you had the lapse, we can be more effective in working to decrease the chance it will happen again. So even though I don't want you to feel pressured or irritated, I guess I'd rather risk that than worry that I'm not doing everything I can to help you move toward that life that feels more fulfilling and meaningful. I apologize if it feels like I'm pressuring you, but I'm only doing it because I care about you and think you deserve better. Does it feel like I'm judging you or criticizing? [For more information on responding to clients who have not completed home practice, see Strategy 4C, pp. 67–71.]

Also, do your best to remain open to the client's response—including any objections. Remember to include a balance of acceptance (reflection/validation/affirmation) along with any push for change. You often might end up agreeing to compromise—by agreeing to small increments in desired behavior or other types of shaping. (See Strategy 5, pp. 71–77.) You also will sometimes decide that continued pressing of the issue might not be worth risking a rupture in the relationship. Of course, you do not want the client to engage in a high-risk situation and potentially lapse back to dysregulated behavior. But if that should happen, you could always deal with the lapse in treatment. If the rapport is damaged to the extent that the relationship is ruptured and/or the client quits treatment, you will lose your ability to help the client—which is more permanent than a potential lapse.

STRATEGY 1E: Reflect and validate what the client brings, but sometimes (maybe often) place additional focus on the *negative*.

Placing focus on the negative means that the therapist should emphasize how difficult (and painful and frustrating and torturous) the process of getting past the dysregulated behavior can be. The focus on this difficulty should continue throughout the process of therapy. In addition, the therapist should also work to reflect and validate any urges and other negative emotions the client may be experiencing—even if the client has not mentioned those emotions. (*Reminder:* Negative emotions can be any emotional experience that feels unpleasant or uncomfortable.)

This substrategy may seem counterintuitive, and it definitely flies in the face of our positive-at-all-costs society; however, it can be helpful in many ways:

1. People often underestimate the difficulty of giving up dysregulated behavior. By focusing on the difficulty beforehand, you decrease the likelihood that the client is caught off guard by the actual experience. Focusing on the negative can also normalize the experience, so the client is less likely to interpret urges and negative emotions as signs of deterioration or lack of progress.

2. Some clients go through a "honeymoon" period in which the excitement about starting treatment or initial abstinence leads to marked decreases in urges and increases in positive emotions. Sadly, this stage always passes, and urges and negative emotions inevitably return. In fact, since the dysregulated behavior served as a method for coping with negative emotions, abstinence from the behavior will often lead to *increased* negative emotions until new coping is learned. By focusing on ongoing difficulty (including negative emotions and urges), you can decrease the surprise and discouragement clients may feel when urges and negative emotions return—or even increase.

3. Getting past dysregulated behavior can feel torturous, and clients will naturally question whether the therapist fully comprehends the extent of their suffering. By focusing on the painful emotions and urges, you show that you understand how overwhelming and intolerable the experience can feel. You thus increase the chance the client will think you know what you are talking about when you express belief in the client's ability to overcome the target behavior. Otherwise, you risk the client's thinking that you only believe the treatment will work because you do not understand the extent of the client's difficulty.

4. Individuals who are suffering tend to perceive the suffering as less intolerable if they believe other people can understand and empathize with their suffering—in other words, when they feel less alone in their struggles (e.g., Neff, Kirkpatrick, & Rude, 2007). Focusing on the negative can help clients feel less alone in their struggles and therefore perceive their negative emotions as less intolerable.

5. Because clients have used dysregulated behavior to "turn off" negative emotions, they often have trouble experiencing, tolerating, and processing those emotions. By placing focus on these emotions, you help clients become aware of the emotions and start to process the emotions

more adaptively. (You are helping the emotions feel less intense and overwhelming. You are also helping the client strengthen emotional muscles—which help emotions feel easier to tolerate.) In addition, these clients have often heard messages that they shouldn't feel or display negative emotions. They have often been told that they overreact and/or that negative emotions are a sign of weakness and/or that choosing to be positive is the healthiest route. A purposeful focus on negative emotions can help clients realize that these emotions are not dangerous, shameful, or a sign of pathology.

Even during times when the therapist is not focusing on negative emotions, she should at least acknowledge and validate them. This can be done through various methods, including double-sided reflections or validations. Double-sided communication can include the following. (Pauses in the following examples can be slight pauses, or they can be several minutes of conversation about the negative emotions before segueing to a different focus.)

Double-Sided Negative Emotions/Positive Emotions

- *You miss your gambling buddies and felt really lonely on Saturday. That does sound sad. (Pause) Then Sunday, you felt happy when you got to tell your brother you had gone 2 weeks without gambling.*
- *It's natural to have strong urges and feel anxious after giving up one of your main ways of coping. (Pause) You also mentioned that you feel a little excited.*

Double-Sided Negative Emotions/Affirmations

- *You miss your gambling buddies and felt really lonely on Saturday. That does sound sad. (Pause) I'm impressed that even though you felt lonely and missed hanging out with your buddies, you were able to keep working toward your values and go another week without gambling.* [If needed, the therapist might follow up with "Tell me how you got through the weekend."]
- *It's natural to have strong urges and feel anxious after giving up one of your main ways of coping. (Pause) I'm not happy that you had to go through that discomfort, but the fact that you've felt strong urges and anxiety—and yet were still able to get through the weekend without acting on the urges—is a positive sign for your success. Good for you!*

Double-Sided Negative Emotions/Facts

- *You miss the friends you did drugs with—and you felt really lonely on Saturday. That does sound sad. (Pause) Unfortunately, the alternative is risking continuing to give dirty urine samples and then spending the next year in jail.*
- *It's natural to have strong urges and feel anxious after giving up one of your main ways of coping. (Pause) Of course, with your diabetes, binge eating could get you sent to the hospital again.*

DISCUSSING NEGATIVE EMOTIONS

Therapists often report being concerned that spending time discussing negative emotions might only *increase* clients' negative emotions, especially when the client is feeling depressed and/or discouraged about treatment. Although such questioning is understandable, both research and clinical experience show otherwise (e.g., Greenberg, 2004; Miller & Rollnick, 2012). In fact, spending time on negative emotions often has the effect of *decreasing* the perceived intensity of the emotions—or at least helping the emotions feel more tolerable—even within a single session. Clients who arrive at the session feeling discouraged or depressed will often report feeling relieved after spending time exploring these emotions (although they will also often report feeling surprised at this relief). Clients rarely (if ever) report that the negative emotions have disappeared by the end of the session, but they often report that the emotions feel more tolerable.

For example, let's say a client arrives at a session saying she feels very discouraged, she engaged in the target behavior 3 days last week, she did not do home practice for the second week in a row, and she doubts that the treatment is working. The therapist will likely decide to use a flex session to target the client's disengagement with treatment. (More information about flex sessions can be found in Chapter 12.)

CLIENT: I just don't care anymore. Every day is just the same—get up, go to work, come home, eat dinner, watch TV, and go to bed. There's nothing to look forward to, just drudgery. The only fun I ever have is drinking. And now I'm trying to give that up. It's hard to make myself get up in the morning. I don't have any energy to do home practice. Truthfully, I think the audios are monotonous and not anything that will help. I don't even know if I should keep coming here.

THERAPIST: Sounds like you're feeling really depressed. And hopeless.

CLIENT: Hopeless that things will ever change. Hopeless that I can ever be happy.

THERAPIST: That sounds very depressing. And that can also be exhausting—to feel depressed and hopeless that things will ever change—but then have to get through the day.

CLIENT: Yes. I am exhausted. I'm exhausted all the time.

THERAPIST: Understandably. (*Pause*) Some people say that when they're depressed, they feel like a huge weight is on them all the time. Like doing anything—even getting out of bed—takes a tremendous effort—because they've got this weight on them.

CLIENT: (*looking at floor*) Yeah, that's how it feels.

THERAPIST: No wonder you have trouble finding enough energy to do the home practice.

CLIENT: I don't have enough energy to do anything. I just want to sleep all the time.

THERAPIST: I can sort of tell by your demeanor. You look almost like you're carrying a weight on your shoulders (*demonstrating*), like it's hard to even sit up.

CLIENT: That's exactly what it feels like. Like everything is just heavy. The world is just heavy.

THERAPIST: Some people say that when they're depressed, they feel heavy—but they also feel like they're tied up in knots inside. Others say that they feel almost like there's a darkness inside—like they're carrying around darkness. And other people say they feel almost hollow. Like there's an emptiness at the pit of their stomach. (*Pause*) Does any of this fit you? It's OK if it doesn't.

CLIENT: Emptiness. I feel empty. Heavy and empty. Like I could implode. (*Wipes tears from eyes.*)

THERAPIST: That's a very insightful description. That sounds tortuous.

CLIENT: (*Wipes tears.*) I hate feeling this way.

THERAPIST: Understandably. Depression sucks. And the hopelessness and emptiness can feel scary. Scary that things will be like this forever.

CLIENT: No, it's not even scary. I'm too exhausted to feel scared. Scared would take too much energy.

THERAPIST: The exhaustion overwhelms everything?

CLIENT: (*Nods.*)

THERAPIST: I know this is hard to talk about.

CLIENT: Yeah.

THERAPIST: I appreciate your talking about this with me. I know it can't be pleasant—to say the least. I know it's a really big deal.

CLIENT: (*after pause*) It's actually a little bit of a relief to talk about it.

After *several* more minutes of reflecting/validating, the therapist segued to the client's initial doubts about the benefits of home practice and treatment. The following is an abbreviated version of that portion of the session, without the client's reactions that occurred throughout.

Considering how depressed and exhausted you feel, I can understand how you'd question whether the home practice is working—and even whether coming to treatment is worth the tremendous effort it probably takes to get here. I appreciate your being honest about that with me. A lot of people wouldn't have been, and I'm glad you were. (Pause) I couldn't blame you if you chose to quit coming in. But I hope you don't quit. I know you're suffering a lot right now—and I hate to see that. I get that it feels terrible. But if you stop treatment now, then there's a pretty good chance things won't get better, that you'll continue to feel this way. And I'd hate that even more.

 Remember at the beginning how I said that sometimes you might feel worse before you feel better? And that sometimes you might have weeks when you feel that treatment isn't working? But that that's temporary? Well, that's where you are right now. I'm not trying to minimize how terrible it feels. I'm not saying it's OK. But it does sometimes happen, and I'd like to work with you to get you past this. I know you might not believe it's possible right now, but even though it sucks to feel hopeless, you don't even have to believe in the treatment for it to work. (Pause) So I know I'm asking a lot, but now that I know how hopeless and exhausted you feel, how about we have a do-over? Maybe I gave too much home practice without realizing how overwhelming it felt for you. Maybe we should restart with a whole new routine. You and I can work together to figure out what feels doable for you— something that will be a little challenging but still doable. Even if it means just doing one or two things between now and next week. (Pause) I know it's a lot to ask. I know that even coming here today probably seemed overwhelming. And now I'm asking for more—when getting out of bed probably felt like it was barely possible. So we can go slowly. What do you think? [This vignette was very loosely based on a combination of a few actual clinical situations. During those sessions, the therapists also assessed for suicidal ideation.]

CHAPTER SUMMARY

Strategy 1: Strong Focus on the Therapeutic Relationship

- A strong therapeutic relationship is essential for effective treatment.
- Work to provide active, nonjudgmental reflection, validation, and affirmation throughout treatment. Watch for chances to focus on emotions.
- Communicate authentic respect and positive regard whenever possible.
- Do your best not to argue with clients.
- When you do (gently) push clients, explain why you are doing so and communicate caring.
- Reflect and validate what the client brings, but often place a little extra focus on the negative.
  - Double-sided communication can be used to eventually segue to a more positive focus.
  - Double-sided communication can occur within one sentence or over the course of several minutes.

CHAPTER 4

Strategies 2 and 3

Client Values and Understanding

MMT asks a lot from clients. Giving up dysregulated behavior can feel overwhelming and painful. In addition, the treatment itself requires substantial effort, both in and out of session. Strategies 2 and 3 help build and maintain engagement during this process by focusing on client values, understanding of self, and understanding of treatment.

STRATEGY 2: STRONG FOCUS ON CLIENT VALUES— AND HOW THE TARGET BEHAVIOR (OR MISSING SESSIONS OR SKIPPING HOME PRACTICE) INTERFERES WITH A LIFE CONSISTENT WITH VALUES

A. Communicate that the target dysregulated behavior is *not* bad.
  - The target behavior is problematic because it:
    - ◆ Keeps the client from feeling like the kind of person she/he wants to be.
    - ◆ Keeps the client from living a life that feels meaningful and fulfilling.
B. Communicate that behaviors that interfere with therapy (missing sessions, skipping home practice) are also not bad.
  - They are only problematic in that they interfere with the effectiveness of the treatment— which interferes with the client's progress toward a valued life.
C. Work with the client to identify the client's values and goals. (Essential!)
  - Must be the client's values—not the therapist's. (Especially critical with clients from different cultural groups than the therapist.)
  - Use the destination metaphor.
D. Continue to focus on values throughout treatment.
E. Clients don't have to "admit" they have a problem. (They don't have to label themselves as alcoholics, addicts, overeaters, etc.)

People are more likely to take difficult action if they believe that action will help them move toward a desired outcome. Thus, it is essential that therapists help clients understand how engaging in treatment can help them move toward more desired lives, regardless of the reasons they initially began attending treatment.

STRATEGY 2A: Communicate that the target dysregulated behavior is not bad, and that clients are not bad for engaging in such behavior.

The target behavior has provided the client with relief and even pleasure; therefore, the target behavior has served a purpose. The target behavior is only problematic in that it:

- Keeps the client from feeling like the kind of person she/he wants to be.
- Keeps the client from living a life that feels as meaningful and fulfilling as it could.

Thus, the reason you work with the client to decrease the target behavior is not because the behavior is bad—and not because the client is bad (or wrong or selfish or weak) for engaging in the behavior. Instead, *the reason you work with the client to decrease the target behavior is because the behavior interferes with the client's values and the client's life*. It is crucial that the therapist communicate this point to the client—and that the therapist learns to genuinely accept this point.

To clarify: Getting drunk is not bad. Gambling is not bad. Getting high is not bad. Compulsive computer gaming is not bad. Compulsive sex is not bad. Binge eating is not bad. Binge shopping is not bad. Aggression is not bad. And so on. These behaviors probably provide the client some combination of relief, pleasure, comfort, and more—in the short term. So it is understandable why clients have been engaging in these behaviors. What *is* problematic about these behaviors is that they interfere with clients' lives. They keep clients from feeling like the kind of people they want to be and from living lives that feel satisfying. Here is an example of a therapist communicating these points to a client:

> *While you're in this clinic, we'll definitely work to stop the target behavior. But that's not the main purpose of the treatment. The main purpose is to help you move closer to living a life that fits more with what you want—and to feel more like the kind of person you want to be. So we'll work to stop the behavior—not because it's bad or that you're bad for doing it—but because it gets in the way of your moving toward the kind of life you want and the kind of person you want to be.*

This conceptualization is similar to the approach of "developing discrepancy" in MI, which involves helping clients become aware of discrepancies between their current lives and the lives they want to lead. The therapist then works to help the client realize that the target behavior plays a large role in creating or maintaining that discrepancy (Miller & Rollnick, 2012). Similarly, DBT and ACT focus on helping the client identify and move toward a life worth living or a more valued life (respectively), while framing the target behavior as an obstacle to that life (Hayes et al., 2011; Linehan, 1993a).

By helping the client see that the behavior interferes with her values—as opposed to the behavior being *bad*—you can decrease the chances of the client (1) feeling judged, (2) viewing you as being on an opposing side, (3) closing off or becoming defensive, and (4) quitting treatment. Instead, you increase the chance that the client (1) feels understood, (2) feels valued, (3) feels as though you are both working toward the same goal, and (4) feels motivated to engage in treatment and work to decrease the behavior. Remember, all of the above are *often essential* components of successful treatment.

Some clinicians have reacted to Strategy 2A by arguing that dysregulated behavior *is* bad if it has the potential to cause harm and/or goes against established societal norms (e.g., physical aggression, unsafe sex, compulsive stealing, using substances while pregnant). Such a reaction is understandable; however, *please remember that such a reaction to the client will (1) greatly increase the likelihood that the client will disengage from treatment, and (2) greatly decrease the likelihood that the client will stop or even reduce the behavior.* Most people have ways of justifying their dysregulated behavior, even behaviors such as physical aggression or stealing. Sometimes that justification is simply the fact that the client feels literally unable to stop the behavior, regardless of effort. As a therapist, you must decide whether you want to be the moralistic judge over the client's behavior—or you want to provide treatment that actually has a chance of decreasing/stopping the behavior. If the latter, it is imperative to do your best to refrain from expressing judgment—and instead help the client see how the behavior gets in the way of his life. Such a reaction is not the natural stance of most people, and you will likely have times when you have to work especially hard to be able to view the situation from the client's perspective. Once the client engages in treatment and begins to decrease the behavior, the client will often start to express remorse or regret about ways the behavior has impacted others. At that point, you can then reflect, explore, and affirm such reactions. However, the therapist's job is not to be the judge (at least not if the therapist wants to be effective).

WHAT IF THE CLIENT SAYS SHE IS COMPLETELY SATISFIED WITH HER LIFE NOW?

In other words, what if the client says that the dysregulated behavior is not interfering with the life she wants or with being the kind of person she wants to be? As a therapist, you will not be effective if you try to force your own values on your clients; however, you *can* help clients become aware of discrepancies between their current lives and the lives they want to lead. If the client is attending therapy because of the dysregulated behavior, whether mandated or not, then you automatically have a discrepancy. Just consider the *reason* the client is in therapy.

- If the client is forensically mandated for treatment, then the client's current life may involve fear of jail, meetings with probation officers, being told what to do, etc. The client may want freedom from all of that, but as long as she continues to engage in the behavior, she will remain in the criminal justice system. A primary goal would be to have a life that is free of being under the thumb of the criminal justice system.
- If the client is in treatment because his partner has threatened to leave unless he stops the behavior, then the client's current life may involve the possibility of living without the partner. A primary goal would be to continue in the relationship.
- If the client has been referred to treatment by her place of work, the client's life involves a possibility of losing her job. A primary goal would be to increase job security.

- If the client has been told he will be kicked out of his home unless he stops the behavior, then a primary goal would be to remain in his home.
- Of course, if the client is self-referred for treatment of the dysregulated behavior, then you can just ask the client directly about the negative consequences of the behavior.

The following is an example of a therapist communicating the purpose of treatment to a court-mandated client:

In the next few months, we'll work to help keep you from doing anything that could be used against you and cause you harm. So we'll work to help you stop using drugs, because if you keep using, you could be sent to jail. (Pause) But working on the drug use isn't the only purpose. The overall purpose is to help you move closer to a life that fits more with the kind of life you want. And I don't think being controlled by the courts is the kind of life you want. So we'll work to get you to the point where you're free of the criminal justice system—free of being told what to do, free of feeling like you're under a spotlight, and free of worrying that one wrong move could totally ruin your life. We'll work on helping you stop using drugs—not because it's bad or wrong, but because it gets in the way of your getting free of the justice system, and in the way of living the kind of life that you want to live. (Pause) And if anything else comes up that gets in the way of the kind of life you want, we can work on that, too.

STRATEGY 2B: Behaviors that interfere with treatment are also not bad, and the client is not bad for engaging in such behavior.

Such behavior is only problematic in that it interferes with the effectiveness of treatment—which interferes with the client's progress toward a valued life. When you need to address client behavior that interferes with therapy (e.g., missing sessions, skipping home practice, arriving late), you need to stress that you are not trying to criticize or chastise the client. You are only addressing the behavior because you want the client to be able to have a life that feels more satisfying—and so you are addressing obstacles that can interfere with reaching that life. In short, these behaviors should be addressed the same way dysregulated behaviors are addressed.

Behaviors that impede therapy are often even more critical to address than dysregulated behaviors, a point that is consistent with the principles of DBT (Linehan, 1993a). The reason: If the client continues to engage in the dysregulated behavior while also continuing to attend therapy and complete at least some home practice, you still have a chance of helping her learn new ways of coping so that she can stop the behavior and improve her life. However, if the client does not attend sessions or complete any home practice, you have much less of a chance of helping her to successfully stop the behavior or improve her life.

If you are a human being, you will have times when you feel frustrated with clients' dysregulation. After working your hardest to help a client improve his life, you can sometimes feel as though treatment-interfering behavior is a personal slight. At those times, you are encouraged to briefly self-assess whether you may be addressing the client's behavior in a way that chastises or criticizes him. If so, you are encouraged to work to be nonjudgmental. **Remember:** These clients often have trouble regulating their behavior in multiple realms (which is why they are in treatment for dysregulated behavior!), and these realms may include attending therapy, completing home practice, or other therapeutic endeavors. In addition, these individuals often have more difficulty resisting dysregulated behavior when they experience uncomfortable emotions, and therapy-related tasks may often bring up discomfort. These conceptualizations are different than what many clinicians are taught, so I encourage you to extend compassion to yourself, even if you have to remind yourself dozens (or gazillions) of times about the importance of non-judgmental communication. Such formulations will become more natural over time.

STRATEGY 2C: Work with the client to identify his or her values and goals.

Since dysregulated behavior is problematic because it interferes with life values, the identification of client values is of ultimate importance. Values may involve family, romantic partners, friends, pets (which could arguably fall under the "family" category), careers, health, hobbies, religion/spirituality, community service, feeling good about self, or a host of other potential areas of life.

To reiterate: The values need to be the client's values, not the therapist's. Be careful not to automatically assume that certain goals and values are healthier than others just because they fit your own cultural norms and personal experience. Although this admonition applies when working with all clients, it is especially relevant for working with clients from cultural groups other than your own. When working with clients of different cultural backgrounds, do your best to be aware of your biases (we all have them), and be diligent in working to keep those biases from interfering with the treatment you provide.

Sometimes clients bring up their goals and values without prompting by the therapist. At these times, you can use reflections, affirmations, validations, and open-ended questions to help clarify and gain further information. MMT also uses a direct approach to assess and discuss values. In the intake session, the therapist asks the client the following:

> *If you could have a life that felt more meaningful and fulfilling—like your life was more like the kind of life you want and you felt more like the kind of person you want to be— what would that life look like? What would be different from the life you're living now?*

You do not have to use the terminology provided above. As always, you are encouraged to use language that you feel is appropriate for the client. MMT focuses on helping clients identify and live more consistently with their values, but if a client scoffs at the term *values*, you are free to use other terms to explain the goals of treatment. (More details about setting up the questions and reacting to responses can be found in Chapter 7's description of the pretreatment intake session.)

Once the therapist and client discuss the client's values and goals, the therapist will use these values/goals to explain the course of treatment. To this end, MMT uses a metaphor called the *destination (or castle) metaphor.* The importance of this metaphor cannot be stressed enough, as it will be used throughout the entire course of treatment.

The destination/castle metaphor provides clients with a concrete image of moving toward a life more consistent with their values. Essential messages from the metaphor include:

1. Clients will likely not completely achieve the life they want while they are in treatment, but if they do the work, you are confident they will move much closer to that life. They will also have the skills to continue moving toward that life even after treatment ends.
2. Treatment is hard work, and the home practice can feel time-consuming and tedious.
3. Clients will likely go through difficult and possibly painful periods in treatment. They might even have times when they doubt whether treatment is working and feel worse before they feel better. Those times are both normal and temporary.
4. If the client comes to sessions and does the work, you are confident the client can make marked progress—and have a life that feels noticeably different from the life he has now.

Note: The metaphor was initially called the *castle metaphor*—with a castle being the metaphorical destination. The title was changed to *destination metaphor* when MMT was conducted with professional football players, who we were afraid might think *castle* sounded too cutesy. That said, many MMT clients have liked visualizing a castle. Feel free to work with the client to choose a destination the client would like—or to just use the generic term *destination*.

The Destination/Castle Metaphor

Warn the client that the metaphor might sound cheesy, while also conveying that the metaphor contains an accurate explanation of treatment.

- *Imagine the life you want—a life that feels more fulfilling and satisfying, with you generally feeling like the kind of person you want to be. Now imagine that life is represented by a destination—a house or building or whatever you want* (or a castle).
- *That destination is over here* (hand gesture, with right hand far to right side) *and you've been over here* (left hand stretched out to left side).
- *You've been trying to get closer to that destination off and on—and you may have really tried your best—but the problem is that you haven't known* how *to get there.*
- *We're going to put you in a car [or bus/train, for people who don't drive] and get you moving toward that destination* (move left hand closer to right).
- *If you come to sessions and do the work, I'm confident that by the end of treatment [or in a few months, if applicable], you'll be much closer to that destination* (move left hand closer to right, although still room in between). *You won't be at the destination, unpacked and moved in. But you'll be much closer, and you'll feel like you're much closer. You'll notice a difference in yourself and your life.*
- *And, you'll have a GPS [global positioning system] that will allow you to keep moving even closer to the destination on your own, because you'll have the coping skills to keep going.*
- *It won't be easy. This program is a lot of work, and the home practice can feel tedious and boring at times.*
- *Some weeks you'll feel like you're going 75 miles an hour. Other weeks you'll feel like you're going up a steep hill with the car [bus] overheating. You might even feel like you have to get out and push the car [bus].*

- *In other words, some weeks will feel like you're making progress, and some weeks will feel like you're putting in a lot of effort but barely moving—or not moving at all. There might even be some times when you feel even worse than you do now. If so, that's normal, and it's temporary. I'll work with you to keep moving until you get past that part.*

- *But as long as you come to sessions and do the work, I'm confident that by the end of treatment, your life will feel very different—and you'll look back and be really aware of the progress you've made.*

Since this metaphor is integral to the entire treatment, it is included in this book twice: once above and once as a therapist template in Chapter 8's description of the first session. The description in Chapter 8 also includes details about processing the metaphor with the client.

STRATEGY 2D: Continue to focus on values throughout treatment.

You will continue to use the destination metaphor throughout treatment, and you will continue to remind the client that the overall purpose of treatment is not to stop the behavior. Instead, the overall purpose is to move toward that destination—living a life that feels more satisfying. (You can also list the client's specific goals when you mention the destination.) With this aim, you can reassess goals and values as the sessions progress, and you can tailor sessions (such as the Goals session and the Pleasant/Fulfilling Activities session) to help clients take steps toward the lives they want.

When a client has lapses and feels discouraged, you can remind her that she has moved much closer to the destination in the past few weeks and has just made a U-turn and gone back an exit. *Emphasize that she has not lost all the progress she has made—but instead has just gone back one exit.* However, the client is currently in a high-risk situation, as once one starts to go backward, it is easy to continue heading that direction. Thus, the central point is to work to get the client turned around and moving in the right direction before she continues to go backward. (If you are using a bus as the metaphorical vehicle, you can just say that the client got on a bus that was going the wrong way for an exit, and she needs to get off that bus so that she can get on a bus going toward the destination.)

When a client goes a week or more without completing home practice or without decreasing the target behavior, you can tell him that it's as if he (or the bus) has pulled off to the side of the road and parked for a week. He has not gone backward, but he has stopped moving forward for a while. You can then stress the importance of moving forward again—so he can get to the point where he feels his life is more like the kind of life he wants and he feels more like the kind of person he wants to be.

In other words, regardless of what you are working on in a particular week, you will always communicate that the ultimate purpose of treatment is to get the client closer to that destination—to that life that fits more with the kind of life the client wants and with the kind of person the client wants to be.

WHAT ABOUT MODERATION?

When clients report wanting to continue the behavior in moderation, the therapist can respond honestly and directly. Some people with dysregulated behavior can eventually learn to engage in their target behavior in moderation; others cannot engage in any instance of the behavior without starting to spiral out of control. Although there is no definitive method of predicting which path a client will take, there *is* a prediction the therapist can confidently share: People who refrain from target behavior for at least a few months are more likely to learn and fully master adaptive ways of coping with emotions and urges. Therefore, if a person has the capacity for moderation, that person will more likely be successful if she is abstinent for at least a few months before attempting moderation. This reason is why MMT therapists ask clients to work to stop the target behavior for the first few months of treatment, even if some clients do not want to remain abstinent forever. *Note:* Clients who initially report wanting to work toward moderation often report wanting to remain abstinent by the time treatment ends, but not always.

What about clients who engage in target behavior involving actions that cannot be completely stopped, such as eating or Internet usage? For these behaviors, therapists can work with clients to define certain forms of the behavior from which the client can work to be abstinent. For example, a client in treatment for binge eating might work to refrain from binges, as defined by the client and therapist. The target might eventually broaden to include other eating behaviors that impede the client's life, such as eating by oneself after 11:00 P.M.; however, the binges will remain the primary target. Therapists may also work with the client to set up healthy eating plans and exercise programs as part of some of the MMT skills (e.g., Pleasant/Fulfilling Activities, Steps toward Goals, and/or overall movement toward the destination). Another example: Clients in treatment for compulsive Internet use may define the target behavior as use of Internet for more than 15 minutes in any given time period and/or for anything other than work-related emails. Thus, therapists can find ways to ask for abstinence regardless of the type of behavior.

(For more information about explaining the reason for abstinence, see *H-A3, Why Do I Ask You . . . ?*, in Chapter 8, Session A. For more information about discussing moderation and creating a plan to test moderation toward the end of treatment, see Chapter 6.)

STRATEGY 2E: Clients don't have to "admit" that they have a problem. They don't have to label themselves as alcoholics, addicts, overeaters, problem gamblers, shopaholics, sexaholics, etc.

This myth does not ever seem to die: "Clients must admit they have a problem before they can get better." The only problem is that the myth is totally false. As long as a client realizes that the target behavior is getting in the way of her life, she never has to give herself a label or say that the behavior is a problem.

I repeat: *The client does not have to give herself a label or say that she has a problem for treatment to be successful. She just needs to realize that the behavior is getting in the way of the life she wants to live.*

Some clients do not like labels. And some people do not like to admit that they have problems. (Or maybe the client has a different definition of *problem* than you have, and thus she really does not have a problem.) Regardless, the purpose of treatment is not to get into arguments about something entirely irrelevant to treatment. The purpose is to move the client toward a more valued life and help the client overcome behavior that is interfering with that life.

For example, one client's son gave him the ultimatum that he either attend treatment and quit drinking—or never see his grandson again. The client was angry about the ultimatum and refused to say that he had a problem; however, he grudgingly attended treatment because his grandson was one of the most valued things in his life. After several weeks of sobriety, the client reported that he generally felt better (more energy, fewer headaches, and compliments about his appearance). By that time, he said he wanted to continue remaining abstinent even if his son dropped the ultimatum. However, the client would never say that he had had a problem with alcohol. He just said he realized that alcohol got in the way of his life (seeing his grandson, feeling healthy, etc.), and so he was committed to working to become and remain sober.

This point will sometimes need to be discussed further if a client goes to a support group. Supports groups can be effective ways for clients to make friends who do not engage in the behavior and who will not judge the client for past behavior. In most 12-step programs, participants introduce themselves using labels (e.g., "I'm Lillian, and I'm an alcoholic"; or "I'm Fred. I'm a compulsive eater"). You can alert clients in advance and discuss ways in which they would like to introduce themselves. Most 12-step groups will accept variations from common introductions: for example, "I'm Lillian, and I'm working on being sober"; or "I'm Fred, and I struggle with overeating."

STRATEGY 3: STRONG FOCUS ON HELPING THE CLIENT UNDERSTAND SELF, BEHAVIOR, AND TREATMENT

A. Focus on helping the client understand self and behavior (boiling pot metaphor, Part I).

B. Focus on helping the client understand the treatment.
  - Use Part II of the boiling pot metaphor.
    - Releases pressure and helps emotions and urges feel more tolerable.
    - Helps clients learn to regulate emotions in ways that are adaptive—not harmful.
  - Mindfulness (awareness) exercises also:
    - Help clients build emotional muscles.
    - Teach clients to value their own feelings and reactions.
    - Help clients find the "pause" button.
    - Help clients take back their power so they no longer feel controlled by emotions/urges.
    - Help clients experience positive emotions.

C. Use the peaks-and-valleys diagram.

D. Continue helping the client understand self and treatment (again and again) throughout the entire treatment.

Most people who struggle with dysregulated behavior have attempted to stop or decrease the behavior many times and through many methods. Eventually, people with dysregulated behavior often start believing that their behavior means some combination of the following: They are weak, have an "addictive" or self-defeating personality that is untreatable, have physical reasons that make stopping the behavior impossible, and/or have other qualities that basically mean that something about them is *inherently wrong* and *ultimately untreatable*.

These beliefs can be strong obstacles to treatment engagement. After all, why would a person make the effort to engage in a time-consuming, uncomfortable treatment if that person "knows" he is beyond help? Even clients who initially engage in treatment often have increasing doubts over time, as each moment of difficulty tends to evoke and confirm their underlying beliefs of being beyond help. Thus, the therapist must work with clients to help them gain a nonjudgmental understanding of (1) themselves and (2) the reasons their struggles with dysregulated behavior make sense, based on their circumstances.

STRATEGY 3A: Focus on helping the client understand self and behavior.

During the first MMT treatment session, the therapist will say something like, "Let me tell you how this program conceptualizes people who come to treatment. You can tell me what fits and what doesn't fit." The therapist then explains the *boiling pot metaphor* (biopsychosocial model), making sure to customize the metaphor to fit the client as much as possible. The boiling pot metaphor is the cornerstone metaphor used throughout treatment, so please take time to learn, understand, and practice it (and practice it again) before conducting MMT.

> The explanation that follows in the next section includes words such as *target behavior*. When working with a client, use words that describe the client's specific behavior(s). For clients who are attending treatment only because it is mandated or they are being pressured to do so, you can say, "Clients who have had some of your experiences" or some other phrase that does not force them to say that the behavior is a problem. (See Strategy 2E on pp. 49–50.)

The Biopsychosocial Boiling Pot Metaphor, Part I

Begin describing the boiling pot metaphor along these lines:

- *Some people are born with a tendency to feel emotions a little more strongly than most people feel emotions. [Give examples that fit client's emotions: "What makes some people a little irritated might make them a little more irritated. . . ."]*
- *This is not a negative trait. These people are likely to be especially creative and/or empathic (e.g., Eysenck & Eysenck, 1978; Leung et al., 2014; Post, 1994).*
  - *They are more likely to have careers or hobbies as artists, singers, florists, builders, hair dressers, etc.*
  - *And/or careers or hobbies that help others or involve interaction with others, like teacher, therapist, salesperson, waiter, pet sitter, etc.*
- *It's not a negative thing! But sometimes these people grow up in adverse or invalidating environments. These might include:*
  - *Experiences like physical, sexual, or emotional abuse.*
  - *Experiences with family members who may not feel emotions strongly and so don't understand—who may say things like "Why can't you get over it?" or "Why are you making such a big deal about it?"*

- *Experiences with family members who have trouble tolerating their own emotions and use unhealthy behaviors to cope.*
- *Experiences outside the home, like bullying at school, mistreatment by other caretakers, routinely being excluded by other children and feeling like there's something wrong with them.*

- *These people are put in situations that would be painful for anyone. Since they already feel things more strongly than most, the pain feels even stronger for them. Eventually, the emotions start to feel unbearable at times.*
- *At first, they may tell themselves: "I'm just going to try not to feel" or "I'm just not going to think about it." Sometimes they get pretty good at that—to the point that they might sometimes feel a little numb in general. But over time, they often feel they need something stronger to "turn off" painful emotions. So they start target behavior(s).*
- *The things is: It works. For the short term. They feel better. But using target behavior(s) to "turn off" uncomfortable emotions is like putting an airtight lid on a pot of boiling water:*
  - *The emotions are still there, just like the boiling water and steam are still there.*
  - *And the emotions keep building—just like the steam and pressure keep building in the pot of boiling water. Or sometimes the person may not be aware of emotions building, but instead may just be aware of the urges building.*
  - *Either way, the person may eventually feel like he/she is often under pressure.*
  - *If the emotions and urges are never experienced or processed (if none of the steam is released from the pot), the emotions or urges will keep building until the pot eventually explodes. In other words, the emotions or urges will feel especially unbearable.*
  - *So the person will feel like he/she has to try even harder not to feel—and eventually he/she uses the target behavior again.*
- *And the person feels relief. But the pressure will almost always start building again.*
- *Pretty soon, life can start to feel like a never-ending cycle of urges building . . . target behavior . . . briefly feeling better . . . then urges building . . . target behavior . . . and so on. (Pause) Does this fit you?*

Take a moment to talk about how the metaphor does and doesn't fit. Then continue.

- *These behaviors can seem so effective in the short term that you might have never learned adaptive ways to handle uncomfortable emotions and urges.*
- *If you mainly know one way of reliably stopping pain or discomfort, it makes sense that you would have strong urges to engage in that behavior when experiencing any discomfort, and you would have extreme difficulty stopping the behavior.*
- *In fact, that behavior probably helped you cope at times when you didn't know any other way to cope. The problem is that it causes damage over time.*

Part II of the boiling pot metaphor continues in Strategy 3B to explain how MMT addresses the biopsychosocial model.

The therapist uses the boiling pot metaphor to help clients understand that their struggle with dysregulated behavior is not a permanent character flaw, not a sign that they are beyond help, and not a sign that they do not deserve happiness. Instead the metaphor and related explanations are aimed at helping clients realize that their behavior is understandable, based on their circumstances.

This point should be emphasized throughout: *The client's behavior (and difficulty stopping the behavior) is understandable based on the client's history and current circumstances. None of us can say with any certainty that we would behave any differently if we had had the same combination of biology, life history, and current circumstances.*

Once the client begins to understand that her behavior can be understood and explained, she is more likely to be open to the possibility that she might not have a permanent, untreatable flaw. In addition, once the client realizes that *you* (the therapist) can understand and explain her behavior, she is more likely to trust that you can help her *change* her behavior.

You will likely have to return to this point again and again (and again) as the client's old beliefs of being permanently flawed are reactivated during difficulties. Keep in mind that you will need to reflect, validate, and affirm throughout your conceptualization of the client, your explanation of the treatment, and your delivery of the treatment. The fact that the client becomes open to the possibility that she can change her behavior does not keep her from having difficulty making the change. It does not keep her from having recurring doubts or from sometimes questioning whether the pain of stopping the behavior is worth the effort. Thus, the therapist will need to continually validate the difficulty of the process.

Clients tend to react positively to the boiling pot metaphor. Clients also seem receptive to the continued use of the metaphor throughout treatment, which provides an effective way for therapists to communicate key elements of treatment without getting bogged down in details. That said, aspects of the explanation will have to be modified at times. The following section provides suggestions for flexibly customizing the explanation to fit potential questions and issues.

Potential Questions/Issues with the Boiling Pot Metaphor

The biopsychosocial boiling pot metaphor describes vulnerable temperament as being "born with a tendency to feel emotions more strongly than most people feel emotions." What if the client does not seem like the kind of person who feels emotions more strongly than most?

The therapist can be tentative about that part of the metaphor, while also working to give examples of emotions that are most likely to fit the client.

> *Some people are born with a tendency to feel emotions a little more strongly than most people feel emotions. From what you've said, I'm not sure if this fits you, so I'll explain a little more, and then you tell me. What makes some people a little irritated might make them a little more irritated. What makes some people a little sad might make them a little more sad. This is not a negative trait. In fact, these people are likely to be especially creative and/or empathic. For example, these people are more likely to have careers or hobbies as [modify some examples to fit client]. Does this fit you?*

If the client says "yes" or agrees somewhat, the therapist can continue with the standard explanation. If the client says "no," then see the next question.

What if the client actually says he does not feel emotions more strongly than most people?

In these cases, the therapist can customize the explanation to fit the client by offering a few possible options.

- The client may have had enough uncomfortable or painful experiences that the environment had the same effects as if the client *did* feel emotions more strongly than most people.
- The client may have grown in up an environment that didn't teach adaptive ways of coping with negative emotions, so the target behavior became the client's way of coping with *any* negative or uncomfortable emotions by default. Once he became accustomed to reacting to negative emotions by trying to turn them off (i.e., putting the lid on the pot), he began experiencing urges to turn off *any* uncomfortable emotions, even if they were not especially strong. The rest of the metaphor will continue to be relevant—with a focus on urges building instead of emotions building.
- The client was born feeling emotions more strongly than many people—but may have gotten so good at "turning off" negative emotions at a young age that his customary state became somewhat emotionally numbed. In fact, he may feel as though he experiences emotions *less* strongly than most people—but instead only feels *urges* more strongly. In this case, the boiling pot metaphor can be modified to again substitute the word *urges* for *emotions* when discussing current functioning.
- Finally, remind the client that therapy isn't an assembly line and clients aren't interchangeable, so all clients should not be expected to fit exactly into the same mold. Assure the client that it is OK if all parts of the explanation do not fit him perfectly.

In the following vignette, the therapist stopped after explaining the strong emotions (temperament) and asked, "Does this fit you?"

CLIENT: Not really. I think I feel emotions about the same as most people do.

THERAPIST: OK, this part doesn't seem to fit, and that's fine. Let me explain a little more, and we can talk about how this all goes together. [Continue explanation without mentioning strong emotions.] People in this program usually have grown up in adverse or invalidating environments. This might include [describe environments]. These people are put in situations that would be painful for anyone. And eventually, the emotions start to feel unbearable at times. At first, they usually tell themselves: "I'm just going to try not to feel or think about it." But over time, they often feel like they need something stronger to "turn off" uncomfortable emotions. So they start engaging in *target behavior*.

Now, you said the part about feeling emotions more strongly doesn't fit. So maybe you weren't born feeling emotions more strongly, but instead you had enough uncomfortable or painful experiences that the experiences still had the same effects—to lead you to want to "turn off" uncomfortable emotions. Or maybe you never learned healthy ways to cope with negative emotions, so the target behavior became your way of coping with *any* uncomfortable emotions—even emotions that weren't strong. Or maybe you once felt emotions a little more strongly, but you started "turning off" negative emotions when you were really young, so now your emotions are almost always pressed down—and you just feel *urges* strongly. No explanation fits everyone, and whether or not you feel emotions strongly doesn't affect how well this treatment will work. Whatever the reason you started using the target behavior to begin with, once you start trying to turn off uncomfortable emotions or urges—the effects are similar. [Continue the boiling pot metaphor, focusing on urges instead of emotions.]

- So even people who weren't born feeling things more strongly may start using their particular target behavior to turn off uncomfortable emotions, or to turn off urges that start after they become accustomed to using the target behavior for coping.
- The problem is that using the target behavior(s) to "turn off" uncomfortable urges is like putting an airtight lid on a pot of boiling water:
- The urges are still there, just like the boiling water and steam are still there—under the surface. [Etc.]

What if the client says she does not have any history of adverse or invalidating environments?

The therapist first works to offer other examples of invalidating environments. If the client continues to deny invalidating experiences, the therapist assures the client that it's OK if that part of the explanation does not fit perfectly. Again, clients should not be expected to fit into a mold like a part on an assembly line. Do your best to customize the answer to what you know about the client. You will likely not give as many examples as offered below; they are included to demonstrate possibilities.

Not all parts of the model fit all people, which is fine. Let's explore further.

- *An invalidating environment doesn't mean your family was uncaring. It could be you had a caring family and great parents—but that your family didn't feel emotions strongly, so they didn't understand when you did. Maybe they had good intentions, but they told you that you needed to quit crying, or stop being anxious, or stop making a big deal about things. They may have accidentally given you the message there was something wrong in the way you felt and expressed emotions.*
- *Or maybe it was the opposite. Maybe you had someone in your family who felt emotions so strongly that seeing you express emotions was upsetting to them—so you may have felt you had to hide your emotions and pretend like everything was OK to protect that person from getting upset.*
- *It could even be that your family had really high expectations—with good intentions, but that somehow you felt that unless you excelled, you weren't as valuable. So you experienced shame and pain when you felt you weren't perfect.*
- *It also could be things outside the home. Maybe you felt excluded or judged by other children or teachers. It could be anything that routinely hurt your feelings or led you to believe that parts of yourself were wrong and needed to be hidden. Or maybe for some reason you set such high standards for yourself that you felt you were never living up to expectations, and so you were afraid you would disappoint others or feel disappointed in yourself.*
- *[If the client still denies any invalidation] Maybe you were born feeling emotions*

so strongly that even the standard stresses and disappointments of daily life just seemed too difficult to bear—and you didn't need anything particularly adverse. Or maybe there's some other explanation. Every part of the model doesn't have to fit perfectly—especially since this part deals with your past and not your current situation. The treatment will still work just as well regardless of whether or not you had adverse experiences in your past.

STRATEGY 3B: Focus on helping the client understand treatment.

MMT contains mindfulness practices that may feel uncomfortable, unfamiliar, and even weird to some clients. The outside exercises can be time-consuming, and many of the exercises might also start to feel repetitive and even boring over time. Thus, helping the client understand how and why you are asking him to engage in such activities is key in fostering completion of home practice. In addition, by taking time to explain each aspect of treatment, you are demonstrating that you respect the client and view him as an intelligent adult.

The Boiling Pot Metaphor, Continued

The boiling pot metaphor is used as a way to begin explaining MMT. Although the metaphor was artificially split in this chapter to demonstrate the two components (helping the client understand self/behavior and helping the client understand treatment), you will actually explain it as one component in one session. The boiling pot metaphor is used to help explain MMT overall, as well as many MMT practices. Thus, the metaphor is used throughout treatment.

After asking the client whether the boiling pot explanation feels like it fits (and having any necessary discussion about the client's response), the therapist (you) will segue into explaining the treatment:

- *In the first few weeks of treatment, we're going to open a steam hole in the lid of the boiling pot—so you can release some of the steam and pressure. [This refers to the mindfulness practices.] That way, the feeling of pressure can start to be released, and your emotions and urges can start to feel less overwhelming. Little by little, the urges will be easier to tolerate without feeling like you need to act on them.*
- *Some exercises might seem weird, but they'll help you start to experience whatever you're feeling, which will let some of that steam out of that pot.*
- *Eventually we'll also help you learn healthy ways to adjust the heat of the burner underneath the boiling pot—in other words, to adjust the intensity of your emotions and urges. Sometimes you'll be able to keep the heat from being turned up so high to begin with, and sometimes you'll be able to turn the heat down—not turn it off—but turn it down.*
- *But first we have to let some of the pressure out of the pot.*

This explanation is provided in the first session along with the rest of the boiling pot metaphor—and then used throughout treatment. You will not provide additional details about mindfulness practice right away, as clients will be more likely to remember the details after practicing the first mindfulness exercise. You will repeat the explanation again (and again and again) when clients question the value of the practices, have trouble completing the practices, and/or are assigned new practices. This explanation also works in explaining the purpose of the Daily Log and other awareness exercises that are not traditional mindfulness exercises.

Explanations of How Mindfulness Exercises Are Beneficial

During Session A, the therapist leads the client on a mindfulness exercise called the *Color Body Scan,* in which the client is guided in experiencing physical sensations throughout the body. Afterward, the therapist tells the client that this and other awareness exercises are important to treatment in several ways:

1. *Being purposely aware of what you experience can open a steam hole in the lid of the boiling pot—so some of the pressure is released.* That's a big deal on its own—being able to walk around without feeling so much pressure. Eventually, your emotions and urges will also start to feel less intense and more tolerable.

2. *By purposely experiencing and tolerating your reactions, you'll start building your emotional muscles*—so eventually your emotions and/or urges won't seem so heavy and overwhelming. If I had to carry around a 30-pound weight all day, I'd be exhausted and in pain by the end of the day—and my arms would be sore for days. But if I lifted weights regularly for a few months, I could carry around the same weight all day—and even though it weighed exactly the same, it would feel much lighter and more bearable. I wouldn't be exhausted, and my muscles wouldn't be sore. Doing these exercises—purposely experiencing your reactions—is like lifting weights. You can build emotional muscles so your emotions and/or urges will eventually feel a lot lighter and less painful.

3. *The exercises retrain your brain to believe that your reactions are valuable.* Sadly, I think you've somehow learned to believe that at least some of your reactions are wrong somehow, that you might have to hide or try to change parts of yourself and your reactions. But if you spend time each day intentionally experiencing your reactions without trying to change them, your brain will get the message that those feelings and reactions must be valuable—and that *you* are valuable. These exercises reach the primitive part of your brain that doesn't always respond to logic.

Note: The above three points are usually enough for the first session. Again, you will repeat them often throughout treatment. In addition, you will eventually share the following:

4. *These practices can help you find your "pause button."* You've probably become so accustomed to using the target behavior as a way to cope that you sometimes engage in the behavior as an automatic reaction. Many people will say they felt like they barely even realized they were going to engage in the target behavior—but that something happened, and they reacted first and thought later. These exercises help you learn to be aware of the emotions and/or urges instead of acting automatically, and then tolerate the urges long enough to press the "pause button," so you can decide how you want to react.

5. *These exercises can also help you take back your power.* Most people who come here say that no matter how hard they work to try to stop the target behavior, the urges sometimes get so strong that they feel like they have no control. It can almost feel like someone else has the remote control for your behavior—like the urges have control of you. These exercises can help you take back your power—so instead of feeling controlled by your urges, you can be in control of how you react to them. Even when you have unpleasant emotions and urges, you can have the power to decide whether or not you want to act on the urges.

6. *Finally, the exercises will help you experience more positive emotions.* You've become used to trying to turn off unpleasant emotions. The problem is that you can't turn off some emotions without at least turning down all emotions. So over time, you might have noticed you don't feel positive emotions as often or strongly as you'd like. You might not even be sure what will bring you pleasure and what you want out of life. By purposely experiencing all of your emotions and reactions, you can eventually start experiencing positive emotions more often and strongly. You can also become more aware of what brings you pleasure and fulfillment—so you can eventually start feeling better about yourself and your life in general.

Strategy 3C: Use the peaks-and-valleys example.

The peaks-and-valleys example gives the client a concrete, visual representation of (1) the time-limited nature of strong urges, (2) the fact that the average intensity and frequency of urges will eventually decrease if the client does not act on them, and (3) the fact that each time the client gets through a peak urge without acting on it, she gets a little closer to having less intense and less frequent urges. The peaks-and-valleys example is consistent with the concept of *urge surfing* in MBRP (Bowen et al., 2010). Urges tend to come in waves. As long as the client can "surf the wave" or get through the peak of the urge without engaging in the target behavior, the urge will eventually subside on its own, just like waves eventually subside back into the ocean. (Because the peaks-and-valleys example is introduced in the second session, it is described in full in Chapter 8.)

Strategy 3D: Continue helping the client understand self and treatment again (and again) throughout the entire treatment.

This strategy seems self-explanatory—and it is, to an extent. However, the importance and necessity of continuing to repeat the above explanations cannot be overemphasized. You will use the boiling pot metaphor at the beginning of treatment to help clients understand them-selves and the treatment. You will use it multiple times throughout treatment to remind clients that the home practice is serving the function of (among other things) letting steam and pressure out of the pot. You will also use it to gently remind clients that avoidant behavior is another way to put the lid on the pot. The main avoidant behaviors to address include the target behavior(s), missing sessions, and failing to complete home practice. Other avoidant behaviors (excessive sleep, self-imposed isolation, engaging in secondary dysregulated behaviors) should never be a primary focus of treatment (pick your battles!); however, you may also mention that these behaviors serve to put the lid on the pot if you feel they may be impeding the client's movement toward his valued life.

You will also need to remind the client about the other benefits of mindfulness practice (see above), the peaks-and-valleys example, and the destination metaphor many times throughout treatment. Thus, it is important for you to memorize the basic gist of each explanation. It is also important to memorize the benefits of mindfulness practice so you will be able to reel off the list (or at least different items from the list) whenever relevant and needed.

Here's a reminder. MMT's mindfulness and other experiential exercises . . .

1. Release feelings of pressure (open a hole in the lid of the boiling pot and release steam and pressure so emotions and/or urges feel less overwhelming).
2. Help build emotional muscles so emotions/urges feel lighter and easier to tolerate.
3. Teach clients to believe that their own feelings and reactions are valuable.
4. Help clients find the "pause button," so they are less likely to react automatically in ways that hurt themselves in the long run.
5. Help clients take back power so they no longer feel controlled by emotions/urges.
6. Help clients experience more positive emotions.

Note: Other MMT exercises will also help decrease the heat of the burner under the boiling pot to turn down the intensity of the emotions and urges. (Benefits of other specific exercises are explained when each exercise is introduced.)

CHAPTER SUMMARY

Strategy 2: Focus on Client Values—and How Target Behaviors Interfere with a Values-Consistent Life

- Communicate that the target behavior is *not* bad. It is only problematic because it impedes the client from (1) feeling like the kind of person she/he wants to be, and (2) living a life that feels as fulfilling and meaningful as it could.
- Similarly, behaviors that interfere with treatment are not bad. They are only problematic because they interfere with the client's moving toward a valued life.
- Work with the client to identify values and goals, and use the destination metaphor to explain the purpose of treatment. Continue to focus on values throughout treatment.
- Clients don't have to "admit" that they have a problem in order for treatment to be effective.

Strategy 3: Strong Focus on Helping the Client Understand Self, Behavior, and Treatment

- Compassionately explain the biopsychosocial conceptualization of the client and the client's behavior. Use the boiling pot metaphor and validate throughout.

- The boiling pot metaphor also provides a broad initial explanation of treatment: Treatment exercises are geared to (1) release pressure and help emotions and urges feel more tolerable (open a hole in the lid), and (2) help clients learn to regulate emotions adaptively (turn down the heat of the burner to turn down the intensity of the emotions/urges).

- MMT's exercises also:

  - Help build emotional muscles.
  - Teach the client to value his own feelings and reactions.
  - Help the client find the "pause" button.
  - Help the client take back power so she no longer feels controlled by emotions/urges.
  - Help client experience positive emotions and increased awareness of her own values.

CHAPTER 5

Strategies 4 and 5

Home Practice and Shaping

In MMT, the work conducted in session is only one component of treatment. In order to move toward lives that fit their values, clients must also practice and master adaptive methods of coping across various situations in daily life. Strategies 4 and 5 offer guidelines for helping clients gain the greatest possible benefits from their time between sessions.

STRATEGY 4: LOTS OF STRUCTURE AND HOME PRACTICE

A. Foster habit.

B. Set up home practice explicitly.

C. Review the home practice at the beginning of every session.

- Ask to see home practice directly or segue into asking.
- Review the home practice in detail.
- If client did not do the home practice . . .
    - ◆ Validate the difficulty and tediousness.
    - ◆ Find out what got in the way.
    - ◆ Tell the client you are not judging or criticizing.
    - ◆ Work on a plan to increase the client's chance of completing the home practice in the upcoming week, including shaping when applicable (see Strategy 5, p. 71).

Assigning daily home practice to clients with dysregulated behavior might sound counterintuitive. However, when clients with dysregulated behavior are assigned home practice once a week, they often wait several days before beginning the practice, even if they initially had intended to complete the practice sooner. This procrastination is usually due to a combination of forgetting, general avoidance, time management difficulties, and/or anxiety about experiencing emotions that might arise from the practice (e.g., Díaz-Morales, Ferrari, & Cohen, 2008; Sirois & Kitner, 2015). In such circumstances, clients often end up either (1) completing the practice in a rush at the last minute (which might not deliver the full benefits) or (2) feeling so overwhelmed that they do not complete the practice at all.

STRATEGY 4A: Foster habit.

When clients are assigned a few minutes of practice every day, they know that if they procrastinate more than a day, they will miss at least some of their assignment. Thus, they will have more incentive to start practice right away. In addition, daily (or almost-daily) practice fosters habit. Performing habitual behavior requires less effort and conscious intention than performing behaviors that are not habitual (e.g., Lisman & Sternberg, 2013). Examples include getting dressed in the morning, bathing, brushing teeth, etc. These behaviors often become almost automatic, so they require less planning and exertion to perform than less regular behaviors. Once the assignments become daily habits, clients are less likely to forget or feel the need to procrastinate. (How many times have you forgotten to bathe?) Another benefit of habits: When clients become overwhelmed with uncomfortable emotions and/or urges, they are more likely to engage in coping strategies that have become habitual than to engage in strategies that require greater cognitive resources to plan and implement.

STRATEGY 4B: Set up home practice explicitly.

The therapist will spend time teaching the client about each new topic and going over the home practice in detail. To ensure that clients remember the details about home practice, MMT provides worksheets with specific instructions and with areas for clients to mark each practice they complete. (Worksheets are at the end of each session guideline, starting with Chapter 8.) MMT also provides a sheet that summarizes all of the home practice for each week. Thus, each week the client will receive:

a. A Daily Log (to track basic emotions, urges, and target behavior; see H-A4 in Chapter 8),
b. A Tracking Sheet (to track the number of times the client engages in the practices; see H-E2 in Chapter 9),
c. Any additional home practice (if applicable), and
d. A Home Practice Summary of all the home practice for the week (see H-A5 in Chapter 8).

The therapist will explain worksheets related to new material as the material is addressed in session. The therapist will also briefly review the Home Practice Summary toward the end of each session. (For more details about how to introduce the mindfulness exercises and additional assignments, see the relevant session in the session guidelines: Chapters 8–12.)

STRATEGY 4C: Review the home practice at the beginning of every session.

Therapists must set the standard of reviewing the home practice at the beginning of every session. Most sessions will begin with the therapist taking a moment to talk to the client as a human being (in other words, listening to what the client brings into session). Once clients are accustomed to the home practice review occurring toward the beginning of every session, they will often hand you the home practice as soon as they sit down (or tell you they did not do the practice—which is discussed later). However, most clients do not automatically hand over the home practice until they have attended sessions for a few weeks, and some clients do not ever hand over the practice until they are requested to do so. In these cases, you have two options, the choice of which will depend upon your therapeutic style.

Asking for the Home Practice Directly or Segueing into Asking

First Option

Some therapists ask for the home practice as soon as the client sits down. If you choose this approach, take care not to mechanically begin reviewing the practice. After being handed the home practice, give the client an opportunity to answer your greeting and just be a human being for a moment. Then you can refer to the Daily Log (of emotions, urges, and target behavior) to show your interest in the client and give the client a chance to talk about occurrences during the past week. You can start by glancing at the Daily Log and then forming a relevant question or reflection. For example:

> (after briefly glancing at the Daily Log) *You had quite a week! Tell me about it.*

Or:

> *So, you had a lot of anxiety and sadness at the beginning of the week, and then you started feeling some hope toward the end of the week.* (Pause for client response)

Or:

> *Looks like you had a rough week with high stress and high urges—especially on the weekend. What was going on?*

Even if the Daily Log contains incidents of the target behavior, you will not immediately focus on that behavior. Instead, you will first mention the client's emotions and urges—to help convey that you view the client as a full person and not just someone defined by the presence or absence of target behavior.

> *Looks like you had a rough week. I see that Monday you were already feeling a lot of sadness and loneliness—and Tuesday you also started feeling strong anxiety, and your urges went to 9. But you were able to keep from engaging in the target behavior. I hate that you were suffering, but I'm glad that you were able to get through the day without the behavior.*

Then Wednesday, pretty much all of your negative emotions went to 10—and you did engage in the behavior. And you've had high urges every day since, but you haven't done any target behavior for the last 2 days. That's impressive. It can be difficult to stop once you've had a lapse, especially since I see you're still feeling a lot of sadness. (Pause) *How are you feeling right now?* (Pause) *[Reflect/validate the client's current emotions.] I appreciate your being honest with me about your use. Tell me a little bit about what's been going on this week.*

Note: You will likely segue to a functional analysis of the target behavior (see Chapter 6, p. 84)—but you will first need to take a moment—even if briefly—to focus on the client's current emotions and overall experiences. You will also conduct at least a brief review of the rest of the home practice prior to any formal functional analysis. If the client also did not complete the home practice, you will choose which behavior you will target for the functional analysis (i.e., the target behavior or a lack of home practice; see discussion of functional analysis on pp. 84–86).

Second Option

Instead of immediately asking the client for the home practice at the beginning of the session, some therapists prefer asking clients about themselves or their weeks—and then naturally segueing to asking for the home practice as the client is talking. You can do this by "jumping" in at a pause with a reflection (or validation or affirmation) of what the client just said, and then segueing to requesting the practice. For example:

> CLIENT: . . . then I went to that new grocery store, which took forever because they didn't have enough help . . . and then I finally got my hair cut, which felt like a big step for me . . .
>
> THERAPIST: (*jumping in at a pause*) I know you were anxious about making the appointment, so good for you for going! Can I see your Daily Log so I can have an idea of what else was going on around that time? (*Looks at log.*) Yes, you were experiencing high anxiety that day—but also some happiness, which I like to see. You also had strong anxiety toward the end of the week. What was going on? [Client answers; therapist validates.] Your urges also got stronger those days. How did you get through the days without acting on them? [Therapist can reflect/validate/affirm and then move on to reviewing the Tracking Sheet.]

Another example:

> CLIENT: My week was OK. My roommate was out of town 3 days, so that was weird. I did find out that the new season of my favorite show is about to be out, so I'm excited about that . . .
>
> THERAPIST: (*jumping in*) It's exciting to have a season of a favorite show to watch! And I can understand how it would feel weird for your roommate to be out of town since you're so used to his being around. Can I see your Daily Log to help me know what you were feeling during that time? (*Pause*) Yeah, you felt a bit lonely, but also less anxious. [Client

responds; therapist reflects/validates.] And you didn't engage in the target behavior again this week. That's a big deal. (*Slight pause*) Let's see your Tracking Sheet and other home practice.

Never let the session progress without asking for the home practice. Otherwise, you will send the message that the home practice is not that necessary after all.

Reviewing the Home Practice in Detail

Therapists should always take at least a little time to review the home practice (which includes the Daily Log, the Tracking Sheet, and potentially another assignment). Do not just glance over the practice and move to the next topic; otherwise, you will be conveying a sense that the practice is not worthy of time or attention. Once the client gives you the home practice, reflect and ask questions about what you see on the Daily Log, the Tracking Sheet, and any additional assignment.

When reviewing the audio mindfulness practices (which the client tracks on the Tracking Sheet), start by asking open-ended questions about the client's experience with the practice. Reflect and validate (normalize) any difficulty, and be sure to affirm any adaptive steps (i.e., any incidents of engaging in the practice). For example:

THERAPIST: You did the audio practice all 5 days. Yay for you! How was it?

CLIENT: It was fine. I got tired a few times and had to work to stay awake.

THERAPIST: That's pretty common. Were you able to stay awake through it all?

CLIENT: Yeah, but I had to work at it.

THERAPIST: I'm glad you did. Was there anything about the experiences that surprised you?

CLIENT: Just that some days it was easy, and some days I wasn't able to do it as well.

THERAPIST: What do you mean by "wasn't able to do it as well"?

CLIENT: Well, some days I just had trouble focusing.

THERAPIST: Your mind wandered a lot.

CLIENT: Yeah. And it was frustrating.

THERAPIST: Yeah, it can feel frustrating. Did you notice your mind wandering and then bring it back to the audio whenever you noticed?

CLIENT: Yeah, I tried. But I had to keep doing it over and over.

THERAPIST: That's absolutely normal. Sometimes it may feel like your mind is spending more time wandering than focusing—and that happens to everyone. Those times might not be as pleasant or relaxing, but as long as you bring your mind back whenever you notice it wandering—even if you have to do it every other second—the practice is working just as well as it is when you feel focused and relaxed. Both times you're building your muscles—but you're building them in different ways. The times you have trouble focusing and feeling frustrated, you're building your ability to tolerate unpleasant emotions and urges without feeling like you have to avoid the situation or engage in the target behavior. Because right now, I think there are times when you feel unpleasant emotions and then feel like you have to avoid situations even if those situations could be helpful to you. Or you experience urges and feel like you have to engage in the target behavior to turn them off. By continuing to practice even when you're feeling frustrated or agitated, you're building your muscles so you eventually won't feel controlled by your emotions or urges. You'll be able to choose *not* to engage in target behavior. But that means continuing to do the practice even when it's frustrating or agitating or boring. Kudos for continuing even when you felt frustrated.

Questions you can ask about any of the MMT assignments include (but are not limited to):

- *What was it like to do the home practice?*
- *Did you have difficulty getting yourself to do the practice?* [This question can be especially helpful, as it normalizes difficulties. Otherwise, clients may be hesitant to admit they had trouble getting themselves to even start the practice. This question also allows you to reinforce clients who practice even when they have difficulty getting themselves to do so.]
- *Was there anything that surprised you?*
- *Were there any times when you felt agitated, antsy, or bored? That's common. Tell me about those.*
- *Did you ever find yourself judging yourself for your reactions? Tell me about that.*
- *Did you ever find yourself questioning whether you were doing it "correctly" or trying to get yourself to feel something different than what you were feeling?*
- *Do you have any questions about the practice now that you've done it?*

Potential comments by the client (and therapist reactions) include:

- The client thought the practice wasn't working because his mind wandered, he felt bored or agitated or frustrated, and/or he couldn't relax.
  - *Response:* Normalize, normalize, normalize! Validate and then explain that the practice is still working just as well when the client has trouble focusing or does not enjoy the practicing. (See the example above.) Reinforce the client for completing the practice.
- The client says that the practice seems pointless or doesn't feel like it is helping.
  - *Response:* Clarify what the client means. Then reflect and validate the client's opinion. ("It's understandable that the practices feel weird. Most people expect therapy practices to help them feel better right away, but these practices often don't have immediate effects.") Then explain the benefits again—possibly in detail. (See Strategy 3B, on pp. 56–58.) If the client still questions the benefits, use the therapy relationship. Stress that you have seen the practices work and you have confidence that they will work for the client. Tell the client you are asking her to trust you and do the practices for a few weeks before deciding whether or not she wants to continue. (After all, what does she have to lose other than a few hours of time? And if the practice "works," her life could be changed.)

- The client says she finds herself judging herself or trying to get herself to feel a certain way when doing the practice.
  - *Response:* Normalize and validate. Encourage the client to do her best not to judge herself for judging—but instead to notice herself judging, gently bring her mind back to the practice, and remind herself that there is no wrong or right way to feel. Encourage the client to allow herself to experience whatever she experiences.
- The client says he falls asleep during practice.
  - *Response:* Find out where he is doing the practice. It is best not to do the practice while lying in bed or any place the client normally sleeps. If the client is already lying down somewhere other than a standard sleeping spot, ask the client to move to a comfortable chair for a few days until he becomes accustomed to staying awake.

If the Client Did Not Do the Home Practice, Take the Following Steps

1. Reflect and validate the difficulty.
2. Repeatedly tell the client you are not judging or criticizing.
3. Find out what got in the way of doing the practice.
4. Work on a plan to address the obstacles and increase the chance of completion.

Reflect and Validate the Difficulty and Tediousness of the Home Practice

It's understandable that someone would have difficulty getting into the groove of doing the home practice. The client is busy, and the practice takes time out of the client's already busy day. Plus it can feel monotonous. And boring. And so on.

Repeatedly Tell the Client That You Are Not Judging or Criticizing

Clients often have strong urges to avoid any talk about not doing home practice, as they fear you will be disappointed in them and think they are "bad clients." Anyone who has ever failed to complete an assignment in school will know the fear of being chastised, so the client may often interpret *any* discussion about the uncompleted practice as criticism. You need to emphasize that you are not judging or criticizing—and then explain *why* you are discussing the lack of practice: You want to find out what got in the way of the practice so you can work together to increase the chance of practice completion the following week. You can also ask for the client's reaction:

> *Does it feel like I'm judging or criticizing? If it does, it just means I'm not expressing myself effectively—because I'm really not judging you. I'm just trying to find out what got in the way so we can work together to make a plan to address the obstacles this week. Thanks for working with me on this.*

You may also reflect and validate the potential discomfort in talking about lack of home practice completion. Be sure to affirm the client's willingness to talk about the topic.

Find Out What Got in the Way of Doing the Practice

Don't just assume you know the reason the client did not do the home practice. You will need to ask and give prompts—to increase the chance that the client doesn't censure her response. You want as much detail as possible, so you can tailor the solutions to fit the client's specific obstacles.

> *Let's talk about what got in the way of your doing the home practice. I'm not judging you, and I don't mean to sound like I'm criticizing or chastising you—because I'm not. It's just that we need to figure out the obstacles so we can create a plan to increase the chance you can do the practice this week.* (Pause for a response)
>
> *Here are some common obstacles people often have. Did you forget—just not think about it after leaving here? Or maybe you thought about the home practice but then kept telling yourself you'd do it later—until the week finally ran out. Or you tried to make time to do it, but just had trouble finding time in your schedule or finding privacy to do it. Or maybe you thought it didn't seem like it could really help and so you didn't feel like doing it. Does any combination of those fit you?* (Pause for answers.)
>
> *Thanks for talking about this. I know it can be uncomfortable being put on the spot like this, so I appreciate your explaining this to me. So you forgot. Is it that you literally didn't think about it at all after you left this room last week? Or is it that you thought about it a few times, but decided you'd do it later—and then forgot to do it later?* [The therapist will then address the client's obstacle with the relevant strategy(ies) in Step 4. Always end by reminding the client that the home practice is necessary for moving toward the life the client wants to live.]

If the client goes more than a week or two without home practice, you may also conduct a functional analysis (see Chapter 6, pp. 84–86) to better understand the obstacles impeding engagement of the home practice (or other adaptive behavior). In this case, the setup and the functional analysis itself will be similar to that of a functional analysis for dysregulated behavior.

Work on a Plan to Address the Obstacles and Increase the Chance of Completion in the Upcoming Week

Continue to validate and assure the client that you are not judging or meaning to criticize. Common obstacles and very basic potential plans to address them include the following.

OBSTACLE: FORGETTING

Potential Plans

a. Find out what time of day the client would be most likely to complete practice. Ask the client to set a daily alarm or reminder in his phone or tablet for that time.
b. The client can write notes to himself and tape them on mirrors, refrigerators, or other places he sees regularly.
c. The client can leave home practice sheets on the nightstand, the kitchen table, or other places

that are obvious and easy to access. (If the client arrives the following week without doing any home practice, you will know that the explanation is more than just forgetting.)

OBSTACLE: PROCRASTINATING

Potential Plans

a. Work with the client to find the best time of the day (either the same time every day, or a specific time for each upcoming day). Ask her to commit to doing her best to do the practice at that time—especially the first day—even when she feels the urge to procrastinate. Ask her to set phone alarm(s) for the time(s) she chooses. Troubleshoot. ("What happens if your alarm goes off at 6:00 A.M. tomorrow and you think, 'I'm tired after a rough day at work yesterday. I'll start tomorrow'? How will you get yourself to do the practice anyway?")

b. Ask the client to generate reasons she may give herself for procrastinating and then write responses to those reasons. (You may prompt the client with potential reasons and responses.) Example: If a client tells herself that she'll do the home practice later, she can remind herself that she committed to doing the home practice as soon as her phone alarm went off—and that past experience shows that she is unlikely to do the practice later. Another possibility would be to generate positive and negative consequences of putting off the practice when the alarm goes off. Write down the client's response to procrastination thoughts or her list of negative consequences of procrastinating. Give the client the list to refer to when she has urges to procrastinate. You may also have the client record those statements in her phone and commit to listening to them when she has urges to procrastinate.

c. Assess whether the client has additional reasons for procrastinating—which may include not understanding the assignments or being hesitant to experience the emotions that may be elicited. If so, validate the client's experience, and see relevant bullet point below.

d. Get a commitment. Troubleshoot. Use shaping. (See Strategy 5, p. 71.)

OBSTACLE: THE CLIENT HAS A BUSY SCHEDULE AND TRULY HAS TROUBLE FINDING TIME

Potential Plans

a. First, make sure that "I don't have time" really means that the client doesn't have time. The "don't-have-time" response often means that clients have really just procrastinated. If the latter, nonjudgmentally move to the preceding bulleted list.

b. Work with the client to find ways to make time. The guided audios take approximately 6–15 minutes; the informal exercises (BEST Bs) take 2–3 minutes each and can be practiced while waiting for someone, while on mass transportation, or even before going to sleep at night. Help the client carve out times to practice (which may change depending on the day). Ask the client to generate ideas. Offer suggestions, including doing practice during lunch hour (while sitting in a car or in the office), doing BEST Bs during breaks, doing BEST Bs while sitting/ standing on mass transit, waking up 15 minutes earlier, delaying bedtime for 15 minutes, or giving up some other activity (e.g., a few minutes of a TV show, time on the Internet, or other activities you may discuss with the client). Remind the client that he is only in treatment for a limited time, so these few months are the only chance he has to work with you to move toward the life he wants (the destination). Would it be worth giving up TV for 15 minutes a day for a few months if that's what it takes to make progress toward the life he wants?

c. Get a commitment. Troubleshoot. Use shaping. (See Strategy 5, p. 71.)

OBSTACLE: THE CLIENT HAS TROUBLE FINDING PRIVACY

Potential Plans

a. Work with the client to generate ideas of ways to create privacy.

b. Employed clients: If the client has a private office, she can practice there. If not, ask the client to do the practice in her car while parked in a safe place during lunch break or right before or after work. The client can lower the seat to the point that she can barely be seen.

c. Clients at home: Ask the client to go to the bathroom and lock the door. For all anyone knows, the client is using the bathroom for "standard" purposes. In addition, the client can find a safe place to park while running errands and do some of the practice then. Clients may also decide to stay up later or get up earlier than other people in the household (if possible) and do the home practice then. Again, it will only be for a few months while in treatment, and it could affect the rest of the client's life.

d. Get a commitment. Troubleshoot.

OBSTACLE: THE CLIENT ACTUALLY DOESN'T *WANT* TO DO THE HOME PRACTICE BECAUSE HE DOESN'T THINK IT WILL HELP AND/OR IS RELUCTANT TO FEEL UNCOMFORTABLE EMOTIONS

Potential Plans

a. If the client doesn't want to do the home practice, reflect and validate his skepticism. (A lot of the assignments will seem weird to someone not accustomed to mindfulness practice!) *Thank him for being honest.* Talk through the benefits of the home practice. (See Strategy 3B, pp. 56–58.) Remind the client that this therapy has only been shown to work when clients do the home practice. Use the therapy relationship: Stress that you believe the practice will work. Ask the client to trust you enough to do the practice for a few weeks—and then decide whether he wants to continue. If he doesn't find it helpful, he hasn't lost anything, and if he does, he has gained a lot. Ask for a commitment. Troubleshoot. Use shaping. (See Strategy 5, p. 71.)

b. If the client is reluctant to feel uncomfortable emotions, reflect and validate her reluctance. Then remind the client that the home practice is necessary to move toward the life she wants (the destination). Discuss how the practice can be helpful (see Strategy 3B, pp. 56–58), with a focus on how the practice will eventually make the emotions feel more tolerable. Then move to plans for overcoming procrastination (above). Get a commitment. Troubleshoot. Use shaping. (Strategy 5, p. 71.)

Note: Although shaping is mentioned in most of the preceding plans, it is not explained until the next strategy (Strategy 5). The reason for presenting shaping separately is that it can be utilized to increase any desired behavior (from home practice to days of abstinence), so its utility is not limited to increasing home practice. Thus, the choice was either to describe shaping twice (once in the above plans and once in its own strategy) or to mention it in the above plans but wait to provide a description until the next strategy. I have (obviously) chosen the latter. Please see the following strategy for information on the use of shaping.

STRATEGY 5: ACTIVE SHAPING OF BEHAVIORS

A. The therapist validates and "uses" the relationship when encouraging and gently pushing.
  - The therapist is authentic in explanation: Express hesitation (or perhaps even apologize), but also express care and concern.
    ◆ Remind the client of commitments and values.
    ◆ Remind the client of the boiling pot.
    ◆ Remind the client of the necessity of home practice on the road to the destination (valued life).
B. Involve the client in choosing the extent of the shaping.
  - Ask the client to share perceptions and reactions.
  - Use a confidence scale.
C. Use the Mirror Exercise.

When clients have difficulty engaging in adaptive behavior (e.g., home practice) and/or refraining from maladaptive behavior (e.g., target behavior), therapists are encouraged to complete the steps in Strategy 4: (1) validate clients' difficulties, (2) assure clients that they are not being judged, (3) investigate the obstacles to adaptive behavior or the antecedents of maladaptive behavior, and (4) plan ways to address potential difficulties in the upcoming week.

For difficulty with home practice, therapists may choose from the plans listed in the previous strategy, taking care to modify the plans for each client. For dysregulated behavior, therapists may conduct a functional analysis of the behavior (Chapter 6, pp. 84–86) and then work with the client to plan ways to cope with antecedents and/or modify consequences. For both types of plans, the use of shaping is often also necessary to help the client begin moving toward the desired behavior.

The strategy of *shaping* is used when a client is having difficulty engaging in desired behavior. Shaping involves gradually increasing a desired behavior by planning and reinforcing responses that are similar to the desired response. In MMT, shaping involves working with the client to create a plan that initially includes only a portion of the desired adaptive behavior (e.g., days of homework practice or days without target behavior)—with the intention of increasing the desired behavior over time. As the therapy progresses, you reinforce any incidents of desired behavior, work with clients to plan increases in such incidents, and continue reinforcing each step.

For example, if a client is assigned 5 days of home practice but does not do any, you may work with the client to plan and commit to at least 2 days of practice in the upcoming week. (Strategy 5B, on pp. 75–79, provides more information on how to create such a plan.) Any reports of home practice will be reinforced the following week, and the client will eventually be encouraged to commit to additional days of practice per week—with each increase being reinforced. And so on.

Similarly, if the client engages in the target dysregulated behavior every day, you may work with him to plan for and commit to at least 1 day without any target behavior. Any reports of days without target behavior will be reinforced the following week, and the client will be encouraged to work toward additional days of abstinence from the behavior—with each increase being reinforced. And so on.

Shaping often occurs after the client has not been able to engage in the planned adaptive behavior for more than 1 week. For example:

- If the client does not complete a significant portion of the practice for 1 week, you will go over the steps in Strategy 4C and work with the client to create a plan to complete the home practice the following week—but you may or may not use shaping.
- If the client arrives for a second consecutive week without completing a significant portion of the home practice, you are encouraged to revisit the steps in Strategy 4 while also using shaping.

However, shaping does not always begin at exactly the second week of difficulty. As with all techniques, you will use your clinical judgment and consider the needs of the client to decide exactly when the technique is implemented.

Shaping can be used to increase a variety of desired behaviors: home practice, days (or hours) without the target behavior, actions needed to overcome obstacles to treatment (e.g., seeking medical care for health issues, increasing social support, decreasing avoidance), and so on. Of course, such shaping is usually easier said than done. The following strategies will greatly increase the likelihood that shaping is effective.

STRATEGY 5A: The therapist validates and uses the relationship when gently pushing the client to increase desired behaviors.

Express hesitation (perhaps even apologize), but also express care and concern. Although you will actively reflect, validate, and affirm the client's behavior throughout the entire course of treatment, you need to be especially active in reflecting, validating, and affirming when encouraging (or gently pushing) clients to move toward desired behavior. Otherwise, clients may perceive your actions as critical (of current behavior), coercive, and/or controlling. Clients may also think you just do not understand (or care) how painful or impossible the behavior change feels to them. Thus, without extensive reflection/validation/affirmation by the therapist, clients are likely to feel defensive, constrained, and/or unheard—while also possibly experiencing decreased rapport and decreased hope about their ability to change their behavior. (Most people feel defensive and resistant when they feel they are being criticized and told what to do. The client is not being unreasonable or pathological if he reacts defensively in such a situation.)

Although active reflection/validation/affirmation is essential for shaping, it is not sufficient. When working to nudge a client toward a difficult behavior change, you also need to "use" the therapy relationship and authentically explain why you are nudging. This explanation will usually involve a combination of (1) feeling a little hesitant about pushing the client for fear of harming rapport, (2) wanting the client to have a life that feels more valuable and fulfilling, and (3) caring about the client's well-being. Thus, it is important for you to explain that although you feel hesitant about pushing, you may sometimes do so because (1) you want the client to have a life that feels more valuable and fulfilling, (2) you believe that the actions you're encouraging are necessary for the client to get closer to that life, and (3) you care enough that you're willing to risk her irritation with you if that's what it takes for the client to get past her current situation and move to a life that feels more fulfilling. Here's an example:

> *I feel like I may be pushing you, and I'm sorry if it feels that way. Part of me doesn't want to keep pushing, because I don't want you to feel pressured. But here's the thing: I really want you to get closer to that destination—to that point where your life feels more like the life you want, and you feel more like the kind of person you want to be. And based on what I know about this treatment, I fully believe that the home practice is necessary to get you to that destination. I wish that just coming in here and talking for 45 minutes every week would be enough to get you to the kind of life you want. But I know it's not. So even though part of me wants to quit talking about this, because I like you and don't want to risk your feeling pressured and getting upset with me, I'm going to push a little more, because I care enough about you that I'm willing to risk your getting upset with me. It's more important to me that you get closer to the life you want than it is to keep you from be irritated. (Pause) Are you OK with talking about this a little more?* (Client agrees.)*
>
> *Thank you. I know you're already making a big effort, and I know you're busy and the home practice can feel tedious and time-consuming. So I appreciate your working with me on this. Let's talk more about the upcoming week.*

Note: This strategy is not advising you to be disingenuous. Of course you should not say you care about the client or the treatment outcome if you do not do so. However, knowing that you have chosen to become a mental health practitioner, I doubt that I would be going out on a limb to assume that you care about clients' well-being and you care about providing effective treatment. Thus, it's not far afield to believe that you will care enough about each client to truly want to increase the client's well-being and decrease any obstacles to that well-being. You do not have to feel intense warmth and concern about a client in every moment to care about the client's well-being and treatment outcome. (I am not necessarily saying that you *won't* feel intense warmth and concern for your clients. I am just saying you do not have to be experiencing such feelings in every moment to truthfully tell a client you care about her and want the best for her.)

Other strategies to help build motivation and actions when clients have trouble taking adaptive action:

● *Remind clients of their commitment and values:* In the first session, you warned clients that they might have weeks when they did not think treatment was working or when they felt a little worse for a short time before they felt better. You then got a commitment that they would stay in treatment a minimum amount of time and work to do the home practice even if they had these reactions. If clients later have trouble engaging in adaptive action (home practice, attending session), remind them that you warned them in the first session that they might have doubts and difficulties, and that they committed to doing the practice and attending treatment anyway.

Remind them that their experience is normal and expected, and it does not mean that treatment isn't working. Also remind them of their values and the reasons they gave for committing to treatment in the first session (and following sessions).

- *Remind clients of the boiling pot metaphor.* (Yes, this ubiquitous metaphor has shown up again. And the next bullet point contains another one.) Any time clients do not do the home practice or other adaptive action, whether because of procrastination and/or explicitly not wanting to experience emotions, they are avoiding actions that may evoke discomfort. In other words, they are putting the lid on the boiling pot a little more tightly—thus trapping the steam and pressure inside the pot to build further. Although it makes sense that they would have urges to continue behaviors that have helped in the past, they are actually causing uncomfortable emotions and urges to increase. In contrast, by completing the home practice and other adaptive actions, they will release steam from the pot—which will help decrease uncomfortable emotions and urges over time.

- *Remind clients of the necessity of home practice on the road to their destination.* As clients work to stop their primary coping behavior, they can easily become mired in day-to-day hassles and lose sight of the overall purpose. Thus, you will often need to remind them of the ultimate purpose of the treatment: to help them move toward lives that feel more satisfying and valuable to them. The home practice is an essential component of helping clients move down the road toward that life. (After all, if people could get to the life they want without doing the home practice, you would not have assigned the home practice to begin with.) You can refer to the destination metaphor when explaining why you are nudging the client to take adaptive action. (See example on previous page.)

In addition, the destination metaphor helps you discuss the lack of home practice in a way that can decrease feelings of shame and potential defensiveness. For example:

We're working to get you closer to a life that feels more like the life you want—so you feel more like the kind of person you want to be. And you've made progress just by coming here and talking about the stuff you've talked about. It's like here's the destination (reach right hand far to the right). *You started out here* (reach left hand far to the left) *and you've moved forward* (show movement toward right hand). *But in the last couple of weeks, it's like you've pulled over to the shoulder and sat idling for a while.* (Demonstrate.) *You haven't gone backward—and that's important to remember. You haven't lost any progress you've made. But for the last few weeks, you haven't been moving forward either. You've just sort of been hanging out. And the problem is that if the weeks keep going by and you continue sitting by the side of the road [depending on the client, you might add "or just barely moving forward"], you're never going to get much closer to the life you want. Sooner or later, you're going to start feeling discouraged. And then there's a big risk you'll make a U-turn and lose the progress. That would be a shame, because you deserve more than what you have now. But you haven't lost any progress yet. So let's talk about how to get you back on that road* (bring your hands up again to demonstrate) *and start moving forward again.* (Pause) *Does this feel like I'm judging you or criticizing you?* (Client answers.) *Good. Because I'm really not.*

STRATEGY 5B: Involve the client in choosing the extent of the shaping.

Ask the client to share perceptions and reactions. People are more likely to engage in a behavior if they feel they have some control of at least some aspect of the planning. Consistently, one key to successful shaping is to directly involve the client in choosing the extent of the plan. For example, suppose a client did not complete any home practice the previous 2 weeks. (For purposes of simplicity, I will focus on home practice. But this strategy can be used to increase any adaptive behavior.) After completing the first three steps listed in Strategy 4C (validate the difficulty, remind the client that you aren't judging, find out what got in the way of the adaptive behavior), you will work with the client to create a plan for doing the home practice the upcoming week. This plan will include shaping.

When shaping a client's behavior, you collaborate with her to decide a minimum number of times that she will commit to engaging in home practice the following week *regardless of potential obstacles.* (Because MMT assigns multiple tasks—such as the audio and the BEST Bs—you may conduct a shaping plan for each task.)

The plan will include fewer instances of the behavior than you would ultimately like the client to perform; however, after a week or two of the client's not doing the home practice (or doing far less than assigned), your main goal will be getting the client to *keep her commitment* as to the amount of times she will engage in the practice the upcoming week. It is more important in the long term for the client to be conditioned to keeping therapy commitments than it is for her to do the full home practice that particular week. Thus, if you err, you want to err on the side of getting the client to commit to too few instances of the practice instead of too many. You can work with the client to add additional days of practice over time.

To work with the client in forming a plan:

1. Tell her that since she had trouble completing the home practice the previous week(s), you want to start over with a plan that she knows she can accomplish. Normalize this approach. It is not uncommon for clients to have to start with small amounts of home practice and build over time.

2. Explain that you want to work together to decide on a number of times she is willing to commit to doing each assigned task *no matter what happens.* Choose one task to discuss (e.g., the audio practice).

   ■ Stress that "no matter what" truly means that she needs to choose a minimum number of times she guarantees that she will do the practice, regardless of anything else that happens in her life. Even if she gets sick, has visitors, feels depressed, has a water pipe break, has a fight with a friend, hears that space aliens have landed on Earth and are taking over the city, or *whatever*—she will still do the amount of home practice she committed to doing.

   ■ It *is* OK to end with a ridiculous example—to stress the importance of "no matter what," while also potentially decreasing the chance that the client might feel pressured.

3. If the client hesitates, suggest a number one or two times higher than what the client did the week before. (Usually stick to one time more for each task unless the client did not do any practice the week before.) Ask the client if she is OK with that number for this week. For

example, if the client practiced the audio exercise one time the week before, you would suggest that she practice the audio exercise at least two times in the upcoming week.

4. If the client suggests increasing her practice by more than one or two instances, suggest that she choose a lower number. Remind her that she needs to pick an amount that she can guarantee doing *no matter what*—and list possible obstacles again. Tell her that the most important thing is that she pick a number she *knows* she can do. Tell her she can always do more than the minimum if she wants, but stress that she is not expected to do so. Choose a lower number and ask her if she is OK with committing to that amount.

5. At the top of the Tracking Sheet for the upcoming week, write the number the client chose in the appropriate column (e.g., write *2 times* in the Audio column).

6. Return to number 2, above, and go through this list again for the other exercises (e.g., BEST B) if applicable.

7. Check with the client throughout the discussion for her perceptions and reactions. Ask if she is feeling pressured. Ask what she thinks about the discussion. At the end, summarize and ask if she is OK with everything. Again remind her that she is committing to do each agreed-upon task *no matter what*—and give her one more chance to decrease the number.

8. Troubleshoot. Affirm (a lot).

Here is an example of a dialogue that might follow after you validate/reflect, assess and address obstacles, and authentically explain why you are pushing/nudging:

THERAPIST: Since you've had difficulty doing all the home practice the last couple of weeks, let's regroup for a moment. The Color Body Scan was assigned five times and you did it once. Now once is still better than not at all, so I'm glad you did it at all. I know you're making an effort. But I'd like to see a little more this week—just to make sure you keep moving down the road toward the life you want. I don't want you to get stalled or move so slowly that you get discouraged. Let's not go for five times. Let's pick something lower. What number of times can you guarantee that you'll do the audio *no matter what*—no matter if you get sick, if your boyfriend comes to town, if you get extra shifts at work, if you don't feel motivated, or if Godzilla appears from the ocean and destroys the entire country except for your apartment and this office? How many times can you guarantee that you'll do the audio, no matter what?

CLIENT: Ummm, I think I can do three.

THERAPIST: Three is a lot. I know you're really busy right now, and you were only able to do it one time in the last 2 weeks. So I want to remind you that you are guaranteeing to do the practice at least this number of times, even if you get sick, you get depressed, you feel overwhelmed—no matter what. It's better for you to pick a lower number and make sure you do it than to pick a higher number and risk not doing what you committed to doing. I still know you're making an effort. Do you want to keep three, or do you want to make it two for this week—just in case? And we can move it to three next week if you want. What do you think?

CLIENT: Ummm. Yeah, two would probably be better. Let's do two.

THERAPIST: Sounds like a good idea. I hope you know I wasn't doubting you. I just know that a lot of unexpected things can happen, and sometimes it's better to be safe than sorry.

CLIENT: That's OK. I didn't think you were doubting me.

THERAPIST: Good. So you'll commit to two—even if Godzilla attacks? (*Client chuckles and agrees.*) How are you feeling about this whole thing?

CLIENT: Good. I know I need to do the home practice. I just need to get myself going on it.

THERAPIST: Do you feel pressured? Like you have to say you'll do the practice to make me happy? (*Client says she doesn't. Therapist affirms.*) Now let's talk about the BEST B. The regular assignment is at least once a day—so seven times a week, and you did it three times last week. Again, at least that's something. It's not that uncommon for people to start slow and build up. It doesn't mean that there's anything wrong with you. So for this week, how many times do you feel you can guarantee to do the BEST B, no matter what?

CLIENT: I'm not sure.

THERAPIST: It takes 2–3 minutes a time. You did it three times last week. What would you think about four or five times this week?

CLIENT: Five. I can do five.

THERAPIST: OK, five. That's almost twice what you did last week. So that means doing it every day this week except for 2 days. Are you sure that feels doable—like you're completely sure you'll do it, or would you rather start with four?

CLIENT: No, five feels like a good number. I can definitely do five.

THERAPIST: Five it is! So we have audio at least two times and the BEST B at least five. What about moving to the pleasant or fulfilling activities. Are you up for adding at least one of those?

You might also choose to focus on the audio and BEST B and postpone the pleasant activities to another week. Once you have the final plan, you will troubleshoot.

THERAPIST: So we have the audio at two times, the BEST B at least five times, and a pleasant or fulfilling activity at least two times. That's a big increase from last week. I commend you on being willing to take this step forward. Let's troubleshoot: What might get in the way? What happens if your phone alarm goes off on one of the nights you've set, and you just feel like watching TV and shutting off the world? How will you get yourself to do the audio?

CLIENT: I'll just remind myself that I committed to doing it and that this is my only chance to get better. And I'll think about having to tell you whether I did it or not next week. (*Laughs*)

Note: Some clients will never get to the point of doing five audio practices and seven BEST Bs per week. If, after several weeks of shaping and other strategies, clients seem to peak at consistently completing audio practices three/four times and BEST Bs at least five, *then strongly consider changing the assignment to those criteria.*

Use a Confidence Scale

Use a confidence scale (e.g., Miller & Rollnick, 2012) whenever you want to increase the chance that a client will engage in an activity—whether that activity be completing home practice, attending therapy, or getting through a period of time without the target behavior:

> THERAPIST: We've talked about the importance of the Daily Log. On a scale of 1–10, how confident are you that you'll come in here next week saying you completed the Daily Log every day?
>
> CLIENT: I'll try, but it's hard to get myself to do things when I get in a rut. I'd say 6.
>
> THERAPIST: (*matter-of-fact*) OK, a little more than half. I know you've been having a lot of trouble getting yourself to do the Daily Log, and you only did it 1 day last week. Why a 6 and not 4 or 5?
>
> CLIENT: Well, I just feel bad coming in here and not doing what it takes to make progress. I do need to stop smoking, so I need to get myself to do what it takes to make the treatment work.

Notice that by asking why the client did not choose *a lower* number, the therapist got the client to explain the reasons he *is* motivated. He said he feels bad when he doesn't do the Daily Log, and he wants to do the work necessary to be able to quit smoking. In other words, the therapist got the client to talk himself into feeling more committed. Once the client starts making statements focused on change, the therapist can reflect, validate, and affirm to continue the conversation.

Here's another example of a confidence scale:

> THERAPIST: On a scale of 1–10, how confident are you that you'll get through this next week without any target behavior—if *1* is absolutely no confidence and *10* is 100% confidence?
>
> CLIENT: Ugh. I don't know. Maybe a *2*.
>
> THERAPIST: (*matter-of-fact*) OK, 2's pretty low. But I also know you said your urges feel almost unbearable. Why a *2* and not a *1*?
>
> CLIENT: Because I'm *so* tired of the way I feel after the behavior! I want to stop feeling that way.

Use of a confidence scale can help increase confidence and commitment by encouraging the client to explore and explain why he is motivated to engage in an activity the therapist wants to increase. Confidence scales can (and should) be utilized heavily within the first weeks of treatment—and again whenever the therapist feels the client needs an extra boost of motivation.

Finally, therapists often ask how to respond if a client picks the lowest number on the confidence scale. That happens very rarely, but if it does happen, just take a moment to reflect and validate the client's feelings of hopelessness. You then get the chance to explain that levels of confidence or hope toward the beginning of treatment have no bearing on whether or not the treatment will work. As long as the client comes to sessions and does the home practice, he has just as much likelihood of moving forward as he would if he felt high hope.

Note: All credit for MMT's use of confidence scales goes to MI's "confidence ruler" (Miller & Rollnick, 2012).

STRATEGY 5C: Conduct the Mirror Exercise.

The Mirror Exercise is a guided visualization to help clients realize the consequences of repeatedly telling themselves that they'll start doing the home practice or stop the target behavior "tomorrow." Notice that the previous sentence does not include the word *procrastinate*, because clients may not perceive themselves as procrastinating when they decide to do the practice "tomorrow" or stop the behavior "next week." Instead, they often believe that they will be more motivated or have less difficulty at that future time. They may also repeatedly convince themselves that they just need to have "one last day" or "one last weekend" of fun before giving up the behavior.

The exercise is a variation of the ghosts of Christmas present, past, and future in the tale of Ebenezer Scrooge from *The Christmas Carol;* however, the Mirror Exercise consists only of visualizations of the future. The client is instructed to visualize himself standing in front of a small bathroom mirror getting ready for the start of his day at various times in the future—after not ever fully engaging in the home practice or stopping the target behavior. This portion of the visualization ends with the client in front of the mirror 5 years in the future, with his target behavior as bad or worse than it was prior to treatment. The client is instructed to be aware of what his life is like after five more years of the behavior—as well as how he feels knowing that he will likely be engaging in the behavior at similar or greater levels for the rest of his life.

The client is then instructed to keep his eyes closed but to "reset" his mental image. He is then guided to visualize himself in front of a small mirror at the same points in the future, but this time after he *did* engage in the treatment and stop (or at least regulate) the target behavior.

The Mirror Exercise is introduced in the semi-flex session, which is usually conducted in the fourth or fifth week of treatment. Thus, the script for the Mirror Exercise is included in the semi-flex session (see Chapter 8, pp. 188–191). The Mirror Exercise can be conducted again when needed to increase motivated action. You are encouraged to record the exercise as you conduct it in session and then provide the recording to the client for playing when additional motivation is needed between sessions and after therapy has been completed.

CHAPTER SUMMARY

Strategy 4: Lots of Structure and Home Practice

- Providing regular home practice is more likely to foster habit. Habitual behavior tends to require less intention and effort, while also eliciting less anxiety.
- Set up home practice explicitly and review the Daily Log in the beginning of every session.
- If the client did not do the home practice,
    1. Reflect and validate the difficulty and tediousness,
    2. Tell the client you are not judging or criticizing,
    3. Find out what got in the way,

4. Work on a plan to increase the chance of completion during the upcoming week, and

5. Include shaping when applicable.

Strategy 5: Active Shaping of Behaviors

- Shaping involves gradually increasing a desired behavior by planning and reinforcing responses that are similar to the desired response.

- "Use" validation, the relationship, and the client's values when encouraging the client to increase the desired behavior.

- Remind the client of her commitments and values, the boiling pot metaphor, and the necessity of the home practice in moving toward a life that feels more fulfilling (destination).

- Involve the client in choosing the extent of the shaping.

- Use a confidence scale.

PART III

MMT Session Guidelines

Part III provides essential guidelines for conducting MMT.

- Chapter 6: Common questions, obstacles, and general issues
- Chapter 7: MMT setup, intake guidelines, and structure of sessions
  - MMT planning and tracking
    - Guide to choosing session schedule
    - Chart for tracking delivery of MMT sessions
    - Guide for tracking guided audios
    - Instructions for tracking emotions, urges, and target behavior (Daily Log)
    - Guide for delivering MMT in various formats and settings
  - MMT intake guidelines—essential for setting up effective treatment
  - Structure of sessions (beginning Session B)
- Chapters 8–12: MMT session descriptions
- Chapter 13: Conclusion

CHAPTER 6

Common Questions, Obstacles, and General Issues

This chapter (1) discusses common questions that often arise in the implementation of MMT, and (2) provides descriptions and examples of concepts mentioned earlier in this book. Despite the range of topics covered, all information in the chapter is vital for conducting MMT.

- Addressing specific needs, values, or behaviors of the client
  - What about client diversity?
  - How do I conduct a functional analysis?
  - Does the client's behavior require more targeted techniques?
  - Does the client want to continue the behavior in moderation?
  - What if the client does not commit to treatment?
  - What if the client presents with an unrelated problem but displays dysregulated behavior?
  - Can clients with posttraumatic stress disorder (PTSD) practice formal mindfulness?
- Therapeutic relationship, therapist characteristics, and therapist disclosure
  - Can focusing on the therapeutic relationship be harmful to clients?
  - Do MMT therapists have to maintain a formal mindfulness practice?
  - Are therapists with histories of dysregulated behavior more effective?
  - What about therapist self-disclosure?
- Additional issues that may arise inside or outside of session
  - What if the Daily Log routinely shows 0's or very low numbers?
  - Should therapists take notes?
  - Why does the Color Body Scan include a color?
  - How do I share the audio files with clients?

ADDRESSING SPECIFIC NEEDS, VALUES, OR BEHAVIORS OF THE CLIENT

What about client diversity?

For therapists to be consistent with MMT principles, they must always conduct the treatment according to its fundamental tenet: The core purpose of MMT is to help the client move closer to being the kind of person *the client* wants to be and living a life that fits more closely with *the client's* values. Thus, every aspect of treatment should always be modified to fit each client's unique combination of beliefs, motivations, obstacles, and experiences in the world. Whether assessing a client's values or helping the client move closer to living those values, therapists should always consider factors related to culture in the most encompassing sense of the word. This tenet is true with all clients, but it is perhaps especially crucial when a therapist works with a client from a culture (race, ethnicity, sexual orientation, etc.) that is different from that of the therapist. Therapists should also do their best to ensure that they do not try to force their own cultural expectations onto their client—whether gently or otherwise. Therapists are strongly encouraged to conduct continued explorations of their own biases—and work to address those biases to decrease the chance that they interfere with treatment.

Through research and in clinical settings, MMT has been conducted with clients who have reported a diverse array of races/ethnicities, religions, nationalities, and overall cultural identities. MMT clients have included those who have identified themselves as Black, Latino/a, White, Arab, Indian, Hawaiian, and Native American. Reported religious affiliations have included Catholic, Christian/Protestant, Orthodox Jewish, Hindi, Muslim, Wiccan, agnostic, atheist, and spiritual but not religious. MMT clients have included those with a variety of reported sexual orientations, gender identities, and socioeconomic statuses. Finally, although MMT has largely been implemented with U.S. citizens, it has also been conducted with clients who were in the United States on green cards, work visas, or student visas (Wupperman et al., 2012, 2015, 2018, 2019a, 2019b). None of this is meant to imply that MMT can somehow magically transcend all cultural issues. Instead, therapists must be diligent in (1) educating themselves about their clients' experiences—cultural and otherwise; (2) working to provide a responsive, accepting atmosphere for clients of all cultures; (3) openly addressing any cultural issues that arise in treatment; and (4) tailoring the treatment to fit *the client's* values instead of their own.

What is a functional analysis, and how do I conduct one?

A functional analysis (FA) involves working to understand the factors contributing to the client's target behavior. As discussed earlier, clients often engage in target behavior in order to change an emotional state with which they're dissatisfied. In such cases, the target behavior is being reinforced by (1) increasing positive experiences (i.e., increasing happiness when a client thinks he *should* be feeling happier), and/or (2) decreasing negative experiences (i.e., decreasing urges, anxiety, sadness, emptiness, etc.). Behaviors that continue or increase after they are reinforced are described as *operantly conditioned*.

Target behaviors can also be *classically conditioned*—which means that they become paired with a stimulus after repeated association with that stimulus. The most famous episode of classical conditioning is the case of Pavlov's dogs. The dogs became so conditioned to receiving food after hearing a bell that they eventually started salivating when hearing the bell—even if no food was forthcoming.

Sometimes clients become so accustomed to using target behavior in association with a previously unrelated thing that they start having strong urges to engage in the behavior any time the other thing happens. For example, if someone is accustomed to eating a sandwich and a donut every time she arrives at work, she may have strong urges to eat a sandwich and a donut when she arrives at work—even if she just had a big lunch and is not at all hungry. She has become classically conditioned to the point that she physiologically expects a sandwich and a donut. In these cases, a person might have strong urges to engage in the behavior even if she is not feeling dissatisfaction about an emotional state. However, if the person does not act on the urge, she may begin to feel extreme discomfort and distress due to the strength of the urge. Thus, instead of distress occurring first and the urges occurring second, sometimes the urges occur first and the distress occurs second.

In an FA, therapists work to understand the antecedents that led to the target behavior. Antecedents include (1) the situational cue and (2) contributing emotions, sensations, thoughts, and urges. (Not coincidentally, the *H-C2: High-Risk Situations Worksheet* in Chapter 8 asks clients for the situation/cue as well as for their emotions, sensations, and thoughts.)

Along with antecedents, therapists also want to know the consequences, which help them identify what might reinforce the behavior. Ask the client for both the positive consequences and the negative consequences. When asking for positive consequences, be sure to suggest a few potential positive consequences in addition to the ones the client reports. This shows that you understand that the client gains benefits from the behavior. It also decreases the chance that the client will feel judged or pressured when you offer suggestions for additional negative consequences.

Always ask for positive consequences first, so you can end with negative consequences, which you will discuss in greater depth. Discussing the negative consequences of target behavior can help the client become more aware of the consequences themselves, as well as more aware of his own emotional reactions to those consequences. Therefore, be sure to offer extensive reflection and validation of the client's description of negative consequences, thereby encouraging further exploration and experiencing of related emotions. In addition, suggest additional potential negative consequences if applicable.

Here is an example of a therapist summarizing the client's positive and negative consequences with reflections and validations:

> *So the positive consequences included feeling happy, feeling confident, getting to spend time with your friends, and feeling like none of your problems mattered at the moment. Those are all really big deals. But eventually, you started* (reads the list of negative consequences) *feeling tired and depressed, and feeling urges to hibernate and shut out the world—which led you to feel even more depressed and like a misfit. You also felt guilty, like you let your parents down. I know that had to hurt especially bad, because I know how much your parents matter to you.* (Pause and then reflect the client's response.) *Sometimes when people engage in the target behavior, they say they also feel bad about themselves later—maybe disappointed, or less confident, or ashamed. Did you feel like that at all?* (Client affirms.) *Tell me about that.* (Client says she felt ashamed and mad at herself.) *I hate to hear that, because I know you already feel ashamed and mad at yourself so much of the time. I hate to hear that those feelings got even stronger.* (Pause and then reflect response.) *A lot of times people say that after a lapse, their urges feel even stronger. Did you feel that way?*

In conducting an FA, a therapist might discover that a client, upon being criticized (*situational cue*), might suddenly feel painful *emotions* of shame and sadness, *sensations* of shakiness, *urges* to engage in the target behavior to "turn off" the discomfort, and *thoughts* that he is a failure and that he just can't stand the urges any more. Once he engages in the behavior, he may feel relief from the painful emotions, thoughts, and urges, while also feeling pleasure and a sense of comfort (*positive consequences*). Thus, his target behavior was reinforced, so he is likely to use the behavior again. However, he eventually may have felt additional shame and sadness, been chastised by his family, felt anxious about the money he spent and what his friends might think, and experienced even stronger thoughts about being a failure (*negative consequences*).

Finally, after assessing the cue, antecedents, positive consequences, and negative consequences, work with the client to plan adaptive ways he might react when faced with such a situation again. Possibilities may include avoiding high-risk situations, learning skills to respond to the situation (e.g., refusal skills), working to tolerate emotions and urges until they begin decreasing on their own, and/or other MMT skills. Affirm any options offered by the client.

FAs can be essential at the beginning of treatment to gain a general idea of the factors contributing to the client's target behavior. They can also help you and the client understand what led to specific incidents of the behavior. Potential questions include the following. (You will likely have to provide prompts for at least some of the answers until the client gains more internal awareness.):

- *When did you start noticing an increase in urges? What was going on at the time?*
- *What were you feeling at the time?*
- *What were your physical sensations?*
- *What were some of your thoughts?*
- *How did you get from that point to the point of deciding to actually engage in the behavior?*
- *What were some of the positive consequences? [Reflect and offer further suggestions.]*
- *What were some of the negative consequences? [Reflect and offer further suggestions.]*

As always, be sure to tell the client that you are not judging, and validate and affirm the difficulty of discussing the lapse. Assure the client that you are asking about the behavior only so that you can work with her to decrease the chance of it happening again. Most clients feel ashamed and uncomfortable when talking about lapses, so you will need to repeatedly stress that you are not judging or criticizing.

What about clients whose specific dysregulated behavior or life circumstances require a more targeted treatment with specific techniques?

MMT was developed to be a transdiagnostic treatment for dysregulated behavior; however, that in no way means that MMT is a "one-size-fits-all" approach. Instead, therapists need to customize the treatment for each client's individual needs and values. Sometimes customization may involve tailoring the treatment for values related to culture or to a variety of the client's other diverse traits and experiences. Other times, customization may involve tailoring the treatment to provide an additional focus on areas related to specific dysregulated behaviors (e.g., nutritional counseling and issues with body image for clients with disordered eating, or issues around medication-assisted treatment for clients addicted to opioids).

The MMT guidelines were set up to provide several avenues for customization.

• MMT's conceptualization and the five basic MMT strategies provide multiple methods for you to (1) gain understanding of clients and their unique values, (2) communicate in ways that foster a collaborative relationship, and (3) tailor each aspect of treatment to move clients closer to lives that are consistent with their particular values.

• Although all MMT sessions should be tailored to clients' values and target behavior(s), several sessions also offer explicit components that allow you to incorporate techniques for specific dysregulated behaviors, if warranted. For example, if a therapist and client wanted to incorporate a focus on nutrition, eating patterns, and body image, they could do so in the semi-flex and flex sessions, as well as in the sessions on adding pleasant/fulfilling activities (Session E), setting and moving toward goals (Session H), and acceptance of self (Session L). The therapist can also monitor such activities in the weekly Tracking Sheet, as any activity that moves a client toward a goal or value can be counted as a pleasant/fulfilling activity.

• Finally, the session guidelines are meant to be just that: *guidelines*. They are not set in stone. You are free to modify sessions and session components based on each client's individual responses and behaviors. For some clients, you may spend more time reviewing the previous week and less time working on the new material. Other clients might need the opposite. In some situations, you may modify techniques or practices, you may take 2 or 3 weeks to get through a session that takes 1 week according to the session guide, or you may add additional flex sessions to the treatment (as long as you continue to assign the basic home practice during those weeks). Such clinical decisions are acceptable and applauded as long as you understand and stay consistent with (1) the core processes that underlie MMT's conceptualization of dysregulated behavior, and (2) the overriding principles and procedures that define the delivery of MMT. These are yet two more reasons why reading Parts I and II, as well as the detailed guidelines for each session, are critical for effective MMT delivery.

• Clearly, clinical judgment and expertise are not just critical; they are essential for providing effective, individualized treatment.

What if the client does not want to stop the target behavior, but instead wants to continue the behavior in moderation?

The answer varies depending on the circumstances. Many clients mandated to treatment by the courts or pressured by jobs or family do not *want* to stop the target behavior; however, they can benefit from stopping the behavior for at least a specified amount of time in order to avoid the negative consequences. Methods for working with these clients are discussed extensively in the five basic MMT strategies, especially Strategies 1–3.

Sometimes clients will report wanting to try to continue the target behavior in moderation, which is understandable considering that the behavior has brought relief, pleasure, and—for some behaviors—social interaction. Despite the widespread belief of the need for total abstinence, some people with dysregulated behavior *can* learn to engage in their target behavior in moderation, even if that behavior includes substance use. That said, many other people cannot ever gain the ability to maintain moderation, and there is no definitive method of predicting which outcome will occur for any given individual.

However, there *is* a prediction you can share: People who refrain from their target behavior for at least a few months are more likely to learn and fully master adaptive ways of coping with emotions and urges, which means that they are more likely to be successful if they do eventually attempt to engage in the behavior in moderation. Thus, therapists can encourage the client to do his best to stop the target behavior during treatment, while also agreeing to revisit the situation as treatment is nearing the end. For clients who are reluctant to commit to abstinence for the entire duration of treatment, the therapist can ask for a shorter commitment. Once clients have stopped the behavior for even a few weeks, they are more likely to be open to committing to a more extended break from the behavior.

Reminder: For clients with dysregulated behaviors related to actions that cannot be stopped entirely (e.g., eating, Internet usage), you can work with the clients to define certain aspects of the behavior as the target behavior. Examples include eating binges (which must be defined) and being on the Internet more than 20 minutes during any given period.

Even after hearing the above explanation, some clients will still want to try to continue the target behavior in moderation without ever going through a period of abstinence from the behavior. In these cases, remember the importance of working toward the client's values—not the therapist's values. Knowing that the target behavior has interfered with the client's values, and knowing that the client will be more likely to learn adaptive coping if he abstains from the behavior during treatment, you will not be going against the client's values if you strive to motivate the client to refrain from the target behavior while in treatment. However, if the client continues to be adamant about wanting to attempt moderation, you are encouraged to keep an open mind. After frankly discussing potential consequences (which may be related to the client's original reason for referral), consider working to create a plan for the client to attempt to engage in the target behavior in moderation. In these cases:

- Define explicit criteria for the frequency and amount of target behavior that would constitute "moderation." For example, the plan might include gambling no more than once every 4 weeks, with the potential total loss never to exceed $50 at any given time in the evening. Or the plan might include drinking no more than twice a week, never more than two drinks on any evening, and never when alone.

- Ask the client if he is willing to view the plan as an experiment. If he is able to stay within the plan for a few weeks, then the odds increase that he will able to continue the behavior in moderation.

- The task would then be to work to redefine the plan if needed, continue to monitor the client's adherence to the plan, and generally proceed as though you were working with a client who had chosen to stop the target behavior—with the *target behavior* now being defined as incidents of the behavior that fall outside the plan (as opposed to being *any* incidents of the behavior).

  - If the client is not able to stick with the plan after a few weeks of attempting, work to remain nonjudgmental while also broaching the matter for discussion. Using basic MMT Strategies 1–3, assess whether the behavior continues to interfere with the client's moving toward a more fulfilling life. If so, gently encourage the client to work to stop the behavior for a specified period of time before attempting moderation, while also affirming the client's efforts and reflecting/validating the client's perspective. Do your best not to appear smug or say anything to convey that you expected such an outcome.

- If the client sticks with the plan initially but then has multiple weeks of the target behavior falling outside the plan, gently reintroduce the potential of working to be abstinent for a few months before attempting moderation. (See the preceding bullet point.)
- If the client is able to continue the behavior in moderation throughout the course of treatment with only one or two lapses from the plan, then pat yourselves both on the back for a successful working relationship.

What if the client agrees to stop the target behavior during treatment but says she wants to work to practice moderation once treatment ends?

At the beginning of treatment, therapists ask clients to commit to refraining from the target behavior during treatment. When clients are reluctant to become abstinent, therapists stress that the commitment is only for the length of treatment. Clients are free to engage in the behavior again after treatment ends without breaking any commitment. Several weeks before treatment ends, therapists will revisit the issue and encourage clients to commit (to themselves) to remain abstinent after treatment. At this time, clients who initially report wanting to resume the behavior in moderation will often report wanting to remain abstinent indefinitely. (Many clients attribute this change to the benefits they've noticed after stopping the target behavior for a period of time; Wupperman et al., 2018). However, not all clients choose this route. If the client has been abstinent for a period of time but reports wanting to resume the behavior in moderation, proceed much as described in the previous section.

- Several weeks prior to the treatment end date, discuss what *moderation* means to the client, and create a plan for the client to attempt to engage in the target behavior in moderation.
- Define explicit criteria for the frequency and amount of target behavior that would constitute "moderation."
- Again encourage the client to view the plan as an experiment as to how his attempts at moderation will work for him. Proceed according to the client's ability to stick with the plan. If the client is not able to stick with the plan, strongly encourage a return to abstinence. Consider lengthening the treatment if you are able to do so. You may have to revisit some of the motivation and commitment strategies described in the five basic MMT strategies.
- If the client *is* able to stick with the plan for several weeks, work together to solidify the plan that will be continued after treatment ends. This plan should include identified warning signs, which can be labeled at three different levels: *caution, high-risk*, and *urgent.*
  - If the client goes more than a week in which she engages in the target behavior at higher amounts or frequencies than in the plan (even if only slightly more), she should be aware that she is on a potential slippery slope. She should consider herself in *caution* territory, and expend more effort on sticking with the plan for the next few

weeks. If she is still not able to stick with the plan, the client should consider herself in *high-risk* territory. At that point, she is encouraged to switch back to abstaining from the behavior at least for a while, and/or to contact a treatment professional for further work on moderation. Finally, if the client then goes additional days of not being able to switch back to abstinence or return to the original plan—and/or if the target behavior suddenly increases dramatically for several days—the client should consider herself in *urgent* territory. In this situation, the client is encouraged to consult with a mental health professional for assistance as soon as possible.

■ Of course, the hope is that the client will stop the cycle at the *caution* or *high-risk* levels. However, communicate that even if the client does have to consult with a mental health professional (whether with you or with someone else), she will likely need a shorter duration of treatment and possibly just one or two booster sessions—as long as she takes action at the soonest point possible.

What if the client does not want to sign the commitments either before or after the clinician plays devil's advocate at the end of the first session?

MMT therapists ask clients to commit to treatment at the end of the first treatment session. If the client does not want to sign the commitments because he does not want to commit to stopping the target behavior, see the previous question for potential responses. Feel free to adjust the commitments to fit any customized plan. If the client has other reasons for not wanting to commit, work to assess those reasons and then respond accordingly. (Basic MMT Strategies 1–3 discuss methods to improve motivation and increase commitment.)

Important: Clients do not have to feel motivated for the treatment and practices to work; however, they *do* have to attend treatment, work with the therapist, and practice the exercises. If the client has not committed to the basic actions required for treatment, the therapist should not continue moving forward with the treatment. You do not want the client to become conditioned to going through the sessions without actually engaging in the session material or in the home practice. Instead, the therapist can consider the sessions to be pretreatment sessions focused on building motivation and clarifying values. (*Pretreatment* does not mean that no treatment is occurring in sessions; instead, it means that treatment specific to MMT is not yet occurring.) Use the basic strategies to work toward getting a commitment. Remind the client that he is committing to "doing his best"—not guaranteeing in stone that he will always perfectly fulfill every item on the Program Commitments sheet (H-A6). The actual treatment can begin again once the client agrees to the MMT commitments.

Contrary to the expectations implied by many questions asked during MMT trainings, instances of clients refusing to commit to treatment are rare. Keep in mind: If the client is in the therapy room, he has already taken steps that most people with dysregulated behavior never get around to taking. Thus, he already has had to realize that he has a reason to be in your office, regardless of whether or not he likes that reason. That reason may be that the client is mandated to treatment by the courts, it may be that the client has been pressured to attend treatment by his job or family or medical doctor, or it may be that the client himself is beginning to realize that the target behavior is interfering with his life. Regardless, that reason is obviously strong enough to impel the client to walk into the therapy room; thus, you can use that reason as a "hook" to help him see the discrepancy between his current life and a life that fits his values. Getting a commitment to work toward that valued life is simply the next step. (This is not to imply that getting such a commitment is always easy. If it were, the first two sections of this book wouldn't cover strategies for doing so. For further information on shoring up motivation, see basic MMT Strategies 1–5, as well as Miller & Rollnick, 2012.)

What if the client presents for treatment for a reason unrelated to dysregulated behavior—but then displays or admits dysregulated behavior over time?

This answer is yet another "It depends." If the client does not express interest in decreasing or stopping the behavior, the therapist must strike a balance between openly expressing concerns about an issue that could affect the client's welfare, while also being careful not to try to force her/his own values onto the client. Therapists may approach the topic by nonjudgmentally (1) helping the client clarify her values, and (2) working to help the client see how the dysregulated behavior may be interfering with a life that feels as meaningful and fulfilling as it could. If the client reports not wanting to address the target behavior at that time, you are encouraged to respect her wishes. If you truly believe that the behavior is interfering with the client's life, you can nonjudgmentally work to continue reflecting, validating, and affirming in ways that might eventually help the client gain clarity on potential courses of action.

If the client expresses interest in decreasing the dysregulated behavior (either on her own or after you have initiated the discussion), the big step is transitioning from your current treatment to MMT. A successful transition requires that the *expectations clearly be set up prior to starting MMT.* If the client is not accustomed to your assigning of home practice or structured exercises within that practice, you will likely have more difficulty getting her to become fully engaged in treatment than you would if she were starting treatment with you from scratch.

Before discussing MMT in depth, you need to decide exactly how you want the treatment to look. Do you want to completely transition from your current treatment focus to MMT? Or do you want to integrate MMT with your current treatment? If the latter, first take a moment to assess whether the current treatment and MMT have consistent core philosophies and conceptualizations. If so, and if you decide to integrate the treatments, you are encouraged to set up a plan by which the client continues engaging in the guided audios, completing the Tracking Sheet, and completing the Daily Log each week—regardless of whether or not a new MMT topic is introduced. (Home practice can only become a habit if it is assigned regularly.) Regardless of how you decide to implement the treatment, it is important that you are explicit in telling the client exactly what she can expect if she chooses to transition to a focus on the dysregulated behavior. Be specific about the structure of sessions, the home practice, and the commitments. Otherwise, you run the risk of the client expecting to continue with a similar style of treatment—and thus having difficulty transitioning to a treatment that might be more demanding than what was expected or wanted. Thus, setting concrete expectations about MMT is essential for an effective transition.

What about clients with PTSD? I've heard that formal mindfulness practices don't work with these clients.

Although this question has repeatedly been asked during MMT trainings, MMT has been conducted with many clients who met criteria for PTSD—in both clinical and research settings. (In one clinical trial, 85% of clients met criteria for PTSD, and many also met criteria for Complex PTSD; Wupperman et al., 2015). When working with individuals who report trauma histories, therapists are advised to (1) provide explanations about the purpose of the practices (so the clients understand what they are doing), (2) assure clients that they have a choice of whether or not to engage in each of the practices, and (3) allow clients to modify any practices to help them feel less uncomfortable or threatened, if needed. For example, although clients are instructed to close their eyes for the mindfulness practices—they also are told that they can leave their eyes open and focus on a spot on the floor or a wall if they feel uncomfortable closing their eyes. Clients are also given the option of lying down or sitting up when practicing the exercise at home, which offers them further choice of how to do the practice. At this point, no client who has been through any MMT trials or been seen by any core MMT therapists has ever had difficulties doing the mindfulness practices due to trauma histories.

THE THERAPEUTIC RELATIONSHIP, THERAPIST CHARACTERISTICS, AND THERAPIST DISCLOSURE

Might the focus on the therapeutic relationship be harmful to clients who are in time-limited treatment and will likely experience negative emotions when treatment ends?

Building a strong therapy relationship can increase motivation, personalize the treatment to fit the client's values, reinforce treatment cooperation, model the ability to adaptively experience and express emotions, provide a corrective experience for processing reactions in an empathic relationship, foster basic mentalization, and help the client feel valuable as a human being (e.g., Castonguay & Hill, 2012; Linehan, 1993a; Moyers et al., 2005; Wolfe et al., 2013). Of course, a strong therapeutic relationship can also increase the chance that the client might experience sadness and even mild grief at the end of treatment. In fact, the therapist prepares the client for coping with such a reaction beginning several weeks before treatment ends—with an especially strong focus in the last 2 weeks of treatment. The key point to remember is that MMT's goal is not to convey the message that the negative emotions are harmful or to shield the clients from ever experiencing such emotions. Instead, MMT works to help clients tolerate such emotions without feeling the need to immediately try to turn them off. Thus, although it would be nice if the clients did not have to experience any sadness at the end of treatment (or ever!), the benefits of fostering a strong therapeutic relationship greatly outweigh any potential drawback.

MMT encourages therapists to express respect and caring to clients. Might clients become dependent on the therapist?

Although the possibility that a client may feel dependent on a therapist exists in any therapy context, such an occurrence is less likely if the MMT therapist follows the core MMT tenets. From the first session, MMT therapists should work to customize the treatment to fit the *client's* values—not the therapist's. The therapist is open in telling the client that the main purpose of treatment is to help the client move toward a life that holds more satisfaction and meaning *for the client*. Although MMT therapists obviously have opinions about how they want the client's treatment to progress, they also are clear that the decisions about treatment goals and the client's "relationship" with the target behavior are ultimately the province of the client.

MMT therapists also work to foster and/or improve the client's interpersonal relationships outside of treatment, which can further decrease the chance the client feels dependent solely on the therapist for support. Some sessions focus explicitly on building social connections (Paving the Road), others allow clients to decide the exact area of focus while also encouraging social connections (Goals, Pleasant/Fulfilling Activities), and still others focus on improving relationships (through Expressing Understanding, the OFFER refusal and assertive skills, etc.).

Finally, when therapists convey caring to the client, they are encouraged to do so in ways that foster the client's movement toward his values, not in ways that imply that the client is fragile or needs to be "taken care of." For example:

> *I know it feels scary, but I care enough about you that I want you to gain the skills you need to get closer to a life that feels more like the kind of life you want. So I'm willing to push you a little to increase the chance that you keep moving toward that life. How are you feeling about this?*

Do MMT therapists have to maintain an ongoing formal mindfulness practice?

Therapists are strongly encouraged to maintain their own formal mindfulness practice; however, they are not required to do so. This decision was made after considerable thought and with one major point in mind: Requiring MMT therapists to practice mindfulness would restrict some clients' abilities to have access to MMT. Although these clients' dysregulated behavior may lead to suffering that could potentially be alleviated by MMT, the clients would be restricted from accessing the treatment if no available therapists maintained a formal mindfulness practice. Although it would be nice to think that therapists might be eager enough to conduct MMT that they would be willing to start a formal mindfulness practice to do so, that possibility does not seem especially likely. Thus, based on all competing factors, MMT encourages but does not require therapists to maintain their own formal mindfulness practice. MMT does require at least some form of mindfulness training, through formal training, reading, or—preferably—both. MMT also strongly advises that therapists practice each mindfulness exercise prior to assigning it to clients.

Some therapists in MMT trials had little to no mindfulness experience when they began MMT training. All therapists were required to (1) attend training in mindfulness and MMT, (2) attend weekly supervision meetings that opened with a mindfulness practice, and (3) practice all MMT exercises on their own before teaching them in session. However, therapists were not required to maintain formal mindfulness practices, based on the rationale above. All therapists were able to deliver MMT adherently, regardless of whether or not they had their own formal mindfulness practice at the time.

Are therapists who have a history with a dysregulated behavior more likely to provide effective treatment for the behavior?

No. If a client ever expresses concern that you may not be able to help him if you have not had a history of struggling with his dysregulated behavior, you can truthfully tell him that substantial research has shown that therapists with histories of the same dysregulated behavior as the client (including addiction to substances) are neither more nor less effective in treating the behavior (e.g., Project MATCH Research Group, 1998).

How advisable is therapist self-disclosure?

Therapists are encouraged to self-disclose when such disclosure can be therapeutic. Selective self-disclosures help build the therapeutic relationship, model respect for the client, foster mentalization, model healthy expression of emotion, and help the client feel supported and understood. Examples include:

- *I can understand how you feel sad. I feel sad just knowing you had to go through it.*
- *I'm excited that you've started doing the home practice.*
- *I know it's not fun to talk about this, but I'm asking you to do so because I believe it's necessary to keep moving forward. I care enough about you that I really want you to get closer to feeling like the kind of person you want to be.*
- *I know you've got a lot going on, but I'm a little concerned about [identify your specific concern], because I'd hate to see you stuck in a life that doesn't feel as fulfilling as you'd like. I think you deserve more.*
- *That does sound stressful! I know I'd feel anxious if I were in the same situation.*
- *Considering your history, it makes sense that you have some of the struggles you've had. If I had the same history, I can't guarantee that I'd be handling things any better—or even that I'd be handling things as well as you are now.*
- *You know, I've had times of practicing mindfulness when my mind seems to spend more time wandering than it does being attentive and aware. I know how frustrating that can feel. [The therapist can share her own difficulty with mindfulness practice or MMT skills as long as she stresses that (1) she persisted despite the difficulties and (2) she fully believes the mindfulness practice/skills work.]*

Note: In general, it is best not to share whether you have ever struggled with the client's category of dysregulated behavior. Although such disclosure may initially foster rapport and a feeling of being understood, it may also impede therapy in at least a couple of ways. First, the treatment can begin to focus too much on the therapist, as the client may then begin asking you repeatedly how you handled situations similar to those of the client (and once you have shared that you have experienced similar difficulties, it may seem inconsistent for you to suddenly refrain from sharing your experience). Second, the client may compare his progress to yours—which may be detrimental if the client feels he is not as successful in moving past the behavior as you were.

If the client asks you about your own history of target behavior, you can explain that your clinic discourages such disclosures, as it could draw the focus of treatment to the therapist instead of the client—and potentially impede the client's treatment. Stress that regardless of whether you have ever struggled with the target behavior, you have had the training and experience to *know how to help people who struggle with dysregulated behavior* move past the behavior to create lives that fit their values. (You may also process why the client asked the question and assure the client that he did not do anything wrong by asking, although that is your call.)

ADDITIONAL ISSUES THAT MAY COME UP INSIDE OR OUTSIDE OF SESSIONS

What if the client's Daily Log routinely shows 0's or very low numbers for emotions and urges—despite your suspecting or knowing that the client experienced higher levels of emotions and urges during the week?

Such a discrepancy may be caused by some combination of the client's lack of awareness of her emotions; her belief that negative emotions are somehow bad, weak, or shameful; her culture's discouragement of the expression of certain emotions; her wanting to suppress or avoid negative emotions; her forgetting what she experienced by the time she completed the Daily Log, etc. Gently broach the subject by asking the client about her previous week. As the client tells you about situations during her week, you can ask her what she was feeling during the situations, validate those emotions, and then mention that the Daily Log does not reflect those emotions. For example:

> THERAPIST: Sounds very stressful! What were you feeling at the time?
>
> CLIENT: I was mainly angry—at her for what she did, and at myself for trusting her.
>
> THERAPIST: That makes senses, although I understand why you would want to give her the benefit of the doubt. (*Pause*) I notice on your Daily Log, your anger that day was listed as 0.
>
> CLIENT: Really. Hmmm. I'm not sure what happened.
>
> THERAPIST: I'm wondering if maybe you're so used to trying not to feel uncomfortable emotions that by the time you filled out the log, you weren't even aware you had felt it. We've talked about how you may have gotten the message that your emotions aren't valuable—to the point that you might not value some of your own reactions and not give yourself credit for feeling the emotions you feel. I wonder if that might have played a part in this as well.
>
> CLIENT: That could be. I'm not sure.
>
> THERAPIST: Is there any other reason you can think of?
>
> CLIENT: Not really. I think sometimes by the end of the day, I don't even remember what I've felt.
>
> THERAPIST: That's normal. And there's nothing wrong with that. (*Pause*) While you're in here, I'd like you to do your best to be aware of what you feel and record it in the log. That lets out some of the steam from the boiling pot, while also retraining your brain to value your reactions and be more aware of your values in general. What do you think?

Should therapists take notes?

Do your best to model mindfulness by being fully present in the room with the client whenever possible. You are encouraged to limit your amount of note taking to information that you feel is utterly necessary to write down that moment. You are also strongly encouraged not to have a desk, table, or any furniture between you and the client.

Why does the Color Body Scan include a color? Why isn't it just a body scan?

During initial stages of the development of MMT, several clients experienced substantial difficulty focusing their attention on a standard body scan—to the point that noncompletion was a pressing issue. Some clients with higher levels of emotion dysregulation also reported distress when doing the scan. Adding the choice of a color seemed to noticeably improve completion of the practice. Clients also reported increased abilities to attend to the practice, as well as decreased distress. Thus, the Color Body Scan became a staple. However, feel free to tell the client that he can choose "clear" as the color or forgo the color altogether at any time. In other words, the client can choose to do a more standard body scan (or you can choose to modify the instructions over time to transition to a more standard body scan).

How do I share the audio files with the clients?

For the Color Body Scan in Session A (*TS-A4: Color Body Scan*) and an exercise in the semi-flex session (*TS-SF1: Mirror Exercise*), you have the option of recording the practices on your own or downloading an already-recorded version from the publisher's website (see the box at the end of the table of contents). If you choose to record the audios yourself, you may record them directly on the client's phone if the client is willing, or you may record them on your own device and then text or email them to the client. (You will need to ask the client to sign a consent form giving you permission to send the file through the medium you choose.)

For all of the guided exercises, including the two listed above, you can access already-recorded audio files on the publisher's website. These audio files can be given one at a time to clients via printable handouts that are on the website; these handouts provide a separate web address for each audio. Clients can stream the audios online or download to their preferred device. More information about the schedule of assigning the audios can be found in a section in Chapter 7 ("Tracking Guided Audios," p. 99).

CHAPTER SUMMARY

This chapter provides answers for questions that commonly arise in the implementation of MMT. You are encouraged to consult with this chapter for information about:

- Client diversity.
- Functional analyses.
- Clients whose behaviors require more targeted techniques.
- Clients who want to continue the target behavior in moderation.
- Clients who do not want to commit to treatment.
- Clients presenting with unrelated problems but displaying dysregulated behavior.
- Questions about the therapeutic relationship, therapist characteristics, and therapist disclosure.
- Additional issues that may arise in sessions.

CHAPTER 7

MMT Setup, Intake Guidelines, and Structure of Sessions

This chapter provides essential information on (1) the planning and tracking of treatment, (2) the components of an effective intake session, and (3) the general structure of MMT sessions.

BASIC MMT PLANNING AND TRACKING

MMT has been delivered as:

- A stand-alone treatment for clients who want treatment solely for dysregulated behavior;
- A first-step treatment to address dysregulated—and potentially treatment-interfering—behavior prior to transitioning to additional treatment (which may be delivered by the same therapist or may require referral to another therapist, depending on therapist qualifications); and
- An intervention integrated with theoretically consistent treatments for co-occurring disorders—when targeting each disorder sequentially does not seem optimal.

Session Schedule

In its standard form, MMT is a 20-week individual therapy that consists of one 90-minute session followed by nineteen 45- to 50-minute sessions. The 20 sessions include 16 core sessions and four "flex" sessions; the topic(s) and timing of flex sessions are chosen by therapists based on client needs. In addition to the 20-week version, modified versions of MMT have been conducted in 12 weeks and in 16 weeks. Finally, MMT has also been conducted without time limits for clients who were not bound to a specific schedule.

The order of most MMT sessions can be customized depending on the needs of the client. For this reason, MMT sessions are labeled with letters instead of numbers (i.e., Session A, Session B), since therapists might get confused if a change in session order resulted in mismatches between session numbers and week numbers (e.g., if Session 10 occurred in Week 6).

Despite the flexible order of sessions, the first five sessions are meant to occur in a somewhat standard order, regardless of the duration or mode of delivery. The first five sessions include four standard topics (Sessions A–D) plus a semi-flex session in which the therapist can choose from a list of topics. Early sessions focus on building rapport, clarifying values, and helping clients gain the capacity to experience neutral stimuli. In the third or fourth week, clients also begin visualizing upsetting situations and working to experience the resulting emotions, thoughts, and urges without engaging in habitual avoidant behavior.

Subsequent sessions continue to focus on the above topics, while also targeting additional skills relevant to dysregulated behavior, including (1) mindful regulation of emotions; (2) mindful communication, acceptance, and empathy; and (3) integration and generalization.

The MMT 20-session schedule (Figure 7.1, p. 113) provides an overview of all 20 sessions.

When MMT is delivered as a time-limited treatment, therapists are encouraged to conduct the 20-week version of MMT if possible, as that version contains all the core topics while also offering flex sessions to provide an additional focus on the client's unique needs. With that rationale, this book contains outlines and descriptions of the 16 core sessions and four flex or semi-flex sessions. However, constraints due to setting or payment do not always allow a 20-session schedule. For these situations, guidelines for offering MMT in 16-week and 12-week schedules can also be found at the end of this chapter. (See Figure 7.2, pp. 114–115.)

Tracking the Delivery of MMT Sessions

After the fifth week (Sessions A–D plus the semi-flex), therapists are encouraged to modify the order of sessions based on client needs. To keep track of the sessions delivered, a blank MMT Session Chart is included at the end of this chapter (TS-2, p. 117) and also available to download and print (see the box at the end of the table of contents). As shown in the sample MMT Session Chart (TS-1, p. 116, also at the end of the chapter and available to download), therapists keep track of the date, the session letter and name, and the week number (i.e., the number of weeks the client has been in treatment). In the sample Session Chart, the client was having trouble saying "no" when friends tried to persuade him to engage in the target behavior. Thus, the therapist chose to move the session on mindful refusal skills (Session I) sooner than it is listed in the standard template. The therapist felt that working on responding to thoughts was not as pressing for the client, so the session on thoughts (Session G) was moved to a later slot than it occurs on the standard template. You are strongly encouraged to download and use TS-2 (or your version of an MMT Session Chart) to keep track of sessions and audios as you conduct MMT.

Tracking Guided Audios

MMT includes seven guided audio practices. New audios are assigned to the clients every 2–3 weeks. The audios are provided on the publisher's website for therapists to download (see the box at the end of the table of contents), but therapists can also give clients access to them one by one. Printable handouts are provided on the website with information to direct clients to each audio practice. Each time the therapist provides the client with the link to a new audio, it can be tracked on the Session Chart (described above). Some guided audios are similar to the mindfulness practices conducted in MMT sessions; however, those sessions do not usually occur at the same time as the relevant guided audio is assigned to the client. Please remember that this is intentional; you have not made any mistakes about session order.

Clients are instructed to do their best to engage in the audio practices at least five times each week. The link to the second audio is given to the client in the third session if he has practiced the Color Body Scan (Audio 1) at least four times each week during the previous 2 weeks. If he has not done so, the link to the second audio is given to him in the fourth session. Each time a new audio is assigned, the client is asked to do his best to practice the new audio at least twice in the upcoming week. The client can then choose which audio to use for the other three (of five) assigned practices. In subsequent weeks, the client is instructed to use whatever combination of audios he chooses. The seven audio practices include:

1. *Color Body Scan* (Audio 1; Chapter 8, TS-A4; first week)
2. *Body Movement* (Audio 2; third or fourth week)
3. *Mirror* (Audio 3; approximately 2 weeks after previous audio; recorded by therapist in semi-flex session or available online in generic version)
4. *Mighty Tree* (Audio 4; approximately 3 weeks after previous audio)
5. *May You Be* (Audio 5; approximately 3 weeks after previous audio)
6. *Thoughts* (Audio 6; approximately 3 weeks after previous audio)
7. *Sounds* (Audio 7; TS-M1; Chapter 11; approximately 3 weeks after previous audio)

Tracking Emotions, Urges, and Target Behavior

The Daily Log (H-A4) is assigned to the client after every session for the entire course of treatment. You are encouraged to download the Daily Log from the publisher's website and customize it to fit the client's specific target behavior. If the client is working on more than one target behavior, then each behavior has its own column. Example: The log may have (1) one column for urges to play computer games, (2) one column for whether the client played computer games (and for how long), (3) one column for urges to smoke, and (4) one column for whether the client acted on the urge to smoke (and how many cigarettes). If the client has multiple dysregulated behaviors, the Daily Log does not need to include every behavior. Start by picking two target behaviors that you and the client have identified as most problematic to the client's life (unless the client only wants to target one behavior). If necessary, additional behaviors can be added to the log once the client gains self-efficacy and builds skills to tolerate negative emotions and urges. The MMT exercises were developed to contribute to such an outcome, regardless of whether all behaviors are listed on the log. Finally, feel free to customize the emotions tracked on the Daily Log to be pertinent to each client. Further information on the Daily Log is provided when it is introduced in Session A (Chapter 8).

Delivering MMT in Various Formats and Settings

Group-Based Delivery

Due to the extensive customization of treatment to fit each client's values, it is recommended that MMT be delivered in individual sessions if possible. That said, some clients in pilot trials of group MMT have reported benefiting from the motivation, support, and feedback provided by other group members (Wupperman et al., 2019a, 2019b). In addition, some settings only have resources to offer treatment via group delivery. The following guidelines apply when modifying MMT for group delivery:

- It is crucial that the group leader meet with each member for an individual group-intake session prior to the first group session. The leader will not have time to learn necessary information about each client's motivations otherwise. During the session, the leader can assess the client's goals and values, assess how the target behavior interferes with the client's life, prepare the client for the weekly home practice, and give the client a chance to ask questions.
- The group needs to remain small, with a maximum of six to eight participants.
- The minimum amount of time required for weekly group sessions is 1 hour and 40 minutes. Thus, the group can be conducted as:
  - A 2-hour group with a 10- to 15-minute break
  - Two 45- to 60-minute groups conducted on the same day with a break in between
  - Two groups conducted on different days (with the home practice review occurring on one day and the new topic being presented on another day)
- Each session schedule should include a (1) weekly review, (2) brief mindfulness exercise, (3) new topic, and (4) wrap-up. Therapists should be sure to transition to the new topic *at least* 40 minutes prior to the end of the session.
- For homework reviews, each client should be given a certain amount of time to be the center of focus, depending upon the number of people attending group that day. (For example, if five clients are in group with 35 minutes allotted to review home practice, you would give each member approximately 6 minutes for home practice—leaving a minute between for transition.) When transitioning from one client to the next, therapists can explain that they would like to hear more from each client, but that they have to move on after a certain number of minutes to ensure that there is time to teach the new skill. Therapists have reported success with setting a timer prior to each person's review to ensure that they do not lose track of time. This also helps therapists transition to a new client when a currently speaking client runs out of time. It can be easier to segue away from a client once the client hears the timer than it can be to interrupt a client with no external prompting.
  - Clients will not have time to review their week in detail, so you can ask to see their Daily Log and Tracking Sheet—and then prompt them to briefly share information about their practice, whether or not they engaged in the target behavior, and any highlights of the week. If the clients did not complete their home practice, you can use the allotted time to assess the difficulties and plan solutions (Strategy 4).
- Therapist are cautioned not to allow too much time for processing of the weekly mindfulness exercise. Clients tend to like processing these exercises, and such processing can often take

15–20 minutes. Although such processing can be helpful, if it occurs regularly, it can take away from time needed for learning new skills, processing of the home practice, and/or focusing on clients' other concerns.

- Sometimes clients may respond to other group members in the confrontational ways they are accustomed to hearing in many treatment groups. Thus, the therapist must stress from the beginning the importance of nonjudgmental communication. If any clients become confrontational and judgmental toward another group member, validate that they are probably accustomed to hearing such language in other groups, while also gently reminding them that language in the MMT group must remain nonjudgmental.

- **Note:** Most mental health professionals have experienced groups in which clients are given home practice worksheets from various therapies without following the protocol of the treatment or reviewing the worksheets in the following session. I do not know whether or not providing MMT worksheets to clients without follow-up will provide any benefit to those clients; however, I do know that such treatment is not MMT. Thus, you are encouraged to offer MMT as a full treatment as opposed to just going over the handouts during session.

- MMT is designed to be delivered in a "closed" group format, which means that members start in the first week and remain together throughout the remaining weeks. Some colleagues are currently discussing trials allowing new participants to enter later in the treatment as long as those participants attend two introductory sessions to learn the basics of Sessions 1 and 2. However, such schedules have not yet been evaluated.

Inpatient and Incarceration Settings

In settings where patients are forced to remain on the premises and may not have access to their own audio playback devices, special accommodations must be made to give patients access to the guided audios when possible. Options may include:

- Scheduling an extra group session in which individuals attend just to listen to the audio or to a person who reads the scripts.
- This could take the place of a standard group, or it could be offered as an additional group that does not require a trained mental health professional to lead.
- Allowing a specific room and an audio-playing device to be "checked out" by individuals who want to listen to the guided audios when the schedule allows.
- Allowing audio devices with earphones to be checked out and used in the library or other room.
- The least optimal option: If providing access to the audios or someone reading the scripts is not possible, the individuals can be assigned nonguided mindfulness practice to take the place of the guided audios.

In addition, therapists will need to customize sessions to fit clients who cannot leave the premises. (For example, several of the items from the Coping Toolbox and Pleasant/Fulfilling Activities should be removed.) However, many of the exercises will be relevant without any revision, and all can be relevant with only moderate revisions.

Integrating MMT with Other Treatments

Therapists are free to integrate MMT with other treatments. Prior to doing so, first take a moment to assess whether the other treatment and MMT have consistent core philosophies and conceptualizations of clients and behavior. Second, set up a plan by which the client continues engaging in the guided audios (or other forms of structured mindfulness practice), completing the Tracking Sheet, and completing the Daily Log each week—regardless of whether or not a new MMT topic is introduced that week. You are encouraged to periodically check to make sure that you are staying consistent with the tenets of each treatment.

Intake Guidelines

Although you will not begin conducting MMT until the first treatment session (Session A), the intake session(s) is crucial for starting to build the all-important therapy relationship. Your interaction with the client during the intake(s) will set the client's expectations about you and the treatment, which may determine whether the client is receptive or even present for the treatment.

Since MMT can be customized to target a variety of dysregulated behaviors, the assessment measures and intake procedures will vary dramatically based on the client's target behavior and the therapist's treatment setting. Therefore, instead of including specific details, this section provides general guidelines that are essential in setting the stage for the effective delivery of MMT.

Start by Greeting the Client and Telling Her or Him What to Expect

After greeting the client and introducing yourself, briefly tell her what to expect during the next session(s); let her know that the actual treatment will not begin until the second or third session.

> *First, I'm going to give you the spiel about what to expect, and then you can have a chance to ask any questions. OK?* (Client nods.) *In today's session [or in the next two sessions], I'm going to be bombarding you with questions. Some of the questions will be relevant to the reason you're here, and some may not apply to you at all. But they'll all be basic questions I have to ask to get a general idea of who you are and how to customize the treatment to work best for you. If any questions feel intrusive, feel free to tell me—and I'll be happy to stop and explain why I'm asking. By the end of this session [or the next session], I should have a basic idea of the bigger picture. So the next session is when we'll start the actual treatment. At the beginning of that session, I'll explain my perspective and get your feedback to make sure it fits. And then we'll start working together to address the reason you're here. I wish we could start working right away, but for treatment to be effective, I need to have a session [or two] of me just getting information from you. Are you OK with that?* (Client responds.) *Do you have any questions for me before I begin?* (Client responds.) *OK, tell me a little bit about why you're here.**

Use This Time to Begin Gaining an Understanding of the Client as a Human Being, While Also Starting to Build the Essential Therapy Relationship

Please review Strategy 1 in Chapter 3.

- Actively listen for opportunities to reflect, validate, and affirm. (These responses are important throughout treatment, but they are crucial when first meeting the client.)
- Be alert for discrepancies between the client's current life and a life that fits her values, and start considering how the target behavior may be an obstacle to the life the client wants.
- Of particular importance is to reflect and validate any affect, as well as any dissatisfaction with the current life and any desire to make changes.
- *Work to find at least one thing to affirm within the first 10 minutes of the session.* (Do not be fake. Keep in mind MMT's conceptualization of clients—as well as your knowledge of people in general, and look for statements and actions to affirm.) Here are two examples:

    It took courage to come here today. A lot of people tell themselves they're going to get help for their behavior, but then never have enough courage to actually start treatment.

    I know it's difficult to talk about this. I appreciate your effort.

For Clients Who Are Court-Mandated or Pressured into Treatment by Others

THERAPIST: That sounds very frustrating. I can understand how you'd be upset about being forced into treatment when you feel like you don't have a problem.

CLIENT: It *is* frustrating. I know 20 people who engage in [target behavior] more than me. But they arrested me.

THERAPIST. No wonder you're upset. (*Pause for response.*) I want to thank you for talking with me about it. I know you don't want to be here—and even though I didn't have anything to do with that decision, I could still understand if you refused to talk to me or took your frustration out on me. So I appreciate your being so polite and talking with me.

For People with a History of Abuse/Trauma/Etc.

Considering all you've been through in your life, it would be understandable if you disliked the entire world and refused to care about anyone—if you just shut out the world and engaged in [target behavior] all the time with no consideration for anyone else. Truthfully, that might be easier in the short run. I think it would be sad, but I couldn't judge you for it. So the fact that you're here, wanting to do this work, is a big deal. I hope you give yourself credit for that.

During the first few minutes of this session, clients will mention their target behavior as at least part of the reason why they are there. Although the conversation will sometimes provide a natural springboard for discussing specifics about the behavior (i.e., frequency, amount, antecedents), the first few minutes will usually focus on broader issues, such as why and how the behavior is troubling to the client, as well as general information the client wants to share with the therapist. The therapist should not immediately jump to asking multiple specific questions about the target behavior. Instead, therapists can use this time to focus on understanding the client, understanding how the target behavior may interfere with the client's life, and building therapeutic rapport. Specific details about the behavior can be discussed later in the session.

If the client is pressured or mandated to treatment, he may bring up the event(s) that prompted such pressure or mandate (e.g., the arrest, a partner giving the client an ultimatum, parents threatening to throw the client out of the home). Be sure to ask for at least some details. The description will give you the chance to reflect and validate events that likely provoke strong emotions. Work to reflect/validate reactions that will not potentially impede the client's progress. For example, validate the client's frustration, hurt, fear, etc. However, do not vilify someone potentially valuable to the client and important for motivation. Here's an example of a client whose partner pressured her to attend treatment for target behavior:

- Helpful therapist response: "You're understandably angry. I can see how that would feel intrusive."
- Unhelpful therapist response: "You're understandably angry. He seems like a control freak."

Saying that you understand how the other person's behavior could feel intrusive is not the same as labeling the other person as a control freak. The first allows the therapist to eventually reflect that (1) the client seems to care about the person even while being angry at him, and (2) the person might not be hurting the client intentionally, but that doesn't make the client's anger any less reasonable.

Finally, if the client does not mention any reaction to the event(s), you can hypothesize what the client might be feeling—and then reflect and validate the responses the client gives you.

> THERAPIST: Your dad talked about your [target behavior] in front of your whole family? I can imagine how embarrassing that felt.
>
> CLIENT: Yeah. Everyone just looked at me like I was some sort of freak. I just shut down.
>
> THERAPIST: That sounds painful. I can see how you'd almost want to disappear at a time like that. (*Client agrees.*) I can also see how you might feel a little angry.
>
> CLIENT: I was so mad! He had no right to talk to me like that in front of everyone else.
>
> THERAPIST: I think you're justified in feeling mad. So maybe part of you wanted to disappear and part of you wanted to snap at your dad for talking about it in front of everyone?

Another scenario:

> THERAPIST: I can only imagine what it was like when you heard you were under arrest.
>
> CLIENT: I couldn't believe it at first.
>
> THERAPIST: Sounds terrifying. I bet your heart felt like it was about to stop.
>
> CLIENT: (*Nods.*) It felt like there was no way that it could really be happening.

THERAPIST: Like a nightmare.

CLIENT: Like a nightmare. A nightmare that just keeps going on.

THERAPIST: A nightmare that had to be extremely distressing. And sad. You seemed really sad when you mentioned your children knowing about it.

CLIENT: I never thought I'd have to tell my kids that their mother got arrested.

THERAPIST: It seems like that hurt most of all. (*Client nods.*) You clearly care a lot about your kids and want to be a good mother. I can see that. So I can understand how it would feel devastating to have to talk to them about all this. (*Client responds, and further discussion ensues.*)

THERAPIST: (*Later*) I commend you for how much you care about your kids. I'm sorry you're having to go through so much pain, and I want to work with you to help make sure that you get through this as soon as possible without anything happening to draw it out or make it worse.

Eventually Segue to Asking for Further Details about the Target Behavior

Once you have built some rapport, you can focus on more specific details about the target behavior(s). Since MMT can be modified to fit various target behaviors, listing exact questions for each possible behavior is beyond the scope of this book (and possibly beyond the scope of your patience as a reader). General areas of focus, to be modified for the behavior, include:

- How often does the client engage in the behavior (e.g., amount per day, week, or month)?
- What is the amount or intensity of the behavior in an average episode (e.g., amount/type of drinks per episode, amount/type of food per binge, amount of time surfing the web)?
- How often and in what amount did the client engage in the behavior in the past week?
- What is the client's history with the target behavior?
- What are common antecedents or cues to the behavior (e.g., certain days of the week, certain emotions, certain situations, interactions with certain people)?
- What are the standard short-term consequences (which are usually positive)? What are the standard longer-term consequences (which are often negative)?

Remember: Clients usually have had many experiences of being judged for their behavior, so they may be reluctant to talk about details and feel intense shame when doing so. They may also underreport in the intake interview out of shame and fear of your reactions. (That is normal.) It is critical to remind the client that you are not judging and are only asking so you can customize the treatment. Be sure to validate and affirm clients for providing the information.

Ask What the Client Wants to Work on during Treatment

Remember: The reason for addressing dysregulated behavior is not because the behavior is bad, but because it impedes the client from moving toward a more valued life. (See Strategy 2A in Chapter 4, pp. 43–45.) Thus, the client's values are a primary focus throughout treatment. However, some clients who attend therapy for dysregulated behavior are more comfortable discussing their desire to stop the behavior than they are discussing their values. Further, clients who are forced or pressured into treatment might not want to discuss their target behavior *or* their values—and they often do not believe they need therapy. Therefore, a practical approach is needed to effectively broach a conversation about what the client wants in life. Focus on the fact that almost everyone has things about their lives they wish were different and would like to change, which allows you to frame such an admission as common instead of something endorsed only by people who need therapy. From that starting point, you can work to find out what specific things would have to change in a client's life for her to feel that she is living more closely aligned with her values.

The two key points to cover/query include:

1. *Normalize.* Communicate that wanting to change things about one's life is universal and normal—not a sign that something is wrong with a person or that the person is unhappy.
2. *Elicit values.* Assess what would need to change for the client's life to be more consistent with his values.

If you could have a life that felt more fulfilling—if you were living more of the kind of life you wanted and being more like the kind of person you wanted to be—what would that life look like? What would be different from the life you're living now? [Write down a list of the client's answers.]

Here is an example of the components put together:

Everyone has things about their lives they wish were different—that they'd change if they could. That's normal; it doesn't mean that there's anything wrong with a person; it just means they're human. (Slight pause) You'll be coming in here for the next few months—and we'll work on the [target behavior], because that's why you're here. But we also have time to work on other things. So I'd like you to think about things you might like to work toward. Imagine that you had a life that felt more satisfying and fulfilling—like you were living more of the kind of life you wanted and feeling more like the kind of person you wanted to be. You have to be realistic—you won't be the ruler of the world or anything like that. But what would that life look like? What would be different from the life you're living now? Some things people say in answer to these questions is that they'd like to work toward improving certain relationships, take classes, take up hobbies, make a different kind of friends . . . and so on. What are things about your life that you'd like to work toward while you're here?

Clients will often provide vague answers, such as "be less depressed" or "be happier." In these cases, just accept the client's answer (write it on the list), and also ask for specifics. For example:

You said you'd like to be happier. What might your life look like if you were happier? What would need to happen or change for you to feel at least a little happier?

Or:

What might your life look like if you were less depressed? Would you make new friends? Would you have more hobbies? Would you volunteer? What would be different?

If the client gives an answer that seems unrealistic ("I would be earning my living as an actor"), just rephrase it to find a related possibility that is more feasible.

That's a possibility—and it often takes a lot of luck as well as training. What's something you can do that could move you closer to making a living as an actor—that would also give you some pleasure before you're making a living at it? Something like taking an acting class? Or volunteering to help out at a community theatre?

The same strategy works if the client chooses a long-term goal such as becoming a therapist:

That makes sense since you said you like to help others. Now, becoming a therapist takes years of training. What's something you can do now that might move you closer to being a therapist or some other job that helps others—that can also help you gain a sense of fulfillment now? What about taking a class? Or doing some sort of volunteering?

For a single client who wants to be in a healthy romantic relationship:

Of course, I can't guarantee you'll be in that relationship by the time you end treatment, because that partly depends on things beyond our control. But we can work to help you feel better about yourself—so you're more likely to attract someone who will treat you well. We can also work to find ways for you to interact with people with similar values—which will increase the chances of your becoming involved in a healthy relationship.

If the client has difficulty generating ideas: Offer suggestions based on what you know (or guess) about the client. Set up suggestions by saying that a lot of people choose some of the following areas they would like to change in their lives, then ask if any fit the client:

- Improving relationships with certain others (partner, children, sibling, parent)
- Taking classes (for fun or to further education)
- Getting a job (or a job they like better)
- Having more friends (or friends who don't engage in the target behavior)
- Having a certain hobby
- Volunteering
- Working out regularly
- Having a healthy romantic relationship
- Changing housing
- Engaging in religious or spiritual activities
- Engaging in creative activities
- Feeling less depressed or anxious

For clients mandated or pressured into treatment, the main (and sometimes only) goal will often be the reason the client is attending treatment. For example, to . . .

- Keep her job.
- Get free from probation.
- Save the relationship with a partner who gave an ultimatum.
- Keep parents from throwing him out of the house and/or refusing to pay for school.
- Keep from ruining her health.
- Get the criminal justice system off his back.

Finally, if a client continues to deny wanting to address any life issues in treatment, don't try to force the client to generate answers. You will have a chance to discuss this issue again in Session A, after you explain your conceptualization of the client. Some clients feel less guarded after they hear a nonjudgmental conceptualization, and they may be more likely to share vulnerabilities at that time.

Once you've compiled a list of potential areas to address, thank the client for sharing, and reiterate that although treatment will address the target behavior, you will also work to help the client move toward a life that feels more satisfying and fulfilling. Tell the client that you will explain more about how that will happen when you start the actual treatment.

The rest of the intake session(s) will include the standard questions that you feel are relevant and/or that your setting requires. Work to actively reflect, validate, and affirm client responses throughout.

Toward the End of the Final Intake Session, Remind the Client That You Will Begin Treatment the Following Session

Thank the client for her patience in answering all your questions. Remind her that you will start the next session by sharing your conceptualization and getting her feedback—and then you will start the actual treatment.

- Tell the client that you will be teaching her new ways to cope so that she can start moving toward a life that's a better fit with her values.
- Let her know that there will be home practice every week.
- Express confidence you feel about working together.

> If you are unable to incorporate all of the preceding suggestions into the amount of time you usually use for an intake, you are strongly encouraged to add an additional pretreatment session that will give you the chance to do so.

STRUCTURE OF SESSIONS

The following suggested structure applies to all sessions beginning with the *second treatment session (Session B)*. The timelines can be somewhat flexible to allow you to modify sessions based on the client's needs. Despite this flexibility, you are encouraged to stay within the maximum allotted time for each section when possible.

Although the structure of sessions should be explained briefly during the first session, take a moment to remind clients about it again at the beginning of the second week. Otherwise, clients may expect to talk about their own choice of topics throughout most of the session, consistent with how therapy is depicted in most television shows and movies. You then run the risk of surprising or even offending the client when you have to interrupt him to ask about home practice or teach the new topic. Knowing what to expect in each session will allow both you and the client the opportunity to organize your time most efficiently.

Of note is that some clients may present with new pressing concerns almost every week. As a caring therapist, you may feel tempted to spend most of the session discussing the client's latest concern(s) instead of moving on to the new topic. Please remember that the topics are designed to help clients acquire the abilities to more effectively navigate pressing concerns and decrease the chance that such concerns will continue to interfere as strongly with their lives. Therefore, you are encouraged to utilize your clinical skills to validate and communicate compassion(!), while also conveying the importance of maintaining the general structure of the session. Otherwise, the client may experience momentary relief from these concerns without ever gaining the ability to more effectively navigate and/or overcome similar concerns in the future.

SESSION STRUCTURE: BRIEF OUTLINE OF SESSION B AND BEYOND

- The first 20 minutes: Greet the client and review the previous week.
  - Listen to the client's experiences and concerns; show the client you are interested in him/her as a human being.
  - Review and discuss the Daily Log and home practice.
  - Address any issues with home practice and/or target behavior.
- The next 20–25 minutes: Introduce and discuss the current session topic.*
  - Customize your explanation of the topic to fit the client's needs, values, and concerns.
  - Discuss the client's understanding of and reactions to the topic.
  - Assign the home practice for the next week. Use shaping when needed.
- The last 5 minutes: Wrap up and conduct any additional planning for upcoming week.
  - Summarize any plan you have discussed for potential high-risk situations.
  - Wrap up session.

*Some sessions will include a mindfulness practice as part of the session topic. Other sessions will include a separate mindfulness practice as a segue from the weekly review to the new session topic, thereby decreasing the amount of time that can be spent on the new topic and/or the weekly review. The specific timeline for each session can be found in the session summary at the beginning of every session.

The First 20 Minutes of the Session

The first 20 minutes of each session will include a review of the previous week, including the Daily Log, the other home practice, and any incidents of target behavior. Although the specific home practice will change throughout the treatment, the following guidelines are largely applicable to all sessions from Session B onward. At times, after particularly eventful weeks (e.g., the client expresses doubts about treatment, lapses into target behavior, has difficulty with home practice), therapists will not have time to focus on all the areas listed below. In these cases, therapists should briefly mention each area and then choose which area or areas is/are important enough for more detailed focus. (Therapists may also choose to conduct a flex session.)

> The following provides a general outline. Before reading any further, you are strongly encouraged to review Strategy 4C and its subsections, which provide a detailed description of the home practice review, including sample vignettes, ways to seamlessly segue to the home practice review, ways to address problems completing home practice, and ways to respond to client questions (pp. 63–71).

- *Take time to listen to the client's experience.* Take a moment to listen to what the client wants to say and actively reflect, validate, and affirm.

- *Review the Daily Log.* Strategy 4C (p. 63) provides a description of requesting and reviewing the Daily Log and home practice.

  - When the client gives you the Daily Log, briefly reflect/validate days with particularly high emotions.

  - If the client did not complete the Daily Log, bring out a blank log and ask the client about the last day or two, filling in the blanks with the client's responses. Then ask whether the client had instances of target behavior or especially high urges during the week.

  - Mention the days on which the client experienced high urges but did not engage in the target behavior. Validate the difficulty, while affirming the client's ability to tolerate urges without acting on them. Ask the client how he was able to ride out the urges.

  - If the client engaged in target behaviors during the week, nonjudgmentally work to find out what happened. Briefly assess (1) what was going on at the time of the behavior, and (2) whether the client completed the rest of the home practice.

    You engaged in the target behavior on Friday. What was going on then? (Client answers.) That sounds stressful. I want talk about that more in a moment, but first let's check the rest of the home practice.

  - After checking the rest of the practice, you will choose whether to focus on (1) problems completing home practice (if applicable), (2) the episode of the target behavior, or (3) some combination of both.

- *Review the Tracking Sheet and other home practice.*

  - Some general questions you may ask about any of the practices:
    - *What was it like to do the home practice?*
    - *Was there anything that surprised you?*
    - *What did you find the most difficult or particularly helpful?*
    - *Do you have any questions about the home practice?*

  - If the client did not complete the Tracking Sheet or other assignment (or repeatedly does not complete the Daily Log), see Strategy 4C (p. 63).

  - (If applicable) *Consider conducting an FA to gain understanding of antecedents to any target behavior, as well as positive and negative consequences of the behavior.* (See the review of FA in Chapter 6, pp. 84–86.) Stress that you are not criticizing or judging, but only want to talk about the behavior to gain understanding so you can help the client to decrease the chance of it happening again.

- *Actively look for adaptive behavior and effective use of skills; provide affirmation.* Even if the client only completed part of the home practice, you can use shaping to affirm those efforts. You can *always* find something to affirm.

- *Thanks for being honest with me about your target behavior. I appreciate that. Let's talk about what happened.*
- *Was it hard to get yourself to come in today knowing that you hadn't done the home practice? I'm glad you showed up.*

- *Validate difficulties.* Clients are often accustomed to being blamed and shamed for their behavior, so this is your chance to establish your relationship as respectful and caring, while also working to combat shame (which is predictive of additional dysregulated behavior; e.g., Kelly & Tasca, 2016). The most effective way to validate the client without reinforcing harmful behavior is to *validate emotions and urges,* as opposed to the behavior itself.
  - *It's natural to feel discouraged when you work so hard but still have trouble getting though the day.*
  - *You've used the target behavior to cope with stress for years. It makes sense that you would have high urges now. It hurts you in the long run, so we need to help you find other ways to cope. But I know that it's not easy.*

> It is key to explain to the client that the skills she will learn in the educational portion of each session will help her more effectively overcome or cope with many of the concerns she is likely bringing into therapy each week. Therefore, by spending a few minutes on the current concerns and then segueing to the new topics, you are not ignoring the client's pain or dismissing her suffering. Instead, you are treating her with compassion and truly addressing her concerns by teaching her ways to cope more effectively in the future.

The Next 20–25 Minutes: Introduce and Discuss the Current Session Topic

- *Segue to the new topic.* Therapists sometimes have trouble segueing to the new topic if the client is talking; however, it is OK to politely interrupt the client to make the transition. You can do so without sounding uncaring by (1) briefly reflecting what the client just said, and (2) saying that you wish you could continue hearing what the client was talking about, but you need to move to the new topic in order to have enough time to teach the skills the client needs to move toward the life she wants. Here is an example.

  You had a tiring weekend! I wish we could keep talking about this, but I'm going to have to interrupt you to move to the new skill. It's not that I'm not interested—I am, and I wish I could hear more. But if we're going to have enough time to teach you the skills that are needed to help you move toward the life you want, we're going to have to move to the next part of the session.

- *When introducing the new topic, do your best to relate it to the client's current or general needs and concerns.*
  - *You've talked about how hard it is for you to keep from [target behavior] when you feel pressured by friends—which is perfect timing for today's topic. We're going to talk about ways to say "no" when friends try to pressure you.*
  - *You know how you said that sometimes the urges don't feel so bad, but then sometimes they seem like they're utterly overwhelming? Today we're going to talk about ways to plan for those times when urges feel especially overwhelming.*

- *Discuss the client's understanding of the topic and reaction to the skill.*
  - You can assess understanding by asking the client how and when he might use the skill in his own life. Affirm and validate any answer, while also correcting misperceptions.
  - If the client says he does not think the home practice will be helpful, reflect and validate his response, and then (1) further explain how it can be helpful and (2) ask the client to give it a chance and practice for at least 1 week before deciding.
    - Use the therapy relationship to ask the client to trust you for a week. Remind him that he doesn't have to believe in the practice for it to work.

      I realize the practice might not sound like it will make a difference. But I've seen it work for a lot of people. You don't have to believe in it for it to help. It works just as well, even if you're not motivated and don't believe in it—as long as you actually do it. I know it's harder to get yourself to practice if you're not motivated, but it works just as well. I'm going to ask you this: Will you humor me and practice this assignment for this 1 week? We can then talk about it next week and decide what to do from there.

- *Assign the specific home practice for the upcoming week.*
  - Discuss specific times/places/situations in which the client might practice (if you have not already done so).
  - Get a commitment from the client that she will do her best to complete all home practice.
    - Consider asking how confident the client is on a scale of 1–10 that she will do the home practice. Then query with a number lower than what she tells you, which prompts the client to explore why she is confident (e.g., Miller & Rollnick, 2012). See the discussion of a confidence scale in Chapter 5 (pp. 78–79).
    - Troubleshoot potential obstacles: "What might get in the way of your practicing this?" Then problem solve.

The Last 5 Minutes: Plan for Upcoming Week

- *Alert the client that the session is nearing the end.*
- *Anticipate any high-risk situations.* (Optimally, this process was already begun in the previous section of the session.)

  We just have a few minutes left, so I want to check on a few things going on this week for you. I know you usually have more trouble resisting the behavior when your mother is in town, so let's review the plan you came up with earlier.
- *Wrap up and plan for upcoming week.*
  - Provide a brief summary of the session and remind the client of all the home practice.
  - Get commitments from the client to do the home practice and to do her best to abstain from the target behavior (or to work to decrease the behavior) for the next week.
  - End with a statement that lets the client know you'll be thinking of her this week and/or that you look forward to seeing her the following week. (In other words, find an authentic way to let the client know you will not forget her between sessions.)

MMT 20-Session Schedule

Early Sessions (mindful experiencing and tolerating of emotions, thoughts, sensations, and urges—and learning/practicing new responses)

Session A: Discussion of Values; Introduction to MMT (Boiling Pot and Destination); Color Body Scan

Session B: Neutral Experiencing; Mindful Exposure to Current Experiences (BEST B)

Session C: Mindful Exposure, Part I: Intentional Experiencing of Higher-Intensity Emotions/Urges

Session D: Mindful Exposure, Part II: Further Intentional Experiencing of Higher-Intensity Emotions/Urges

Semi-Flex Session: (After Session B, C, or D, based on need) Therapist Chooses Focus of Portion of Session; Mirror Exercise

Mindful Emotion Regulation Module

Session E: Identifying, Scheduling, and Participating in Activities That Are Pleasant and/or Fulfilling

Session F: Urge Roadblocks

Session G: Freeing Yourself from Being Controlled by Your Thoughts

Session H: Identifying, Breaking Down, and Moving toward Goals

Mindful Communication/Relationships Module

Session I: Saying No: OFFER Mindful Refusal Skills

Session J: Mindful Assertiveness Skills: OFFER

Acceptance/Empathy Module

Session K: Freeing Yourself from Being Controlled and Taking Back Your Power, Part I: Acceptance and Tolerance of Situations That Cannot Immediately Be Changed

Session L: Freeing Yourself from Being Controlled and Taking Back Your Power, Part II: Acceptance and Tolerance of Self and Others

Session M: Experiencing and Expressing Understanding (Improving Empathy and Relationships)

Integrating and Generalizing; Planning for the Future

Session N: Paving the Road: Building and Strengthening Connections

Session O: Integrating and Generalizing

Session P: Termination: Planning for Continued Progress toward a Valued Life

Flex Sessions: Clinician Chooses Topic and Timing of the Session

Flex Session #1: Use when needed.

Flex Session #2: Use when needed.

Flex Session #3: Use when needed.

FIGURE 7.1. MMT 20-session schedule.

The following provides templates for offering MMT in 16-week and 12-week schedules. Chapters 8–12 provide detailed session guidelines for each MMT session based on a 20-week schedule, which include descriptions of 16 core sessions, one semi-flex session, and three flex sessions. The templates that follow use the same session labels as provided in the session guidelines.

MMT 16-Week Schedule

In the 16-week version of MMT, there are no longer separate sessions for goals (Session H) or assertiveness (Session J). Two flex sessions are also dropped.

- Instruction on breaking down goals is integrated into the session on Pleasant/ Fulfilling Activities (Session E). Each step the client takes toward a goal can be counted as one Pleasant/Fulfilling Activity on the Tracking Sheet.
- Instruction on assertiveness is integrated into the session on Saying No: OFFER Mindful Refusal Skills (Session I), as both use the OFFER acronym.
- Two flex sessions are dropped, leaving one flex session and one semi-flex session.
  1. **Session A:** Assessment of Goals and Values; Boiling Pot; Introduction to MMT
  2. **Session B:** Neutral Experiencing; Mindful Exposure to Current Experiences (BEST B)
  3. **Session C:** Mindful Exposure, Part I: Intentional Experiencing of Emotions/ Urges
  4. **Session D:** Mindful Exposure, Part II: Intentional Experiencing of Emotions/ Urges
  5. **Semi-Flex Session:** (Placement based on need)
  6. **Session E:** Pleasant/Fulfilling Activities (includes Session H: Identifying, Breaking Down, and Moving toward Goals)
  7. **Session F:** Urge Roadblocks
  8. **Session G:** Freeing Self from Being Controlled by Thoughts
  9. **Session I:** Saying No: OFFER Mindful Refusal Skills (includes Session J: Mindful Assertiveness Skills: OFFER)
  10. **Session K:** Freeing Yourself from Being Controlled and Taking Back Your Power, Part I (Acceptance and Tolerance of Situations That Cannot Immediately Be Changed)
  11. **Session L:** Freeing Yourself from Being Controlled and Taking Back Your Power, Part II (Acceptance/Tolerance of Self and Others)
  12. **Session M:** Experiencing and Expressing Understanding
  13. **Session N:** Paving the Road: Building and Strengthening Connections
  14. **Session O:** Integrating and Generalizing
  15. **Session P:** Termination: Planning for Continued Progress toward a Valued Life
  16. **Flex Session #1:** Use when needed.

(continued)

FIGURE 7.2. Schedules for 16-week and 12-week delivery of MMT.

MMT 12-Week Schedule

If possible, therapists are encouraged to choose the 20-week version of MMT over the 16-week version and to choose the 16-week version over the 12-week version. Although preliminary research has suggested feasibility and acceptability of the 12-week version (Wupperman et al., 2012, 2019b), that research also showed that therapists and clients both thought that clients would benefit by the treatment being lengthened. That said, some setting and payment limitations place restrictions on the durations of treatment. In the 12-week version of MMT:

- Instruction on goals is integrated into the session on Pleasant/Fulfilling Activities (Session E). Each step the client takes toward a goal can be counted as one Pleasant/Fulfilling Activity on the Tracking Sheet.
- Instruction on assertiveness is integrated into the session on Saying No: OFFER Mindful Refusal Skills (Session I), as both use the OFFER acronym.
- Instruction on acceptance of self and others is integrated into the general session on acceptance (Session K), as both use similar worksheets.
- The session on experiencing and expressing understanding (Session M) is dropped.
- The session on building connections (Session N, Paving the Road) is dropped.
- All three flex sessions are dropped, leaving one semi-flex session to be delivered when needed.
    1. **Session A:** Assessment of Goals and Values; Boiling Pot; Introduction to MMT
    2. **Session B:** Neutral Experiencing; Mindful Exposure to Current Experiences (BEST B)
    3. **Session C:** Mindful Exposure, Part I: Intentional Experiencing of Emotions/Urges
    4. **Session D:** Mindful Exposure, Part II: Intentional Experiencing of Emotions/Urges
    5. **Semi-Flex Session:** (After Session B, C, or D, based on need)
    6. **Session E:** Pleasant and/or Fulfilling Activities (includes Session H: Identifying, Breaking Down, and Moving toward Goals)
    7. **Session F:** Urge Roadblocks
    8. **Session G:** Freeing Self from Being Controlled by Thoughts
    9. **Session I:** Saying No: OFFER Mindful Refusal Skills (includes Session J: Mindful Assertiveness Skills: OFFER)
    10. **Session K:** Freeing Yourself from Being Controlled: Acceptance/Tolerance (includes Session L: Acceptance/Tolerance of Self and Others)
    11. **Session O:** Integrating and Generalizing (May include some focus on building connections from Session N)
    12. **Session P:** Termination: Planning for Continued Progress toward a Valued Life

FIGURE 7.2. *(continued)*

MMT Session Chart—20 Weeks (Example)

Client: _____   7 Guided Audios

Date	Session Letter and Partial Name	Week Number
1/16	Intake	Pretreatment
1/23	Session A, First Session (90 minutes)	1*
1/30	Session B, Neutral Experiencing (BEST B)	2
2/6	Session C, Mindful Exposure, Part I	3*
2/13	Semi-Flex Session	4
2/20	Session D, Mindful Exposure, Part II	5*
2/27	Session E, Pleasant/Fulfilling Activities	6
3/6	Session F, Urge Roadblocks	7
3/13	Session I, Saying No: OFFER Mindful Refusal	8*
3/20	Session H, Goals	9
3/27	Flex Session 1	10
4/3	Session G, Freeing Self: Thoughts	11*
4/10	Session J, Mindful Assertiveness: OFFER	12
4/17	Flex Session 2	13
4/24	Session K, Freeing Self, Part I: Acceptance and Tolerance	14*
5/1	Session L, Freeing Self, Part II: Acceptance and Tolerance of Self and Others	15
5/8	Session M, Experiencing/Expressing Understanding	16
5/15	Session N, Paving the Road: Building Connections	17*
5/22	Flex Session 3	18
5/29	Session O, Integrating and Generalizing	19
6/5	Session P, Termination	20

* = Client given link to new audio practice.

MMT Session Chart—20 Weeks

Client: _____   7 Guided Audios

Date	Session Letter and Partial Name	Week Number
	,	

* = Client given link to new audio practice.

CHAPTER 8

Early Sessions

MMT Session A (First Treatment Session)
Discussion of Values; Introduction to MMT (Boiling Pot and Destination); Color Body Scan

(One 90- to 100-minute session or two 45- to 50-minute sessions)

- Greet the client and take a moment to interact with him/her as a person (15 minutes).
    - Briefly ask about target behavior since last session, but do not go into detail.
    - Briefly explain the treatment and program.
- Explain the biopsychosocial conceptualization (10–15 minutes).
    - The boiling pot metaphor, Part I
    - Basic description of how treatment will address dysregulation; boiling pot, Part II
- Review what the client wants to work on during treatment and explain the *destination/castle metaphor* (15–18 minutes).
- Lead the client in the Color Body Scan and process the experience (*TS-A4*; 20 minutes).
- Explain and assign *H-A2: Coping Toolbox* (7–8 minutes).
- Read *H-A3: Why Do I Ask You . . . ?* (5 minutes).
- Introduce *H-A4: Daily Log* and review home practice (5 minutes).
- Get commitments and play devil's advocate; troubleshoot and wrap up (10 minutes).
- Home practice: guided audio (five times), two activities from *Coping Toolbox (H-A2),* and *Daily Log (H-A4).*

Needed for session (all therapists sheets and handouts for this session are at the end of the Session A guidelines):

- Therapist Outline (Therapist Sheet; TS-A1)
- Boiling Pot Outline (TS-A2)
- Destination Metaphor (TS-A3)
- Color Body Scan Script (TS-A4)
- Tracking Sheet (Handout; H-A1)
- Coping Toolbox (H-A2)
- Why Do I Ask You . . . ? (H-A3)
- Daily Log (H-A4)
- Practice Summary (H-A5)
- Program Commitments (H-A6)

SESSION A (FIRST SESSION; ONE 90- TO 100-MINUTE SESSION OR TWO 45- TO 50-MINUTE SESSIONS)

> Prior to delivering Session A, please be sure to conduct an intake session consistent with the MMT intake guidelines (see Chapter 7, pp. 102–108).

Session A is the most structured of all the sessions. It is also arguably the most critical, as it sets expectations about treatment and provides the chance to start building the relationship. Because of the large amount of information therapists must convey and elicit, Session A has a therapist outline for you to bring into the therapy room and glance at when needed. (See *TS-A1: Therapist Outline*, end of Session A.) The following section provides a detailed guide for conducting Session A. Please read through the guide and refer to the referenced pages (e.g., for the boiling pot metaphor) prior to conducting MMT. Because some portions of this session will be modified slightly when seeing clients who are mandated or pressured into treatment, this section will include additional guidelines (in boxes) for mandated or pressured clients.

> Although approximate time guidelines are provided for each section of Session A, you are not expected to monitor the exact number of minutes you spend on each section. Here's a more general guideline: The session is progressing according to schedule if the *destination metaphor* is completed approximately 45 minutes into the session (or before the break if the session is delivered in two 45- to 50-minute sessions).

Greet the Client, Take a Moment to Interact with Him/Her as a Person, and Briefly Introduce the Treatment (15 Minutes)

Ask How the Client Has Been Feeling Since the Intake Session(s)

Today we get to start doing the actual work. But before we get started, I just wanted to check in to see how you're doing.

Continue to work to gain understanding and build rapport; *actively* reflect, validate, and affirm.

- *Of particular importance throughout treatment:* Reflect and validate any affect, any dissatisfaction with the current life, and any desire to make changes.
  - Discussing affect builds rapport, models the fact that emotions are acceptable and not dangerous, and helps the client process and habituate to emotions.
  - Awareness of dissatisfaction with the current life gives more of an incentive to make changes that may be difficult.

Briefly ask about any target behavior that has occurred since the last intake session, but do not spend much time on the topic. You already assessed the behavior in one or two pretreatment sessions, and you have not yet taught the client any new coping tools. Spending time assessing the behavior again this week runs the risk of discouraging the client before he begins learning new ways to cope. Reflect and validate any negative consequences and/or emotions the client reports related to the behavior, and assure him that you did not expect him to decrease the behavior on his own. Remind him that you will start working to address it today.

Briefly Introduce the Treatment and the Program

Provide a brief overview of what the client can expect from today's session and from treatment in general. Points to address include:

- Tell the client
    - How many weeks or months the treatment will last (if applicable).
    - How long each session will be (and whether the current session will be twice as long as usual or be broken into two parts).
- Explain that you will be talking a lot during the first session because you have a lot of information to provide, but that the client will get to talk more in future sessions.
- Briefly explain that you will be working with the client to help him learn new ways to cope with emotions—so he can feel less controlled by emotions and urges and more like he is living the kind of life he wants to live.
    - If the client is voluntarily attending treatment for target behavior, he will not need clarification of what you mean by "less controlled by urges."
    - If the client is mandated or pressured into treatment, he might not think the target behavior is a problem. In these cases, give an amended explanation of how treatment can be helpful. (See the next box.)
- Briefly explain the structure of future sessions (see the section "Structure of Sessions" in Chapter 7, pp. 108–109).

> *Let me tell you a little bit about what you can expect from coming here. This is a [20/16/12]-week treatment to help you learn new ways of coping with your emotions and urges—so you can feel less controlled by your urges and more like you're living the kind of life you want. Today we'll meet for an hour and a half, but starting next week, we'll meet once a week for 45–60 minutes [modify to fit delivery]. Today I'm going to be talking a lot—much more than usual—because I have a lot of information to give you. I'm even going to glance at this outline (TS-A1) every now and then to make sure I remember everything. Because sometimes I might get so caught up in what you're saying that I might lose track of what I've told you, and it's all important enough that I don't want to miss anything. Starting next week, we'll spend about 20 minutes checking in to see how you're doing and reviewing the home practice and what happened during the week. Then we'll move to learning a new skill and discussing how you can use it in your life. Sometimes I might have to move to the second part of the session even when I'd like to hear more about you and your week. But teaching you the new skills is essential, because that's what's needed to get you closer to the life you want.*

EXAMPLES FOR CLIENTS MANDATED TO TREATMENT OR FORCED BY JOBS, PARTNERS, OR PARENTS

The point is to explain how attending treatment and stopping the target behavior—even for a short time—can benefit the client by decreasing the chance something unwanted will happen.

Let me tell you a little bit about what you can expect from coming here. . . . I know you said you don't have a problem with the target behavior, but let me tell you why I think you can still get something out of coming here. You can tell me whether you agree.

- [Mandated for aggression] *When someone yells at you, it makes sense to yell back. If someone is physically aggressive to you, it makes sense to become aggressive back. It can be automatic. The problem is that you've been arrested for aggression and mandated for treatment. So you're going to be under a spotlight for the next few months, and one wrong move could get you in a lot of trouble. If the police are ever called because of noise—even if all you did was yell at someone who yelled at you first—the police will know you've been mandated to treatment for aggression, and so they'll likely think it was at least partially your fault, and you'll be the one who is arrested. So I'd like to use this time to help you learn how to respond differently when you feel provoked—to give you the power to choose whether or not to yell or to become aggressive, instead of reacting automatically the way a lot of people do when they're angry. That way, even when other people do things that you justifiably get angry at, you can have control over how you respond, so you can react in a way that's not likely to hurt you in the long run—at least until these next few months are over. So you can get the criminal justice system off your back and not have to worry so much about what you do. Does that sound like it would be helpful?*

- [Mandated for alcohol/drugs] *Even if you don't have a problem with drinking, the problem is that you've been mandated to alcohol treatment. So you're going to be under a spotlight for the next few months. [Customize the next part to fit the client.] So if you go out with your friends and have one or two drinks but then get stopped on the way home because of a taillight—and the police officer smells alcohol on your breath—you may get arrested again, even if you were completely capable of driving, because the officer will know you're on probation. Or if the police get called to your home because a neighbor thinks you're playing your music too loud, and the police can tell you seem high, you will likely get in trouble. And the thing is, if you're used to going out drinking with your friends or doing coke while at home—it's sometimes harder to stop than you might think—even if you don't have a problem. So I'd like to use this time to help you learn ways to cope to make sure you don't do anything within the next few months that can be used against you. Once your court case is over, you might want to start drinking and smoking again the way you did before. But what we can do now is work to get the criminal justice system off your back without your accidentally doing something that can hurt you in the long run.*

For more examples and explanations of working with people pressured to treatment by jobs, partners, parents, or the court, see Strategy 2A in Chapter 4 (pp. 43–45).

If the client still questions or disputes, be sure to validate his frustration and ambivalence. *Then remind him that he has a choice.* The choice may be extremely unpleasant or even unfair—but it is a choice nonetheless. He can either attend treatment and work to stop the behavior even if just for a limited time—or he can risk the consequence (losing his job, going to jail, being left by a partner, being thrown out of his home, having probation extended, etc.).

> *Here's the thing. You have a choice. It's not a fun choice. Both options suck. But it's a choice. You can choose to come here and work to stop the target behavior for a little while—for the months until you [find a new job/work things out with your partner/are off probation/show your parents you don't have a problem/etc.]—or you can say that this whole thing is unfair and choose to risk [losing job/losing partner/extending probation/ being thrown out of home/etc.). I can't tell you which option is right for you. You know what fits what you want more than I do. I, personally, hope you choose the first option, because I would hate for [relevant negative consequence] to happen. But the whole thing may seem so unfair that you choose the second option. Maybe the second option seems less bad than the thought of having to stop the target behavior and having to come in and talk to me every week. I couldn't judge you for that. But I hope you choose the first option— because I'd like to work with you to help you get past all this.*

Explain the Biopsychosocial Conceptualization (10–15 Minutes)

Although the boiling pot metaphor was explained in Strategy 3, it is so central to MMT that it is explained again here. An outline is also provided for you to take into the therapy room to use as a cheat sheet. (See *TS-A2: Boiling Pot Outline.*)

The Boiling Pot Metaphor, Part I

After briefly telling the client what he can expect in treatment, the therapist segues to the biopsychosocial model (with modifications to fit the client). The boiling pot metaphor can help clients understand that their experiences make sense based on their circumstances. Remember: By showing that you understand their behavior, you increase the chance that they will believe you can help them change their behavior.

> Please read the following explanation again and practice describing it in your own words. The explanation includes words such as *target behavior*. As always, you are encouraged to instead use words that describe the client's specific behavior(s).

Biopsychosocial Boiling Pot Metaphor

- *Let me tell you how I view what's going on with you based on what you've told me.*
- *Some people are born with a tendency to feel emotions a little more strongly than most people feel emotions. [Give examples that fit.] What makes some people a little irritated might make them a little more irritated . . .*

- *This is not a negative trait. These people are likely to be especially creative and/or empathic. (You can also say passionate or driven instead of creative if applicable.)*
  - *They are more likely to have careers or hobbies as artists, singers, florists, architects, builders, hair dressers, etc.*
  - *And/or careers or hobbies that help others or have interaction with others, such as teacher, therapist, volunteer, salesperson, waiter, etc.*
- *It's not a negative thing! But sometimes these people grow up in adverse or invalidating environments. These might include:*
  - *Experiences like physical, sexual, or emotional abuse;*
  - *Routine experiences with family members who may not feel emotions so strongly and so don't understand—who may say things like, "Why can't you get over it?" or "Why are you making such a big deal?";*
  - *Experiences with family members who have trouble tolerating their own emotions and use unhealthy behaviors to cope; or*
  - *Experiences outside the home, like bullying at school, mistreatment by other caretakers, routinely being excluded by other children and feeling like there's something wrong with them.*
- *These people are put in situations that would be painful for anyone. Since they already feel things more strongly than most, the pain feels even stronger for them. Eventually, the emotions start to feel unbearable at times.*
- *At first, they may tell themselves: "I'm just going to try not to feel or think about it." Sometimes they get good at that—and sometimes feel a little numb in general. But over time, they often feel they need something stronger to "turn off" emotions. So they start using their target behaviors.*
- *The thing is, it works—for the short term. They feel better. But using target behaviors to "turn off" uncomfortable emotions is like putting an airtight lid on a pot of boiling water:*
  - *The emotions are still there, just like the boiling water and steam are still there—under the surface.*
  - *And the emotions keep building—just like the steam and pressure keep building in the pot of boiling water. Or sometimes the person may not feel the emotions building, but instead may only be aware of the urges building.*
  - *Either way, the person may eventually feel like he/she is almost always under pressure.*
- *If the emotions and urges are never experienced or processed—if none of the steam is released from the pot—the emotions or urges will keep building until the pot eventually explodes. In other words, the emotions or urges will feel especially unbearable.*
  - *So the person will feel like he/she has to try even harder not to feel—and eventually he/she uses the target behavior again.*
  - *And the person feels relief. But the pressure will almost always start building again.*
- *Pretty soon, life can start to feel like a never-ending cycle of urges building . . . target behavior . . . briefly feeling better . . . then urges building . . . target behavior . . . and so on. (Pause) Does this fit you?*

Take a moment to talk about how the metaphor does and doesn't fit. Modify if necessary. See Strategy 3A in Chapter 4 (pp. 51–56) for ways to modify the metaphor to fit specific clients—and how to respond if clients say the metaphor does not fit.

- *These behaviors can seem so effective in the short term that you might have never learned adaptive ways to handle uncomfortable emotions and urges.*
- *If you mainly know one way of reliably stopping pain or discomfort, it makes sense that:*
  - *You'll have strong urges to engage in that behavior when experiencing any discomfort, and you'll have extreme difficulty stopping the behavior.*
  - *In fact, that behavior probably helped you to cope at times when you didn't know any other way to cope. The problem is that it causes damage over time.*

> The point that should be stressed throughout this explanation: The client's behavior (and the difficulty with stopping the behavior) is understandable based on the client's biology, history, and current circumstances. None of us can guarantee that we wouldn't be having the same difficulties if we had had the same biology/history/circumstances as the client. You will likely have to return to this point again and again throughout treatment as the client's old beliefs of being beyond help resurface during difficulties.

Provide Basic Description of How Treatment Will Address Dysregulation; the Boiling Pot Metaphor, Part II

After explaining Part I of the metaphor and attending to the client's reactions, continue with a brief overview of how MMT will address the cycle of the boiling pot:

- *In the first few weeks of treatment, we're going to open a steam hole in the lid of the boiling pot—to release some of the steam and pressure—so your emotions and/or urges can start feeling less overwhelming.* [This refers to the mindfulness practices.] *Little by little, the urges will be easier to tolerate without feeling like you need to act on them.*
- *Some exercises might seem weird—but they'll help you start to experience whatever you're feeling, which will let some of that steam out of the pot.*
- *Eventually we'll also help you learn healthy ways to adjust the heat on the burner underneath the pot—in other words, to adjust the intensity of your emotions and urges.*
  - *A lot of people who come here say they feel like someone else has the remote control over their emotions and/or urges; that they may be feeling OK one minute—but then feel overwhelming urges the next minute.*
  - *They feel like emotions and/or urges have control over them. Do you ever feel like that?*
  - *This treatment will help you take back the remote control—so you can have control over how you react to your emotions and urges (instead of having them control you).*
  - *But first we have to work on letting some of the pressure out of the pot.*

See Strategy 3B in Chapter 4 (pp. 56–58) for a fuller description of how to broadly describe the treatment.

Review What the Client Wants to Work on during Treatment and Conduct the Destination (Castle) Metaphor (15–18 Minutes)

Review the list you created in the intake sessions(s) and briefly assess whether the client wants to add or change anything. If the client did not share any areas of life he wanted to work on during the intake, he may be more willing to share now that you've explained the conceptualization. If not, then just agree that the treatment objective is simply to keep the client from experiencing negative consequences related to the target behavior. Remain open to adding additional objectives as treatment progresses.

Explain the Destination/Castle Metaphor

After assessing values, use the destination/castle metaphor to explain how MMT will help the client move closer toward a more valued life. (You can decide whether you want the destination to be a castle, a grand structure that is unnamed, or any destination of the client's choosing.) Review Strategy 2C (pp. 46–48) for a description of the destination metaphor. Because the metaphor is so central to MMT, a template is also included with the therapist sheets at the end of Session A (*TS-A3: Destination Metaphor*). The destination metaphor is one of the two core metaphors (along with the boiling pot) that are used throughout treatment. Please familiarize yourself with the metaphor before conducting Session A. The metaphor provides clients with a concrete image of moving toward a life more consistent with their values. Essential messages within the metaphor include:

1. Clients won't necessarily achieve all their goals in treatment, but they will move much closer to the life they want and will have the skills to keep moving toward that life. *Example:* Clients won't necessarily be married to the love of their life, but they can make changes that will improve their chances of meeting someone who treats them well and of having a healthy relationship in the future.

2. Treatment is hard work, and the home practice can feel time-consuming, tedious, and boring. Therefore, if clients eventually complain that the home practice is tedious and boring, you can say, "Yes, it can feel tedious and boring! Remember, I warned you about that in the first session. But the practice is essential to keep you moving toward the destination."

3. Clients will likely go through difficult and painful periods in treatment. They might even have times when they doubt whether treatment is working and briefly feel worse before they feel better. Those times are normal and temporary. So, if clients ever feel discouraged or doubtful, you can remind them that it's normal and expected—and that you even warned them about it in the first session.

4. If the client comes to sessions and does the work, you are confident he can make substantial progress—and have a life that feels noticeably different from the life he has now.

Keep these four points in mind as you go over the destination metaphor.

Process the Destination Metaphor

After going over the metaphor, reflect/validate/affirm the client's response. You may need to give double-sided reflections: Reflect and validate hesitation or anxiety about the client's ability to succeed in treatment, but then segue to reflecting and affirming change talk. *Change talk* may include the client's desire to move toward a valued life, his dislike of his current life, his willingness to make an effort, etc. Express confidence that the client can make progress regardless of whether or not he believes it himself—as long as he attends treatment and does the work. Then segue to the Color Body Scan.

Deliver the Color Body Scan (20 Minutes)

You can lead the client through the Color Body Scan by reading from the script (*TS-A4*), or you can play the audio file (*Audio #1: Color Body Scan*) that can be downloaded from the publisher's website (see the box at the end of the table of contents). You will also give the client a copy of the audio for home practice by (1) using the client's phone to record the exercise while you read it, (2) recording the exercise with your own phone or other device and sending the audio file to the client (after getting signed permission), or (3) downloading and printing the supplemental client handouts on the publisher's website that provide a dedicated web address for each audio (see the box at the end of the table of contents).

To set up the Color Body Scan, warn the client that it might not be what she expects. Then turn your chair or body to face away from the client while reading the script.

> *I'd like to lead you in an exercise that might seem a little weird. But I'm going to ask you to bear with me and do it anyway. I can explain it afterward. Are you OK with that?* (Client answers.) *I'm going to turn my chair around so you don't have to worry about being looked at while you have your eyes closed.*

Ask the client to sit up as straight as comfortable, with both feet on the floor and her hands in her lap. Read *TS-A4: Color Body Scan Script*. After the Color Body Scan:

- Ask questions aimed at evoking a curious, nonjudgmental attitude toward the client's experience of herself and the practice. Reflect and validate responses.
- Tell the client that her experience might change throughout the week, being sure to normalize and share the possibility of difficulty.
- Briefly touch on how the exercise can be helpful by . . .
  - Opening a steam hole in the lid of the boiling pot and releasing some of the pressure,
  - Building emotional muscles so that emotions and/or urges feel less overwhelming (especially when the client has urges not to do the practice or to let her mind wander—but instead stays with the practice anyway),
  - Retraining the brain to believe that the client's emotions are valuable—and thereby helping the client gain a greater awareness of what she values.

Here's an example of a post-exercise discussion:

THERAPIST: What was that like for you?

CLIENT: Good. I liked it.

THERAPIST: What did you like about it?

CLIENT: It was relaxing.

THERAPIST: Yes, a lot of people find it relaxing. What else did you notice?

CLIENT: That's really the main thing.

THERAPIST: Did you ever find yourself thinking you "should" be feeling a certain way or find yourself judging your reactions?

CLIENT: A few times I thought I should be feeling more centered or something. I thought I might be doing it wrong. Then I reminded myself what you said about not judging.

THERAPIST: It's interesting you found yourself thinking you might be doing it wrong even though I said there's no right or wrong way to do it. Almost like you're so accustomed to believing there's a way you *should* be that it seems unnatural to let yourself be how you are.

CLIENT: I guess so. That's a little surprising.

THERAPIST: That's normal. It happens a lot. (*Pause*) Did you notice your mind wandering?

CLIENT: A few times. But then I just started thinking about what you were saying again.

THERAPIST: That's normal, too. Everyone's mind wanders. Good for you for noticing and bringing it back. (*Pause*) I'm going to ask you to do this exercise a few times this week at home. Sometimes your mind might wander a zillion times in one exercise. But the exercise is working just as well when your mind wanders a zillion times as it is when it wanders just a few times—as long as you notice your mind wandering and bring it back to the exercise. When you do this on your own, you might find yourself getting bored or feeling anxious or agitated at being still when you have other things to do. Those reactions are also normal and expected. It's not as enjoyable when you're bored or agitated—or when your mind is wandering everywhere. But as long as you do the practice and bring your mind back when it wanders, the practice is working just as well as when you have a relaxing experience. (*Discuss reaction.*)

There are a lot of ways this practice can be helpful. First, by taking time to purposely experience your reactions, you're opening a hole in the lid of the boiling pot—so some of the pressure can start to be released. That's a big step of this treatment. Also, by purposely experiencing your emotions and reactions, you'll start to build your emotional muscles—so your emotions eventually will seem less heavy and overwhelming. That's why it can be especially helpful to practice the exercise when you have urges to skip the practice or to just let your mind wander. By experiencing the urges without acting on them, you're building your muscles for coping with urges—so they start to feel easier to tolerate over time.

Also, the exercise retrains your brain to believe that your emotions and reactions are valuable. Unfortunately, I think you've somehow learned to believe that some of your reactions might be wrong somehow—that you might have to hide or try to change parts of yourself and your reactions. But if you spend time each day purposely experiencing your reactions without trying to change them, you're sending a message to your brain that those feelings and reactions must be valuable—and that *you* must be valuable. You'll also have a better idea of what you value in life—what kind of things bring you pleasure and help you feel like the kind of person you want to be. (*Pause*) Does this make sense?

At this point, ask the client to practice the Color Body Scan at least five times in the upcoming week. Bring out *H-A1: Tracking Sheet* and show the client how to complete the Day column and Audio column. Mark that the client completed the practice on the current day, since she completed the audio practice in session.

If the client appears reluctant to do the practice four additional times, validate the potential difficulty, while also working to get the client to agree. However, you do not want to get into a battle; therefore, you can also work to find a mutually agreed-upon number of times to practice. (See Strategy 5 in Chapter 5, p. 71.)

The Color Body Scan was inspired by the body scan meditations in *Mindfulness-Based Stress Reduction* (e.g., Kabat-Zinn, 2002, 2005), *Mindfulness-Based Cognitive Therapy for Depression* (Segal, Williams, & Teasdale, 2002), and *Mindfulness-Based Relapse Prevention for Addictive Behaviors* (Bowen et al., 2010).

Explain and Assign *H-A2: Coping Toolbox* (7–8 Minutes)

The *H-A2: Coping Toolbox* provides ways to "mindfully distract" oneself from urges until their intensity begins to subside. Over time, the client will learn new ways of experiencing and responding to emotions and urges; however, at the beginning of treatment, the client will often need concrete methods of "riding out" high-urge episodes without acting on the urges.

> The purpose of *H-A2: Coping Toolbox* is to help clients ride out high-urge episodes without doing something (e.g., acting on the urges) that will cause negative consequences. Be sure to warn the client that she won't always feel better after doing an activity from the toolbox. As long as the client gets through the episode without engaging in the target behavior, the toolbox did what it was supposed to do. Sometimes a client might do one activity in the toolbox and then feel that the urges have decreased enough to be bearable. However, sometimes she may have to do two or three (or five) activities before she feels she can tolerate her urges. Again, as long as she can get through the episode without acting on the urges, she has used the toolbox effectively.

Introduce *H-A2: Coping Toolbox* by explaining the above concept and reading the directions on the worksheet. Then ask the client to:

- Read through the list and put a star by anything she has done within the last few months or anything she might be willing to do at some point. (Stress that this isn't a commitment.)
- Use the blank lines to write down anything she can think of that is not listed.

By marking some items, the client will more easily find feasible items when she is experiencing high urges and not feeling regulated enough to read through an entire list.

- Briefly review the list with the client, making comments and affirming the marked items.
- Assign the home practice: Do one item (or more) from *H-A2: Coping Toolbox* at least twice in the upcoming week. Explain that since the purpose is to help clients get through urges without doing something that slows progress toward their destination, the best time to use the toolbox is when the client is experiencing urges. However, the client is instructed to practice skills from the list even if she does not experience urges. Once she is accustomed to using skills from the list during low-risk times, it will be easier for her to choose and engage in the skills when she has higher urges and feels less regulated.
- Tasks from the Coping Toolbox are recorded in the third column of *H-A1: Tracking Sheet*.

Read *H-A3: Why Do I Ask You . . . ?:* Tailor to Client's Target Behavior (5 Minutes)

Read the *H-A3: Why Do I Ask You . . . ?* sheet aloud. Ask the client to do her best to refrain from the target behavior for the next *x* weeks (the number of weeks depends on length of treatment and your own demands). It is imperative that you ask the client only to commit to work on stopping the behavior for a limited time, as clients are more likely to believe they can stop the behavior if they have an end date. Tell the client that she can start the behavior again once the agreed-upon time ends, if she chooses, although you can also say that you might revisit the issue at that time. (By the end of treatment, most clients report feeling so much better that they want to keep working on abstaining. Some clients want to work to resume the behavior in moderate amounts—which is discussed in Chapter 6, pp. 89–90.)

> If the client has already expressed an intent to refrain from the target behavior, you may choose not to spend time reading through H-A3, as that may seem as though you are discounting the client's expressed intent. Instead, you may just mention the main point and then provide H-A3 along with the other handouts.

What if the client does not want to stop?

If the client's dysregulated behavior includes actions that cannot be completely stopped, such as eating or using a computer, then define an aspect of the behavior that can be stopped (see Chapter 4, Strategy 2D, p. 49). If the client says she would like to continue the target behavior in moderation at this time, refer to the reasons given on the sheet as to why you ask her to do her best to refrain for a few weeks. You can also shorten the amount of time you request, as you can always ask for another commitment once that timeframe ends. Here is an example: If the client says she can't commit to doing her best to stop the behavior for 6 months, ask if she's willing to commit to 3 months—or even 1 month or 1 week. Then get another commitment at the end of that time period. However, start by asking for a commitment that lasts the length of treatment—or a few months if the treatment does not have an end date. (If this issue comes up earlier in the session, just introduce *H-A3: Why Do I Ask You . . . ?*)

At this time, you will also encourage the client to remove any items directly related to the target behavior from her home if possible. Items may include alcohol, drugs, cigarettes, specific binge-cueing food, computer games or gaming consoles, pornography, etc. Ask the client to either discard these items (throw them down the commode or in a receptacle outside the home) or to give them to someone who does not live with the client. Validate the difficulty of doing so. Do not pressure the client if she refuses; just tell her that you will check in regarding the topic in the future.

Introduce *H-A4: Daily Log* and Briefly Review Home Practice (5 Minutes)

H-A4: Daily Log is the final portion of home practice to be introduced. You will need to download the Daily Log and customize it to the client's target behavior prior to the session. You will then assign the customized Daily Log every week for the rest of the treatment. Since you will be using the log that you downloaded throughout the rest of treatment, a copy of it is not included in the handouts at the end of subsequent sessions.

> *The log should be customized for the client's specific behavior(s).* Each behavior should have a separate column for urges and for whether or not the client engaged in the behavior. If the client is working on more than one behavior, then choose two behaviors to monitor and give each its own column. Example: The log may have (1) one column for urges to watch porn on the Internet, (2) one column for whether the client watched porn (and for how long), (3) one column for urges to smoke, and (4) one column for whether the client acted on the urge (including how many cigarettes).

Key elements to communicate when assigning the Daily Log include the following:

- *On a scale of 0–10, if 10 is the highest you've ever felt the emotion or urge, and 0 is absolutely none—write the highest you felt the emotion or urge during that day. If most of the day your anger was 4, but for 20 minutes or so it was 8, you'd write 8.*

- *You don't have to be perfectly accurate or take a lot of time on this. You can do this in 2–3 minutes. Just briefly think about your day and write the number that comes to mind. If you're not sure whether an emotion was a 6 or a 7, just take your best shot. The purpose is to get a general sense of what you feel over time—not to be perfect.*

- *Do your best to do this every day. By taking even a couple of minutes to be aware of your emotions and urges, you're releasing more steam and pressure out of the boiling pot. You're also taking another step toward retraining your brain to value your reactions.*

- *This also helps us both understand what you're experiencing during the week and helps me tailor the treatment so that it's the most helpful for you.*

After assigning the Daily Log, briefly review the home practice for the upcoming week.

- *H-A5: Home Practice Summary* lists everything the client is assigned.
- Also explain the last column in the *H-A1: Tracking Sheet*. The column is for clients to record anything they might like to share with the therapist: difficulties with practices, experiences that surprised them, or anything else. The column is entirely optional.
- Ask when the client might do the Color Body Scan and the Daily Log each day. Help the client generate ideas. (Many people find it helpful to set a daily alarm in their smartphones to remind them to do the practice. Others prefer sticky notes around the home.)

Get a Commitment and Play Devil's Advocate: Customize Items 1 and 5 (5 Minutes)

Go through *H-A6: Program Commitments* with the client. Before asking the client to sign, explain:

- *I am asking you to do your best to keep these commitments. Keeping these commitments will keep you moving down the road toward the life that's more like the life you want.* [Note: You can also use details specific to each client.]
- *Attending sessions is essential. If you're not in session, I can't help you to keep moving toward the life you want. If you miss home practice, you won't be doing what has been shown to be necessary to move down that road.*
- *I know you are human, and I won't judge you if you have difficulty. I'd love for you to come in next week saying you didn't do the target behavior at all. But I won't think less of you if you did engage in the behavior. You might still be doing your best but just not have the skills to stop yet. If you have instances of engaging in the target behavior this week, we'll find out what happened and work to decrease the chance of it happening the next week.*
- Most critical: *It's going to be hard. The home practice is time-consuming and can feel tedious. And giving up the target behavior can feel unbearable for a while. You might have weeks when you feel like the treatment's not working. There's even a chance you might feel a little worse before you feel better. But, if you come to sessions and do the work, I'm confident that by the end of treatment, you can be a lot closer to that destination—and you'll be able to notice a huge difference in yourself and in your life.*
- *Knowing all this, do you want to sign the program commitments?*

If the client refuses, reflect/validate while working to understand her reluctance. Assure her that the commitments are just agreements to work toward the life she wants. Stopping the target behavior during treatment is a way to move toward that life, not an admission of a problem.

After the client signs, give the signed page (*H-A6*) to her. Tell her that the commitment is to herself even more than it is to you, so she gets to keep the signed commitments as a reminder.

Play Devil's Advocate

Now is the time to play devil's advocate:

I told you this would be extremely difficult—that the home practice would be time-consuming and tedious . . . that giving up the target behavior would likely feel almost unbearable for a while . . . that you might feel worse before you feel better. Why would you commit to this?

Devil's advocate is necessary for two reasons. First, the client *will* likely have times when she questions whether the treatment is working and/or is upset because she feels worse (or at least as bad) as when she started treatment. When these things happen, you can (1) validate the pain and difficulty, but then (2) remind her that you warned her about these obstacles in the first session—and that she committed to treatment anyway. Second, the client's answer(s) will give you material to use whenever her motivation falters. For example:

CLIENT: It's the third week, and I don't think I'm feeling better. I just don't know if it's worth it.

THERAPIST: I know you're making a lot of effort. I understand being discouraged. (*Processes response.*) The thing is, the way you're feeling is normal. Remember in the first session, when you signed the commitments, I told you that you might feel worse before you felt better, and that you might go through stages when you wonder if the treatment is working? I told you that some weeks would feel like you were going uphill about a mile an hour with the air conditioner broken—or even like you have to get outside and push the car. And you committed anyway, because you said you were sick of feeling bad about yourself, and you'd try anything to stop the target behavior. So even though I hate that you're going through this, I'm asking you to keep your commitment to staying in treatment for [number] weeks. I'm confident you'll get past this rough patch and get to the point where you're feeling better about yourself and not feeling controlled by the target behavior. But the only way to do that is to stay in the treatment and do the work.

If a client seems tentative about committing to treatment, you have the option of toning down devil's advocate slightly. However, you do not want to tone it down much, as preparing the client in advance is important. If the client does not agree to commit, the next step would be to work on the client's ambivalence. (See Chapter 6, pp. 90–91.)

Troubleshoot, Wrap Up, and Remind the Client of Home Practice (5 Minutes)

Ask the client what might get in the way of doing the home practice for the week. Will he have difficulty finding time or privacy? Does he tend to procrastinate? Might he forget? Once you've identified potential obstacles, briefly discuss ways they might be addressed (e.g., setting a standard time, finding private time, reminding himself what he wants out of treatment, setting a daily alarm on his phone). Revisit asking the client to remove any items directly related to the target behavior from his home if possible. Ask him to do so right after he arrives home. End on a personal note. Express confidence, affirm the client's courage, or say anything else that is genuine and fits your style as a therapist.

First Session: Therapist Outline

(One 90- to 100-minute session or two 45- to 50-minute sessions)

- Greet client and interact with client as a person

  - Briefly check on target behavior in the last week

  - Explain what to expect in treatment

- Biopsychosocial conceptualization: boiling pot metaphor

  - Mindfulness lets out steam; releases pressure

  - Eventually helps turn down heat on stove; turns down intensity of urges and helps gain freedom from feeling controlled

- Review what client wants to work on; castle/destination metaphor

(Approximate halfway mark of 90-minute session or split between two sessions)

- Color Body Scan and discussion

- Coping Toolbox

- Read "Why Do I Ask You . . . ?"

- Introduce Daily Log; review assignments on Tracking Sheet

- Get commitments, devil's advocate, troubleshoot, and wrap up

Boiling Pot (Biopsychosocial) Metaphor: Therapist Bullet Points

- Some people born feeling emotions more strongly than others.
  - Not a bad thing. Often creative and/or understanding/interpersonal focused.

- Sometimes raised in adverse environment:
  - Routinely put in situations emotionally painful for *anyone*.
  - Since already feel emotions more strongly, pain feels *unbearable*.

- So they try to turn off pain. (*Makes sense* if pain feels unbearable.)
  - Sometimes tell selves, "I'm not going to feel or think."
  - Eventually may feel they need something stronger: <u>*target behavior.*</u>
    - ◆ Works at turning off uncomfortable emotions and urges in short term.

- Problem 1: Never fully learn healthy ways to cope with emotions.
- Problem 2: "Turning off" emotions is like putting a lid on a pot of boiling water:
  - Emotions still there; just like boiling water and steam still there.
  - Feel better briefly, but steam/pressure keeps building, like urges/emotions keep building.
  - Person may almost always feel under pressure from urges.
  - Eventually pot explodes; that's when urges and emotions feel *really* unbearable.

- So person tries harder to "turn off" urges and emotions.
  - <u>Uses target behavior</u> (puts lid on pot) and feels better for short time.
  - But pressure starts building again.
  - Over time, life becomes vicious cycle of <u>target behavior</u> . . . then pressure building . . . then urges feeling unbearable . . . then <u>target behavior</u> . . . and so on.
    - ◆ Might sometimes feel like someone else has remote control for emotions or urges.
  - Does this feel like it fits you?

- First few weeks of MMT, we'll help open a steam hole in lid of the pot.
  - Let out some of the pressure and make urges and emotions easier to tolerate.
  - Some exercises might seem weird—but they help you experience what you're feeling and let steam out of pot.
  - Also retrains your brain to value your emotions and reactions.
  - Later, we'll work to turn down heat on the stove under the pot—turn down intensity of urges and emotions.
  - But first we have to let out some of that pressure.

Destination Metaphor: Therapist Template

(Acknowledge that the metaphor might sound cheesy, while also conveying that it presents an accurate explanation of treatment.)

- Imagine the life you want—a life that feels more fulfilling and satisfying, with you generally feeling like the kind of person you want to be. Now imagine that life is represented by a destination—a house or building [or castle] or whatever you want.

- That destination is over here (*hand gesture—with right hand stretched to right side*) and you've been over here (*left hand stretched to left side*).

- You've been trying to get closer to that destination off and on—and you may have really tried your best—but the problem is that you haven't known *how* to get there. So you've been trying to get there (*show with hand gesture*), not knowing which way to go.

- We're going to put you in a car [or bus/train for people who don't drive] and get you moving toward that destination (*move left hand closer to right*).

- If you come to sessions and do the work, I'm confident that by the end of treatment [or in a few months, if applicable], you'll be much closer to that destination (*move left hand much closer to right*). You won't be *at* the destination, but you'll be much closer, and you'll *feel* like you're much closer. You'll notice a difference in yourself and your life.

- And you'll have a GPS [and/or bus/train route] that will allow you to keep moving even closer to the destination on your own, because you'll have the coping skills to keep going.

- But it won't be easy. This program is a lot of work, and the home practice can feel tedious and boring at times.

- Some weeks you'll feel like you're going 75 miles an hour. Other weeks you'll feel like you're going up a steep hill on a dirt road with the car [bus/train] overheating. You might even feel like you have to get out and push the car [bus/train].

- In other words, some weeks will feel like you're making progress, and some weeks will feel like you're putting in a lot of effort but barely moving—or not moving at all. There might even be weeks when you feel a little worse for a short time. If so, that's normal, and it's temporary. I'll work with you to keep moving until you get past that part.

- But, ultimately, as long as you come to sessions and do the work, I'm confident that by the end of treatment, your life will feel very different—and you'll look back and be really impressed by the progress you've made.

- What do you think about that?

Color Body Scan: Therapist Script

I'd like you to gently bring your attention to my voice. Allow your eyes to close, or, if that's uncomfortable, just focus on a spot in front of you. The purpose of this exercise is not to relax or feel calm; it might happen or it might not. The purpose is to allow yourself to experience *whatever* you experience: to be *aware* of what you are experiencing. If you're like most people, your mind will wander many, many times. That's fine. When you become aware your mind is wandering, give yourself credit for noticing, and then gently bring it back to this exercise.

Now I'll count from three to one. Three: Allow yourself to be aware of the sounds around you. Know that your mind might wander to various noises . . . and that's fine. Just bring it back to the exercise. The purpose is not to go into a trance or to be hypnotized; you won't. The purpose is to allow yourself to be aware. (*Slight pause*) Two: Be aware of the sensations in your feet, legs, and body as they touch the floor or chair. (*Slight pause*) One: Be aware of the sensations in your chest and stomach as you breathe in and out. Just allow yourself to breathe naturally, without trying to control your breathing. (*Slight pause*)

Now I'd like you to allow yourself to be a little playful. Imagine that your breath is a color. When you inhale, this colored breath fills your chest and stomach—so your chest and stomach turn this color from the inside and then outward—and remain this color when you exhale. Try two or three colors and then pick one you'll keep for the rest of the exercise. (*Pause*) Allow yourself to be aware of the sensations. (*Slight pause*)

Now allow yourself to be a little playful again. Imagine that the colored breath fills up your chest and stomach . . . and then goes all the way down your legs and fills up your toes. So your toes turn the color from the inside out—and then stay that color when you exhale. Allow yourself to be aware of the sensations in your toes. Some people say their toes tickle or tingle, some say their toes feel warm or cold, others say they don't even feel their toes at all. Whatever you feel is completely fine. (*Slight pause*)

Now allow your attention to move to the sensations in the bottoms of your feet and heels. Be aware of whether you can feel the fabric or air against them. Maybe you will, maybe you won't. (*Slight pause*) Now your attention spreads up *through* your feet to the top of your feet and ankles. Be aware of any difference in sensations in the tops of your feet compared to the bottoms of your feet. The purpose isn't to try imagine what they look like; the purpose is to be aware of the sensations. (*Slight pause*) Now imagine the color fills up the lower part of your legs: the bones, the muscles, the skin. (*Slight pause*) Some people say they feel relaxed when they do this; others say they feel antsy or bored. Any feeling is fine. There've been too many times in your life when you've felt you *should* be feeling one way or another. This is a time to allow yourself to feel whatever you feel. (*Slight pause*) And now the color fills up your knees—the back of your knees, the joints, and the front of your knees—all radiate with the color. (*Slight pause*)

Now allow your attention to move to your thighs: the bones, the muscles, the skin. (*Slight pause*) Notice whether the pressure feels any different in the back of your thighs compared to the front of your thighs. (*Slight pause*) Notice whether you feel your hands or arms against your thighs. (*Slight pause*)

Now the color fills up the lower half of your trunk—from your waist down. (*Slight pause*) Allow

(continued)

yourself to be aware of the sensations in your lower back (*slight pause*), your bottom (*slight pause*), your front (*slight pause*). Some people feel tension in their lower back. If you come across areas of your body that feel tight or tense, just allow the color to seep through those areas and see what happens. Some people say they're able to release some of the tension when they exhale. If so, that's fine—if not, that's fine, too. Just be aware of the sensations in your lower trunk (*slight pause*), as your abdomen expands and contracts. (*Pause*)

And now, the color goes up through your spine and radiates out to fill the top half of your body: your organs, your rib cage, your muscles, your skin. (*Slight pause*) Be aware of the sensations in your upper back. (*Slight pause*) If you notice any tension, just imagine the color seeping through the muscles. Maybe some tension will leave with the exhale; maybe not. Either way is OK. (*Slight pause*) Now be aware of the sensations in your chest (*slight pause*) and upper abdomen (*slight pause*), your lungs expanding and contracting. (*Slight pause*) Allow yourself to have a sense of curiosity. This is one time there is no certain way you are *supposed* to be reacting—other than experiencing whatever you experience. (*Slight pause*)

Now imagine that when you inhale, the color goes down through your arms and fills up your hands. (*Slight pause*) Focus on the tips of your fingers. Some people say they feel tingly or tickly . . . or warm or cold . . . or even have no feeling. (*Slight pause*) Now, be aware of the feelings in your fingers and the places where your fingers touch each other. (*Slight pause*) And your palms (*slight pause*), and the backs of your hands and wrists. Just be aware of the sensations. (*Slight pause*)

Now the color fills up your lower arms and elbows. Your mind has probably wandered dozens of times during this exercise—if not more. When you notice it happening, give yourself credit for noticing, and gently bring your mind back to your sensations. (*Slight pause*)

And allow your attention to move to your upper arms. You may feel your arms touching your body— or the floor or furniture. Or maybe not. Whatever you're feeling is fine. (*Slight pause*)

And now, the color fills up your shoulders and neck. (*Slight pause*) If you carry any tension in your shoulders or the back of your neck, just imagine the color seeping through the area. (*Slight pause*) Just be aware of the experience: your shoulders (*slight pause*), the back of your neck (*slight pause*), your throat (*slight pause*), the front of your neck. (*Slight pause*) And the color moves up to fill up your face, from behind the face through the skin. (*The following is said slowly, with many very short pauses.*) Your jaw . . . your lips . . . your mouth—maybe you can feel your tongue touching the roof of your mouth or your teeth . . . your nose and the area around your nose . . . your cheekbones . . . your eyes and the area behind and around your eyes . . . your eyelids . . . your eyebrows and brow line . . . your forehead. (*Slight pause*)

And now the color spreads back to include the sides of your head (*slight pause*) and your ears (*slight pause*). And then it spreads through your head to include the top of your head (*slight pause*) and the back of your head (*slight pause*). If there's any tightness, just allow the color to seep through so the area is filled with the color. (*Slight pause*) Be aware of the sensations as your entire head is filled with the color (*Pause*). The top portion of your head almost glows with this color. (*Slight pause*) Be aware of the sensations. (*Slight pause*)

Now allow yourself to be a little playful again. Imagine that as you inhale, the colored breath fills up your head and then puffs out the top of your head through the pores—to make little color cloud puffs above your head. And as you exhale, it comes back through your pores and goes all the way through

(continued)

your body and puffs out your toes. And then as you inhale again, it comes back in through your toes and all the way through your body and out your head again. (*Slight pause*) So every time you inhale or exhale, the color comes in, goes all the way through your body, and then goes out again. Just allow yourself to be aware of what that feels like: the sensations in your body as the breath goes through. And allow yourself to be curious. (*Slight pause*) There's nothing that you are *supposed* to feel or supposed to be. You're just *you*. And you're experiencing whatever you experience. (*Pause*)

Now, gently allow your attention to come back into the room. One: As the breath turns back to the normal color, focus on the sensations in your chest and stomach as you inhale and exhale. (*Slight pause*) Two: Be aware of the feelings of your back, legs, and feet against the floor or chair. (*Slight pause*) Three: Be aware of the various sounds in and around the room. (*Slight pause*) And whenever you're ready, allow your eyes to open. And you might want to stretch a little. . . . (*Therapist stretches before turning chair around to face client.*)

What was that like for you?

Tracking Sheet, Week A

Please write the day and what you did each day in the appropriate column. You can use the "Comments" section to write about anything that occurs during practice so you can remember to talk about it in session.

Day	Audio Practice: At least five times	Coping Toolbox: At least 2 days What skill?	Comments (Optional)
Wed.	Yes	Worked out	Attention wandered many times during audio, and I noticed myself having judgments. But I stuck with it.

Coping Toolbox

Riding out urges without doing something that gets in the way of moving toward the life you want

Do your best to utilize your full awareness when you engage in each activity. Be aware of the physical sensations, sounds, sights, tastes, and/or whatever you choose for your area of focus.

1. Listen to the Color Body Scan or other audio.

2. Say a reminder phrase to yourself. (Ex: *It's difficult, but it will pass.* OR *Just until the next session*.)

   _____

3. Do something creative (draw, take pictures, paint, knit, create a graphic, build something, sew).

4. Write in a journal.

5. Call someone. (Who? Name: _____; Name: _____)

6. Do something to contribute to others. (Call someone lonely; say "hi" to a cashier; volunteer.)

7. Say a prayer to a higher power or the universe. Ask for strength to bear this moment.

8. Focus on sensations. (Take a hot shower or bath. Or take a cold shower or bath.)

9. Engage in physical activity. (Run, sit-ups, push-ups, yoga [DVD or Internet], dance, bike, walk at a brisk pace, or other workout.)

10. Take a walk. Notice shapes or colors around you. Or notice sensations in your feet.

11. Practice mindfulness of *any* activity. (a) Drink coffee, tea, or juice. Drink slowly, focusing on the sensations of taste, smell, and temperature. (b) Put on a comfy sweatshirt or wrap up in your favorite blanket. (c) Pet your cat/dog. Be aware of the feeling of the fur and warmth. (d) Burn incense and be aware of the smell. (e) Play music you like and *really listen*. (f) Sit still and focus on your breathing. (g) Spend time in nature. (h) Etc.

12. Sing along with your favorite songs. (Find them on YouTube if you don't own them.)

13. Cook or bake (for yourself or as a gift for someone else).[a]

14. Play a computer game.[a]

15. Visit someone who doesn't engage in the behavior, or go to a support group meeting.

16. Get on a bus and just ride around the city. Really look at the scenery.

17. Take a moment to imagine how you would feel tomorrow if you act on the urges.

18. Think about moving toward a life that fits your values and who you want to be.

19. _____

20. _____

[a]Only if this activity is not related to the target behavior.

Why Do I Ask You to Do Your Best to Stop
the <u>Target Behavior</u> for the Next _____ Weeks?

Many people have learned to cope with uncomfortable emotions and urges by trying to turn them off—or at least trying to numb them a little. However, that's like putting an airtight lid on a pot of boiling water. The pressure of the steam keeps building, and the urges become more difficult to bear.

In this treatment, you'll learn skills for coping with uncomfortable emotions and/or urges so the pressure decreases and the emotions and urges feel easier to handle. That's like letting the steam out of the pot of boiling water. By fully learning these new skills, you can take back your power so you no longer feel controlled by urges or emotions.

It's important that you work hard to refrain from [target behavior] as much as possible for the next _____ weeks, so you can fully learn the new coping skills. Even if you don't have a problem with [target behavior], the behavior numbs your emotions at least a little—which means that you're still putting the lid on the pot of boiling water. That means the skills are less likely to fully "sink in." In other words, even if you make progress during treatment, there's a higher risk of losing progress after treatment ends. I know I'm asking you to do something difficult. So I won't judge you if you tell me you slipped up. I just ask you to do your best. That means you might be able to stop right away, or you might take a little longer to build up your emotional muscles. It is important for you to be honest about your behavior so I can help you.

Remember: People who do their best to stop [target behavior] during treatment are more likely to have the skills "sink in"—which means they will make more progress in treatment and have a better chance of *keeping their power* even after they've finished treatment.

So whether or not you have a problem, I ask you to work your hardest to stop [target behavior] during treatment. Thank you!

Daily Log

Week date: _____ to _____   Completed each day? (Y or N): _____   Name: _____

Do your best to complete the following log each day. Enter the highest you felt the emotion or urge during the day. (For example, if you experienced anxiety at a 3 for most of the day but at an 8 for an hour, you would enter an 8.) You don't have to spend a lot of time on this.

Day	Frustrated/ Angry 0–10	Sad 0–10	Happy 0–10	Stressed/ Anxious 0–10	Bored 0–10	Lonely 0–10	Satisfied 0–10	Ashamed 0–10	Interested 0–10	Urge 0–10	Act on urge? Y/N Details?	Urge 0–10	Act on urge? Y/N Details?
Mon.													
Tues.													
Wed.													
Thurs.													
Fri.													
Sat.													
Sun.													

Home Practice Summary: Color Body Scan and Coping Toolbox

1. **Practice the Color Body Scan at least five times.**

   Do your best to **practice the Color Body Scan with the audio at least five times** this week. Remember that there is no right or wrong way to feel when practicing. Whatever you feel is fine. Just notice it—and do your best not to judge or try to change what you are feeling. Allow yourself to be curious about whatever you are experiencing. Just keep practicing, and we'll talk about it next week. Be sure to fill in the Tracking Sheet each time you practice with the audio.

2. **Do your best to do something from *H-A2*: *Coping Toolbox* at least 2 days this week.**

   Do your best to give the activity your full awareness. Do *at least two* activities from the toolbox even if you don't have urges this week. This will give you practice using the toolbox so you're more likely to think of it when you do have urges. Using the toolbox is *especially* important when you are having urges. Do your best to keep yourself busy with the activity, so you can ride out the urge without doing something that keeps you from moving toward the life you want. You may feel better when you're doing the activity, or you may not. You may even have to use two or more activities from the toolbox before the urge starts to fade. But as long as you can ride out the urge without using the [target behavior], you're taking back your power and using the activities effectively. Be sure to fill in the Tracking Sheet each time you do something from the toolbox.

3. **Complete the *Tracking Sheet (H-A1)* and the *Daily Log* each day.**

   Fill out the Tracking Sheet and the Daily Log each day. This helps us both keep track of what works best for you, what gets in your way, and how you are feeling through the week.

Note: When you fill out the Tracking Sheet and the Daily Log, please do your best to be honest. You will not be judged about how much or little you have practiced, how strong or weak your urges are, or what behaviors you have or haven't engaged in during the week. The more honest you are on these forms, the more I can tailor your treatment to meet your needs. This will allow me to be more effective in helping you get closer to the kind of life you want to live. Also, please write any comments you have or anything that comes up during practice so we can talk about it at the next meeting.

Program Commitments

1. I commit to *doing my best* to attend session *every week* for ____ weeks.

2. I commit to *doing my best* to be on time every week.

3. I commit to *doing my best* to do the home practice every week.

4. I commit to *doing my best* to be fully honest on everything I report, even though it might be difficult.

5. I commit to *doing my best* to refrain from [target behavior] for the next ____ weeks.

6. Although these steps will be difficult, I realize that they will help me move closer to being the kind of person I want to be and living the kind of life that fits my values.

Name _____ Date _____

MMT Session B (Second Session)
Neutral Experiencing; Mindful Exposure to Current Experiences

- Greet the client and review the week (20 minutes).
  - Assess client's experiences, home practice, and target behavior.
  - Actively reflect, validate, and affirm throughout.
- Introduce new topic: Mindful exposure to current experiences (20–25 minutes).
  - Introduce and discuss *peaks-and-valleys* example of emotions/urges.
  - Hand client *H-B1: Urges and Emotions.*
  - Extended BEST B: Mindful exposure (facilitate awareness and experiencing of **B**reath, **E**motions/urges, **S**ensations, **T**houghts, and return to **B**reath).
  - Assign new home practice: BEST B once per day.
- Wrap up and plan for upcoming week (5 minutes).
- Home practice: guided audio (five times), daily *BEST B (H-B2)*, Daily Log (customized).

Needed for session (all therapist sheets and handouts for this session are at the end of the Session B guidelines):

- BEST B Neutral (TS-B1)
- Urges and Emotions (H-B1)
- BEST B (H-B2)
- Tracking Sheet (H-B3)
- Practice Summary (H-B4)
- Daily Log (Use the version you downloaded and customized.)

SESSION B (SECOND SESSION)

Like Session A, Session B is packed with information. It requires a balancing act between making sure you take enough time to review the client's week, while also making sure you take enough time to explain the new material. This session is the second-most important for providing core material that comprises the basic elements of the entire treatment.

Greet the Client and Review the Previous Week (20 Minutes)

This session provides your first chance to conduct a review of the client's previous week. Thus, it is important to set the precedent of spending a few moments on whatever the client wants to discuss, but then segueing to a review of the Daily Log, which can help you understand the bigger picture surrounding whatever the client is discussing. Remind the client at the beginning about the structure of the session: (1) You will spend about 20 minutes reviewing the previous week, but (2) you will then have to move to the new material in order for the client to gain the abilities to move closer to a life that fits her values.

Please review the detailed instructions on conducting the weekly review in the section on "Structure of Sessions" in Chapter 7 (pp. 108–112). The general order for the review section follows:

1. Review the Daily Log. If the client did not do the Daily Log, have her complete a few days of it while sitting in session.

2. Review *H-A1: Tracking Sheet* (which tracks the Color Body Scan and Coping Toolbox practices).

    The first week of home practice varies widely from client to client. Some clients are especially motivated to complete the home practice during the first week or two, then have sporadic episodes of practice the following weeks. Others complete the practice throughout most of treatment. Many others have trouble completing practice the first week but are able to increase their practice over time (often with the help of shaping). If a client comes in with minimal home practice, (1) find adaptive behavior to affirm ("At least you did one Color Body Scan; that's better than none"); (2) normalize the difficulty of getting started with the practice; (3) briefly assess obstacles; (4) create a plan to address the obstacles (see Strategy 4C in Chapter 5, pp. 63–71); (5) briefly remind the client of the benefits of the practice; and (6) use shaping to find an agreed-upon number of times the client will practice during the upcoming week (see Strategy 5 in Chapter 5, pp. 71–78). If problems with the home practice continue, you will eventually conduct a more detailed functional analysis; however, this session's exploration of obstacles will be much briefer and less structured.

3. If necessary, conduct a *brief* functional analysis of any target behavior (see the section on functional analysis, Chapter 6, pp. 84–86). The first functional analysis will be less structured and detailed than subsequent analyses. The purpose is to help you and the client gain a general idea of antecedents, consequences, and possible alternative methods of coping. Be sure to suggest tools from *H-A2: Coping Toolbox* as alternative methods.

If the client has instances of target behavior and also doesn't complete any (or most) of the home practice, you may not have time to focus adequately on greeting the client, reviewing the week, and addressing both the target behavior and the home practice. In the early stages of treatment, it is more imperative to spend time on the home practice than on the target behavior. Consistent with the rationale of the treatment hierarchy in DBT (Linehan, 1993a), clients attend treatment because they don't yet have the ability to regulate their target behavior and move toward more valued lives. The home practice was designed to help clients acquire the ability to tolerate their emotions/urges and regulate their behavior. Thus, if you are pressed for time and have to choose between prioritizing the home practice or the target behavior, mention the target behavior, but spend the bulk of the time on the home practice (especially within the first few weeks, when the client has only begun to learn the new ways of coping).

Introduce and Discuss the Session Topic (20–25 Minutes)

This session introduces (1) the peaks-and-valleys explanation of urge fluctuations and (2) the BEST B mindfulness exercise. Both are central components of the entire treatment.

Provide the Peaks-and-Valleys Explanation

The peaks-and-valleys graphs (Figures 8.1–8.3) provide a concrete, visual explanation of the client's cycle of urges and target behavior, with emphasis on the facts that (1) strong urges are time-limited and tend to wax and wane; (2) an urge will eventually decrease on its own if the client does not act on it; (3) the more the client can ride out urges without acting on them, the weaker the average peaks will become and the less frequently urges will occur over time; and thus (4) each time the client rides out a strong urge without acting on it (i.e., without putting the lid on the boiling pot), she gets a little closer to having less frequent and less intense urges overall.

To explain the peaks-and-valleys graphs, draw each on a piece of paper (instead of just showing clients the graphs in Figures 8.1–8.3). Most therapists draw them on the back of the client's handouts for the upcoming week (in other words, on the backs of the *Daily Log, H-B1, H-B2,* and *H-B3*). As always, modify the explanation to fit what you know about the particular client.

> The following example demonstrates the conversational tone that has been shown to be effective with clients. You are not expected to learn phrases verbatim. Instead you are encouraged to read the example and practice the explanation enough to become familiar with the main points—while always being sure to validate the difficulty of tolerating urges. (For clients who report urges but deny having negative emotions prior to target behavior, focus on urges and minimize reference to emotions, at least during the early sessions.)

Peaks and Valleys

Let's say this is a graph of urges. Urges are often cued by unpleasant or uncomfortable emotions—so it can sometimes feel like urges and emotions are all mixed up together.

Emotions and urges tend to fluctuate. Sometimes, as your emotions and urges start to rise (draws line rising) *[see Figure 8.1a], you may tell yourself that you shouldn't be feeling so upset or you shouldn't be feeling urges. But that actually tends to make it worse, because you still feel the emotions and urges you were already feeling, plus you may also start to become upset that you can't* stop *the emotions and urges—which can make them go even higher. Or maybe you don't feel much emotion but instead mainly feel the urges. Either way, the urges continue to rise.* (Continues drawing the rising line.)

Eventually, the urges often get to a point where they feel unbearable (Figure 8.1b). You may try to white-knuckle it for a while, but sooner or later, you may think, "I just can't take it anymore." Or maybe you think, "It's never going to get better, and it may just keep getting worse. I'm going to have to do something to turn it off sooner or later, so I might as well do it now and get it over with." Have you ever had either of those thoughts?

So you engage in the target behavior [and/or perhaps other dysregulated behaviors], and you feel a release (points to Figure 8.1c). *You feel better—for a while. But sooner or later, the urges start to rise again* (points to Figure 8.1d). *And pretty soon, they're back up where they were before. And then it all feels like it's* really *unbearable. You might try to resist the urges for a while, but then you probably think "I can't handle this anymore" or something similar—and so you act on the urges and engage in the behavior.* (Draws the line dropping again.) *And you feel better for a little while. But pretty soon, the urges start rising. And eventually, life becomes this constant cycle of feeling overwhelming urges and maybe unpleasant emotions, then doing something to turn off the urges, but then the urges slowly building until they feel unbearable again. So life becomes this rollercoaster* (Figure 8.1). *Does it feel like that for you some of the time?*

(Takes a new sheet of paper.) *The thing is, when urges and emotions get up to the highest points* (draws a peak on the graph) *[Figure 8.2a], if you can ride out the urges without doing something to try to turn them off, they'll eventually start to fall on their own [Figure 8.2b]. It will likely feel horrible while urges are at the highest point—like your head is going to explode—but if you find other ways to cope so that you can ride out the urges, the urges and emotions* will *eventually start falling. Over time, if you continue to ride out the high points without doing something to turn off the urges and emotions—the high points will start getting a little lower and last for a shorter time [Figure 8.2c]. And little by little,*

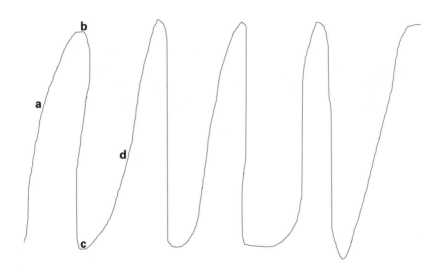

FIGURE 8.1. Peaks and valleys, Example 1.

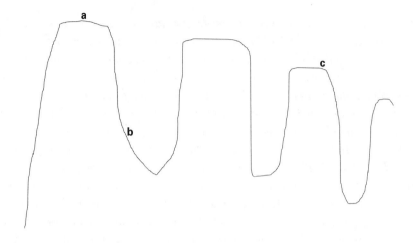

FIGURE 8.2. Peaks and valleys, Example 2.

the urges and any related emotions will feel less and less unbearable. (Draws shorter peaks on another piece of paper *[not shown here].*) *It won't happen as fast as in these drawings— but you will probably notice at least some difference after just a few weeks. Over time, you'll have more instances when the urges are just background, instead of taking all of your attention. Eventually, you can get more like this* (draws Figure 8.3)—*instead of this* (shows client Figure 8.1). *Every once in a while, you might still have a high point—but in general, your urges will be manageable—and sometimes even unnoticeable.*

But the only way you can get from here (points to Figure 8.1) *to here* (points to Figure 8.3) *is to ride out the urges without acting on them—without trying to turn off the urges and unpleasant emotions. I wish there were an easier way. But I'm going to work with you to help you find ways to get through those times. It's hard. It will feel unbearable at times. But every time you get through one of these peaks* (points to Figure 8.2), *you're getting closer to this* (points to Figure 8.3).

After explaining the peaks and valleys of the cycle of urges to the client, ask for the client's opinion, and then work to modify the explanation to fit the client, if necessary. For example, as mentioned previously, some clients report that they don't feel any uncomfortable emotions when they have urges. Clients have even reported feeling fairly content or happy when experiencing strong urges. In these circumstances, one or more of the following could be occurring:

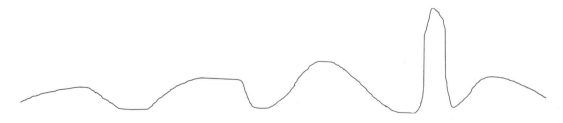

FIGURE 8.3. Peaks and valleys, Example 3.

1. The client may have become so conditioned to responding to certain cues by engaging in target behavior that the cues automatically elicit urges, regardless of the client's emotions. For example, the client may have a history of engaging in target behavior when she watches television. Therefore, she may experience urges to engage in the behavior any time she sits down to watch television, regardless of her emotions. However, when she works to resist the urges, the client will likely *then* experience discomfort. Thus, the emotional discomfort that is difficult to tolerate may occur when resisting the urges instead of prior to the urges. If the client reports that she does not experience discomfort when resisting the urges in these circumstances, validate her reports, and then ask her to experiment by resisting the urges in the upcoming week. She will likely report difficulty doing so, because the urges were difficult to tolerate.

2. Instead of feeling emotions that are usually interpreted as uncomfortable or negative, the client may instead just experience dissatisfaction with her current emotional state. For example, she may think that she should be feeling happier after receiving a promotion, or should feel more outgoing around friends, or deserves to feel more excited about dating someone she likes. Thus, even though the client might already be somewhat happy, confident, and/or excited, she may not feel that she is as happy as she *should* be or is *expected* to be. Thus, the urges and initial discomfort may be based on dissatisfaction with her current level of emotion, and resisting the urges often causes further discomfort.

3. A third possibility might be that the client is so accustomed to avoiding or suppressing negative emotions that she is not aware of uncomfortable or negative emotions until they become strong. Thus, she may be experiencing low levels of uncomfortable emotions and not be fully aware of them—but instead might experience them only as urges.

4. Even positive change can elicit stress, and sometimes even happiness can feel stressful. Clients sometimes report feeling agitated when happy, and many clients report fearing that the happiness will go away. Thus, sometimes happiness can be an uncomfortable emotion until the client becomes accustomed to experiencing and "tolerating" happiness.

Give H-B1: Urges and Emotions *to the Client*

This handout summarizes points made by the peaks-and-valleys example. Thus, you will not need to spend time discussing the handout—which is good, because *you will not have time to discuss the handout.* (You need time to conduct and discuss the BEST B, plus a few minutes to wrap up the session.) Tell the client the handout further explains what you just discussed and can be read as a reminder between sessions. Just for your benefit: The key points of the handout, which you will bring up throughout the rest of treatment, include the following:

*   *When you try to avoid urges/emotions, they get stronger over time.*
*   *Urges/emotions can influence behavior almost before you are aware of what is happening (almost like someone else has the remote control).*
*   *MMT exercises help you become aware of what leads to these urges/emotions—and give you a choice of how to react.*
*   *The first step is to be aware of urges/emotions.*
*   *The second step is to get through the urges without acting on them.*

- *The more you can get through the peaks of urges without acting on them, the weaker the peaks will become over time.*
- *Over time, your "emotional muscles" will become stronger, and the urges will feel weaker, less overwhelming, and easier to bear.*

Introduce the BEST B

The BEST B is a 2- to 3-minute exercise that is intended to help clients:

1. Increase awareness of low-level emotions and urges (when they are less intense and easier to handle), and
2. Begin to build the ability to experience and tolerate the present moment (emotions/urges/sensations/thoughts).

The acronym BEST B stands for:

- **B**reath,
- **E**motions and urges,
- **S**ensations,
- **T**houghts, and
- **B**reath.

The BEST B is introduced under neutral circumstances—thereby providing exposure to neutral emotions. Clients are encouraged to practice the BEST B daily, regardless of urges. They are also encouraged to purposely do a BEST B whenever they experience urges—as a step toward increasing their ability to tolerate the peaks of high-intensity urges without acting on them.

Introduce the BEST B much like the Color Body Scan—that is, without much explanation. Tell the client you'd like to lead her in an exercise that involves an acronym. Hand her *H-B2: BEST B*, but do not give her time to read the handout. Instead, just read the words associated with each letter in the BEST B (above), and tell her you'll explain the practice after you lead her through it. Have the client close her eyes (or focus on a spot on her lap or the floor if closing her eyes is difficult). If possible, turn your chair to face away from the client while reading the script.

Read the *TS-B1: BEST B Neutral—Therapist Script*. After reading the BEST B script, explain that you purposely made the practice longer than it usually will be, just because you needed to explain all of the parts to the client. Tell the client that when she practices it on her own, she just needs to take 2 or 3 minutes. In fact, specifically instruct her *not* to take more than 3 minutes, so as not to feel overwhelmed.

Ask what the exercise was like for the client. Key points to remind the client include the following:

- The client does not need to label every emotion she is feeling during the *E* part (emotions and urges). Stress the importance of just labeling the first one to three emotions that come to mind—and being aware of any related sensations. Spending too much time on that portion or trying to determine all of the "accurate" emotions runs the risk of the client's losing focus and not finishing the BEST B.

- Clients often report that the *T* (thoughts) section is confusing and difficult at first. Clients often find themselves thinking of things unrelated to emotions/urges (e.g., wondering if it's time to get a haircut) and/or thinking about odd topics (e.g., "Why is the sky blue?"). Such thoughts are fine. The purpose is to become accustomed to stepping back and labeling thoughts *as* thoughts—instead of automatically reacting as if they were facts. As long as the client takes time to label a few thoughts, the content does not matter.

- If the client says she wasn't able to think of anything, remind her that "I can't think of anything" is a thought.

- The purpose is not to challenge the thoughts. The purpose is for the client to just start practicing being aware of thoughts as "just thoughts."

- During the last breath, the client is encouraged to commit to herself that she will act in a way that fits the kind of person she wants to be. The specifics of the commitment might change depending on when she does the BEST B. Sometimes she might commit to riding out current urges without acting on them. Sometimes she might commit to continue doing the home practice even when she is tired or bored, and so on.

Bring out *H-B3: Tracking Sheet* and assign the BEST B. For the upcoming week, the assignment will include the Color Body Scan, the BEST B, and the Daily Log. An optimal assignment would be the Color Body Scan five times, the BEST B at least once a day, and the Daily Log every day. However, *work with the client to find an amount she will commit to doing.* Remind the client that the BEST B should only take 2–3 minutes each time. Tell her she does not need to memorize the instructions to the right of each letter. Those are just prompts to remind her about the exercise in case she forgets. Once the client memorizes the basic acronym, she is encouraged to practice the BEST B in a private space with her eyes closed. After a week or two, she can also add a BEST B practice with her eyes open (e.g., while walking, riding mass transit, going about daily life).

Ask the client when she will be the most likely to do the BEST B. Popular times include in the morning right after waking, right before a meal, at night before going to sleep, right before leaving for work/school, and sitting in the car before getting out to go to work/school. Ask if setting her phone alarm would be helpful. Get a commitment.

> The BEST B owes credit to the "SOBER Breathing Space" from *Mindfulness-Based Relapse Prevention for Addictive Behaviors* (Bowen et al., 2010). Although MMT integrates strategies from several empirically supported treatments, the BEST B is one of the skills that is most directly related to its source of inspiration.

Wrap Up and Plan for Upcoming Week (5 Minutes)

- Alert the client that the session is nearing the end. Briefly remind her of ways to cope with any high-risk situation (*H-A2: Coping Toolbox, H-B2: BEST B*).

- Remind the client about the home practice, and get a commitment that she will do her best to ride out urges without engaging in the target behavior (or go longer than usual without the behavior, if using shaping). Wrap up.

BEST B Neutral: Therapist Script

(*Tell the client that this will take longer than the standard 2–3 minutes.*) The first **B** is for **breath.** Allow yourself to be aware of the physical sensations in your chest and stomach as you inhale and exhale. (*Pause*) You'll focus on about three breaths when you do this on your own. (*Pause long enough for 3–4 breaths*)

We've done B for *breath,* now **E** for **emotions and urges.** Gently bring your attention to your emotions and urges. Purposely experience what you're feeling. (*Pause about 3 seconds*) Allow yourself to be open to *all* of your emotions and urges —without trying to control them. (*Pause about 3 seconds*) Mentally label the emotions and urges: "That's stress or anxiety. That's boredom. That's an urge." [*Note: You can suggest a few emotions you think the client might be experiencing. "Perhaps you're feeling some irritation? Maybe some sadness? If so, just label the emotions."*] You don't have to label every emotion you might be experiencing. Just be aware of the first few that come to mind. (*Pause about 2 seconds*) And allow yourself to be curious about what the emotions and urges feel like—including any related physical sensations. (*Pause about 3 seconds*) Emotions and urges won't make your head explode, even if they feel like they will. Urges don't predict the future. You can have emotions and urges without acting on them. You can ride them out—even though it's hard. (*Pause about 3 seconds*) This is your chance to take back some power by purposely experiencing your emotions and urges, and riding them out. (*Pause for about 5 seconds*)

We've done B for *breath,* and E for *emotions and urges*—now **S** for **sensations.** Gently shift your attention to focus *primarily* on physical sensations. (*Pause*) Do a quick mental scan of your body. If any area of your body feels tight or tense, imagine that your breath goes to that area when you inhale—and then surrounds and fills the area. When you exhale, some of the tightness may or may not leave with the breath. There is no right or wrong way. (*Pause for about 5 seconds*)

We've done B for *breath,* E for *emotions and urges, and S* for *sensations.* Now **T** for **thoughts.** Gently shift your awareness to the thoughts that pass through your mind. Most of the time we act on thoughts as if they were facts, but actually our brains generate thoughts based on what we were taught to believe in the past. (*Pause about 2 seconds*) Thoughts don't necessarily equal facts. You can have a thought without acting on it. (*Pause about 2 seconds*) Notice the thoughts going through your mind, and then label each thought by telling yourself, "That's a *thought.*" (*Slight pause.*) Thoughts may be anything: Even thinking "I can't think of any thoughts" is a thought. If you think, "I can't take it any more"—tell yourself, "That's a thought." You might notice thoughts like, "I don't think I'm doing this right," or "I'll stop the behavior next week." Just tell yourself, "Those are thoughts." You may even notice unrelated thoughts like wondering whether it's raining or worrying about the future. Those are all just thoughts. It doesn't matter what thoughts you have, as long as you observe them and label them as thoughts. You're training your brain to respond to your thoughts in a different way. (*Pause about 3 seconds*) Notice your thoughts passing through your mind like clouds floating through the sky. Clouds come and go, but the sky remains the sky—just like thoughts come and go, but your mind remains your mind. (*Pause for about 2 seconds*) Now I'm going to be quiet a few seconds, and just notice the thoughts that pass through your mind. (*Pause for about 5 seconds*)

(continued)

Now we've done *B, E, S,* and *T,* so we're up to the last **B**—which is **breath** again. Gently bring your attention back to your breath for a few breaths. Allow yourself to be aware of the sensations in your chest and stomach as you breathe in and breathe out. (*Pause for about 3 breaths*) Remind yourself of your commitment to work to be the kind of person you want to be. (*Slight pause*) Now, if you choose to do so, make a commitment—right now to yourself—to do your best to act in a way that fits that kind of person. (*Slight pause*) And be aware of what that feels like. (*Pause for about 3 seconds*) Really be aware of what it feels like to make that commitment to yourself. (*Pause for about 3 seconds.*) Now, whenever you're ready, allow your eyes to open. (*The therapist turns chair around and faces the client.*) What was that like for you?

Urges and Uncomfortable Emotions

Urges and uncomfortable emotions can be cued by things around you (people, places, events) or inside you (emotions, thoughts, sensations).

In the past, you've probably tried to avoid thinking about urges and uncomfortable emotions. The thing is, *when you try to avoid urges and emotions, they get stronger over time (like the steam and pressure in the pot of boiling water).* There's more! When you try to avoid urges and emotions, they can affect your behavior almost before you're aware of what's happening. Some people say that they feel almost like someone else has a remote control for their behavior. They might not plan to act on the urges, but then they feel an uncomfortable emotion or an unexpected spike in urges— and suddenly they start [engaging in <u>target behavior</u>] without even thinking about it. And then they often feel worse and regret their behavior afterward.

MMT exercises can help you become aware of what leads to these urges and emotions—so you're not taken by surprise and you can choose how you want to react. In other words, you won't feel like someone else has the remote control.

The first step is to become aware of urges/emotions. To be *unaware* makes it easier to go on autopilot and do things that can cause you pain in the long run. Awareness gives you the freedom to make your own choice about how you want to act.

The second step is to get through the urges without acting on them. Many people think that once an urge/emotion begins, it will keep getting stronger until the person acts on it. Instead, urges/emotions are like waves. They rise to a peak, and then if you ride them out without acting on them, they naturally decrease. Urges and emotions can rise and fall many times a day. They can be uncomfortable or painful to experience. However:

- The more you can get through the peaks of urges/emotions without acting on the urges, the weaker the peaks will become over time.
- Every time you get through a peak without acting on the urges, you build your "emotional muscles," so you will gradually build more strength to cope with the urges.
- Over time, your emotional muscles will become stronger, and the urges will feel weaker and weaker. So urges will feel less overwhelming and much easier to bear.
- But the only way to get to that point is to get through the urges *without acting on them*.

BEST B

Only take about 2 or 3 minutes when you do this on your own.

Breath Focus on your breath for about three breaths; allow yourself to be aware of the physical sensations in your chest and stomach as you breathe in and breathe out.

Emotions/urges Gently bring your attention to your emotions and urges. Be aware of what you're feeling. Label the emotions and urges. ("That's stress or anxiety. That's boredom. That's an urge.") Allow yourself to be curious about what the emotions feel like, including any related physical sensations. Emotions and urges won't make your head explode. You can have an urge without acting on it.

Sensations Gently shift your attention to focus *primarily* on physical sensations. Do a brief scan of your body, and if any area feels tight or tense, imagine that your breath goes to that area and seeps through it. When you breathe out, some of the tightness may or may not leave with the breath. There is no right or wrong way to feel.

Thoughts Allow yourself to be aware of your thoughts. Then label the first few thoughts that come into your head as "just thoughts." Your brain generates thoughts based on what it has been trained to believe in the past, but you can have a thought without acting on it. (Thoughts may be anything: "I can't think of anything" or "I'm not doing this right" or "I can't take it any more" or "I'll stop [the target behavior] tomorrow" or *anything*.)

Breath Bring your attention back to your breath. Allow yourself to be aware of the sensations as you breathe in and breathe out. Now, if you choose to do so, gently commit to yourself to act in a way that fits the kind of person you want to be. Really make that commitment. And be aware of what that feels like.

Remember:

This is your chance to take back some of your power by choosing to purposely experience your emotions, urges, sensations, and thoughts.

Emotions and urges won't make your head explode, even if they feel like they will. Urges don't predict the future. You can have an urge and ride it out without acting on it.

Most of the time we act on thoughts as if they were facts, but your brain generates thoughts based on what you were taught to believe in the past. Thoughts don't necessarily equal facts. Thoughts don't predict the future. You can have a thought without acting on it.

An emotion is just an emotion; an urge is just an urge; a sensation is just a sensation; and a thought is just a thought.

Tracking Sheet, Week B

Please write the day and what you did each day in the appropriate column.

Day	Audio: At least five times	BEST B: Once Daily Where? When?	Comments (Optional)
Wed.	Yes	Bathroom, morning	Noticed getting sleepy in the BEST B. I find it relaxing.

Home Practice Summary: Color Body Scan and Best B

1. **Practice the Color Body Scan at least five times.**

   Do your best to **practice the Color Body Scan with the audio at least five times** before our next meeting. Remember that there is no right or wrong way to feel when practicing. Whatever you feel is fine. Just notice it—and do your best not to judge or try to change what you are feeling. Allow yourself to be curious about whatever you are experiencing. Just keep practicing, and we'll talk about it next week. Be sure to fill in the Tracking Sheet to record your practice.

2. **Do the BEST B at least once a day. (See *H-B2: BEST B*.)**

   Be sure to fill in the Tracking Sheet to record your practice.

3. **Complete the Tracking Sheet and the Daily Log each day.**

   Fill out the Tracking Sheet and the Daily Log each day. This helps us both keep track of what works best for you, what gets in your way, and how you are feeling throughout the week.

Note: When you fill out the Tracking Sheet and the Daily Log, please do your best to be honest. You will not be judged about how much or little you have practiced, how strong or weak your urges are, or what behaviors you have or haven't engaged in during the week. The more honest you are on these forms, the more I can tailor your treatment to meet your needs. This will allow me to be more effective in helping you get closer to the kind of life you want to live. Also, please write any comments you have or anything that comes up during practice so we can talk about it at the next meeting.

MMT Session C (Usually Third or Fourth Session)
Mindful Exposure, Part 1: Intentional Experiencing of Higher-Intensity Emotions/Urges

- Greet the client and review the previous week (15–20 minutes).
  - Assess client's experiences, home practice, and target behavior.
  - Actively reflect/validate/affirm throughout.
- Conduct mindful exposure, Part I (20–25 minutes).
  - Visualization of exposure to urges and uncomfortable emotions.
  - Extended BEST B and alternative reaction:
    - Include visualization of reaction that is inconsistent with urges and consistent with the kind of person the client wants to be.
    - Therapist may provide suggestions *when needed.*
    - Briefly process the experience.
    - Assign new home practice: *High-Risk Situations Worksheet (H-C2).*
- Wrap up session, check emotions/urges, and plan for upcoming week (5 minutes).
- Home practice: guided audio (five times), BEST B (at least once daily), Daily Log (everyday), *High-Risk Situations Worksheet (H-C2).*

Needed for session (all therapist sheets and handouts for this session are at the end of the Session C guidelines):

- Exposure/BEST B (TS-C1)
- High-Risk Examples (H-C1)
- High-Risk Situations Worksheet (H-C2)
- Tracking Sheet (H-C3)
- Practice Summary (H-C4)
- Daily Log (Use the version you downloaded and customized.)

SESSION C (USUALLY THIRD OR FOURTH SESSION)

Many clients do not fully believe that they can experience intense urges without eventually acting on those urges; instead, they assume that their urges must decrease before they can reduce the target behavior. By providing exposure to high-risk urges and emotions, you can help clients start to habituate, which can decrease the perceived necessity of acting on the urges.

Greet the Client and Review the Previous Week (15–20 Minutes)

- Review the Daily Log.
- Review the Tracking Sheet (Color Body Scan and BEST B).

Affirm any incidents of home practice. If the client has not completed the Tracking Sheet but reports doing the practice, ask him for the number of times he did each assigned practice—while also nonjudgmentally stressing the importance of recording the practice.

Ask about the client's experience doing BEST B. Reflect and validate. If he reports trouble finishing once he starts, validate that his experience is common at first. Remind him that:

- The practice only needs to be 2–3 minutes.

- He does not have to be aware of every emotion or thought he is experiencing, but instead he can just be aware of the first two or three that come to mind, and then move on.

- His thoughts do not have to be related to the target behavior or treatment. As long as he labels his thoughts as thoughts—regardless of what the thoughts are—he is training his mind to be aware of thoughts as "just thoughts." He is building his ability to choose how to respond to his thoughts instead of automatically acting on them.

  See Strategy 4C in Chapter 5 (pp. 67–71) for instructions on how to proceed if the client has not completed most or all of the home practice. Use shaping (Strategy 5 in Chapter 5, pp. 71–78) to plan the amount of home practice the client will do the following week. Reminders of the destination metaphor can help the discussion be memorable while also decreasing the chance the client feels judged:

  Remember the destination metaphor? You've started down the road just by coming here each week—and I'm glad you're here. That takes effort on its own. But for you to really get going and make progress toward your destination—toward the life that fits your values—you have to do the home practice. I know it's time-consuming and boring at times, but the home practice is essential for moving closer to the kind of person you want to be.

- If necessary, conduct a functional analysis of instances of target behavior (see Functional Analysis, Chapter 6, pp. 84–86).

If the client's target behavior has not decreased at all, conduct shaping: Get the client to commit to going a longer time without the behavior. For example, if the client has engaged in the behavior every day, ask him to work to go at least 1 day—or at least a certain number of hours—without the behavior. Then plan how to do so: The client can use items from the Coping Toolbox, do a BEST B, or use any other strategies you decide upon together. Get a commitment.

Introduce and Discuss the Session Topic: Mindful Exposure, Part I (20–25 Minutes)

Introduce the session topic of mindful exposure. Clients tend to begin treatment feeling like they are sometimes controlled by urges and/or emotions. MMT will help them gain freedom from feeling controlled. Instead, through MMT, *they* can gain control of *how they react* to urges and emotions. In the current session, clients will start to build emotional muscles by purposely experiencing urges without acting on them or engaging in other avoidant actions. The goal is to help clients separate urges from actions. A key statement to make to clients is: "Urges don't predict the future. You can have an urge without acting on it." This statement should be repeated often throughout the treatment.

Conduct Visualization of Exposure to Urges and Uncomfortable Emotions: Extended BEST B and Alternative Reaction

Ask the client to think of an upcoming situation that is likely to cue urges. Alternatively, you can ask the client to choose a recent situation in which he experienced urges and engaged in the target behavior. (This is more effective if the situation is likely to occur again soon.) Ask the client to choose a situation that does not feel traumatic or intensely distressing—but that is likely to elicit at least some urges or uncomfortable emotions if he visualizes it in the session. Some clients may want to spend several minutes trying to pick the "perfect" situation, which will cause you to be pressed for time later in the session. Assure the client that as long as the situation is likely to elicit *any* urges, the situation will be fine. Examples clients have chosen include:

- Feeling anxious at a social event and/or embarrassed after the event.
- Being criticized by partner, boss, parent, or another person significant to the client.
- Having a fight with an important other.
- Walking past a liquor store or bakery (or any source for the particular target behavior).
- Being rejected—socially, career-related, or otherwise.
- Feeling pressured to complete a stressful task while home alone.
- Being exposed to any paraphernalia related to the target behavior.
- Feeling loneliness or other negative emotions, with easy access to sources of the target behavior (food, substances, the Internet, a casino, computer games, porn, etc.).

Once the client chooses a situation, ask for enough details to help you set up the basic premise in an exposure visualization. Find out what the situation is, who is involved, where the client will be, what the client may be thinking and feeling, etc. You do not have to know every detail, nor will you have time to do so. The main points of the exposure visualization are to guide the client in (1) spending several minutes experiencing the chosen situation, (2) imagining himself doing a BEST B before reacting, and (3) visualizing himself reacting in a way that fits his values (instead of reacting in his habitual manner). As you guide the client through the visualization, use prompts, questions, and reflections to help him stay on track and experience everything that is happening in the situation, including the behaviors of others (if applicable) and the client's own behaviors, emotions, thoughts, physical sensations, and urges.

Tell the client you are going to lead him in a visualization of the situation. Ask him to sit up with both feet on the floor and close his eyes (or focus on a spot on his lap or the floor). Turn your chair around and begin leading him on the visualization. *Note:* The template will need to be customized extensively to the client's situation and reactions, so please familiarize yourself with the template enough that you will be comfortable customizing it while reading it to the client.

Lead the client through the exposure using *TS-C1: Exposure Visualization and BEST B.*

After guiding the client through the visualization and BEST B, ask him what it was like for him. Reflect, validate, and affirm his response. Validate the difficulty of changing conditioned reactions, but also focus on processing the client's (1) reported dissatisfaction with previous ways of reacting and (2) reported desire to change his reactions and/or have the confidence that he can do so. Problem solve any trouble the client may have had identifying alternative methods of coping.

- Ask the client to rate his urges and discomfort/distress. Most of the time, they will be lower than the highest point in the exercise and near the level they were before the exercise. If so, point out how much urges can fluctuate even in the few minutes during session—but also stress that it would have been OK if the urges remained high, since having urges doesn't mean that a person has to act on them.

- If the client continues to report high urges and discomfort/distress, validate but stay matter-of-fact. You want to communicate that urges and negatives emotions are not dangerous or harmful in and of themselves. It is the client's *reaction* to the urges and emotions that have sometimes caused negative consequences; the urges and emotions themselves are unpleasant but not harmful. (In MMT trainings, clinicians sometimes express concern about clients potentially leaving session with high urges or uncomfortable emotions. However, if the client is in treatment for dysregulated behavior, high urges and uncomfortable emotions are probably not uncommon for him. He likely experiences high urges and uncomfortable emotions on a fairly regular basis.) Use a caring but calm tone to talk to the client about what he will do to get through the rest of the day to decrease the chance he will act on the urges.

  - Although MMT has been conducted with clients who reported passive suicidal ideation, it has not been conducted with clients referred for active suicidality. An exception to the above advice would be if the client experienced high suicide urges.

  - In the unexpected event that the client suddenly begins experiencing high suicidal urges, perform a suicide assessment and refer to a treatment protocol for suicidal clients. Instances of sudden suicidal urges after completing this exercise would be highly unexpected.

- Sometimes clients do not experience increases in urges during the exercise. Similarly, some clients say they have trouble visualizing and thus "did not get much" out of the exercise. In these cases, normalize the experience and assure them that the exercise "still worked."

    Some people have trouble visualizing, and that's completely fine. The exercise still worked, because it helped you think about using the BEST B and planning ways of coping that are different than your previous reactions. [The same general response can be given if the client reports never experiencing noticeable urges during the exercise.]

Assign New Home Practice: H-C2: High-Risk Situations Worksheet

Ask the client to do a short BEST B whenever he experiences urges in the upcoming week, and discuss possible opportunities to do so.

I know that urges can be uncomfortable and upsetting, so it's not that I want you to have high urges this week. Even so, in some ways it would be nice if you do have urges, because that will give you an opportunity to practice using the BEST B and a new a way of responding—like you just practiced doing.

(You're encouraged to have an extra copy of *H-B2: BEST B* available in case the client has misplaced his copy.) Segue into the assignment by showing the client *H-C1: High-Risk Situations That May Cue Urges,* and then introduce *H-C2: High-Risk Situations Worksheet.* (Please download the sample sheet from the publisher's website [see the box at the end of the table of contents] and customize it to fit the client's behavior prior to printing. Some examples will not fit all behaviors, and the wording "engage in the target behavior" sounds artificial and sterile.) The instructions are largely self-explanatory:

Complete this sheet when you notice yourself experiencing increased urges. Do your best to complete it as soon as you notice the urges. However, if you can't complete it at that time, then please complete it afterward—regardless of how you respond.

The point to stress is that the client should do his best to do a BEST B whenever he has urges—even if he intends to engage in the target behavior after the BEST B. (Of course, the hope is that the BEST B will allow him to gain enough perspective to choose an alternative behavior.) Ask him to be honest in recording whether or not he engaged in the BEST B in each situation. In addition, stress that you hope he does not engage in the target behavior, but if he does, *those times are especially vital for completing the worksheet* (even after the fact). The client's completion of the sheet will help you understand what happened, which in turn will help you tailor the treatment to be more effective. (The sheet contains the main points of a functional analysis; see Chapter 6, pp. 84–86.)

Check Emotions/Urges, Wrap Up Session, and Plan for Upcoming Week (5 Minutes)

- If the client has done the Color Body Scan eight times total in the past two weeks, give him the link to the new audio exercise (Audio #2). Ask the client to do the new practice at least 2 days, and then choose either of the practices for the other 3 days.
- If the client has not done the Color Body Scan at least four times the previous week and at least eight times total, continue with the Color Body Scan for 1 more week before giving the client a new audio exercise.
- Remind the client about the home practice: audio practice 5 days, BEST B at least once a day (with encouragement to do another when experiencing urges), and *H-C2: High-Risk Situations Worksheet* whenever the client experiences urges.
- Get a commitment that the client will do his best to refrain from the target behavior.

Exposure Visualization and BEST B: Therapist Script Template

A final script cannot be provided, since the visualization should (obviously) be specific to the client's situation. Instead, a (fairly muddled) script template appears below. Direct instructions to the therapist are in parentheses and italic. The underlined portions should be customized to fit the client. The portions that are not underlined can be said largely verbatim (if you choose). Please become familiar enough with the template that you can customize it as you lead the visualization. Start by asking clients to rate their urges to engage in the target behavior on a scale of 0–100. Also ask for levels of discomfort or distress (0–100). Then segue to the template.

Allow your eyes to close if you haven't already. I'm going to count from three to one to help you focus. Three, be aware of the various sounds in and around the room. (*Slight pause*) Two, be aware of the feelings of your feet against the floor and your body against the chair. (*Slight pause*) One, be aware of the physical sensations in your chest and stomach as you breathe in and breathe out. (*Slight pause*) Now, imagine that you're in the situation you just told me about. (*Provide a few details about the situation.*) Really visualize yourself in the situation. Do your best to really picture your surroundings. (*Pause*) (**Skip the rest of this paragraph if the client is alone in the chosen situation.**) Picture the person [people] who is [are] with you. Do your best to see that person [those people] in your mind. Imagine what they are saying to you. Really hear what they are saying—and then imagine how you respond.

Be aware of what you are doing—whether you are sitting or standing, and what is actually happening in the situation. (*Pause*) Tell me what's going on in the situation right now. (*Pause for answer. Reflect what the client said and lead the client a little further in imagining what is being said and/ or done. Give cues based on what you know. Then continue.*) What are you feeling as this happens? (*Pause for answer*) So you're feeling (*list relevant emotion*) and (*list relevant emotion*). Maybe you're also feeling (*list potentially relevant emotions*)? (*Reflect response*) Also be aware of your thoughts. You might be thinking things like (*provide potentially relevant thoughts, such as "I'll feel better after [target behavior]" or "Just this one more time"*). What are you thinking? (*Pause*) So you're having thoughts like (*list relevant thoughts*). What else are you thinking? (*Pause for answer*) OK, so you're feeling (*relevant emotion*) and (*relevant emotion*), and you're thinking (*relevant thought*) and (*relevant thought*).

What are your physical sensations? Do you feel tight or tense anywhere? Or perhaps any heaviness or burning? Or maybe pressure or emptiness? (*Pause for answer*) OK, what other sensations are you feeling? So you're feeling (*relevant emotion*), you're having thoughts that (*relevant thoughts*), and you're feeling (*relevant sensations*). (*If there is another person involved, ask what the other person does and how the client responds during all of this time.*) Now be aware of your urges. Be aware of urges to [target behavior]. Some people say that the urges feel almost like a magnet pulling them to act. What do the urges feel like for you? (*Pause*) What sort of thoughts are you having about the urges? (*Pause*) What sort of emotions and physical sensations are you having? (*Pause*) So your urges feel (*reflect the client's description*), and you're having thoughts that (*reflect thoughts*), and you're feeling (*reflect emotions*). Where are your urges right now on a scale of 0–100? (*Pause*) OK. Where is your discomfort or distress on a scale of 0–100? (*Pause*) OK. Now I'm going to be quiet a few moments to let you continue imagining

(continued)

yourself in the situation. Really imagine what's going on: what you do; what you feel; what it's like to feel the urges rising. If your mind starts to wander, just bring it back to the situation. (*Pause for about 15 seconds—with a prompt reminding the client to focus on the situation sometime in the middle. Then continue.*)

So you're (*describe the situation*). What emotions are you feeling now? (*Pause*) (*Repeat the emotions the client reports.*) What sensations are you feeling? (*Pause*) You're feeling (*list emotions*), and you're having physical sensations of (*list sensations*). In fact, these emotions and sensations might be growing even more intense. You're also having urges. Where are your urges now on a scale of 0 to 100? (*Pause*) You're in this situation, and you're having urges at (*number*), and you keep thinking about [target behavior]. (*Pause a few seconds*) What are you thinking now? (*Pause*) So you're feeling (*list emotions*) and you're thinking (*list thoughts*). (*Pause*) Now I'm going to be quiet again. Continue picturing yourself in the situation and being aware of what's happening. Really imagine what you're doing, what you're feeling, and what the urges are like. (*Pause for about 15 seconds, with a reminder prompt in the middle.*)

EXTENDED BEST B

(*Calm voice*) Continue being aware of the situation and your urges. (**If the client is alone in the situation, skip to the next paragraph.**) Now, I'd like you to imagine finding a way to leave the situation for a moment. Maybe you say that you need to step out to answer a text or return a call. Maybe you say that you need to go to the bathroom. Maybe you find another reason to leave. Whatever the reason, picture yourself leaving the situation for a moment to get some privacy. (*Pause*)

(**Skip to this paragraph if the client is alone.**) Now, instead of acting on autopilot and letting the urges control you, imagine taking a moment to do the BEST B. Picture where you are, and then picture yourself deciding to do a BEST B before making any decision about what to do. (*If the client is alone, ask him or her to move to another room or another part of the room if possible.*) I'm going to guide you through a long BEST B now. Do your best to picture yourself doing the BEST B in the situation—while also being aware of what you're experiencing now as you picture yourself. Does that make sense? (*If the client says no, talk through what you are asking.*) Remember: The purpose is not to try to change your emotions or urges. They may change, they may not. The purpose is just to experience whatever you experience—and to practice riding out the urges so you can stop feeling controlled by them.

First, B for the breath. Focus on your breathing for a few breaths; allow yourself to be aware of the physical sensations in your chest and stomach as you breathe in and breathe out. (*Pause for about 4 breaths*)

Next, E—emotions and urges. Gently bring your attention to your emotions and urges. Purposely experience what you're feeling. (*Pause about 3 seconds*) Allow yourself to be open to all of your emotions—without trying to control them. (*Pause about 2 seconds*) Mentally label the emotions and urges. (*Suggest emotions the client has mentioned.*) That is (*relevant emotion*). That is (*relevant emotion*). That is (*relevant emotion*). That's an urge. (*Pause*) You don't have to label every emotion you might be experiencing. Just be aware of the first few that come to mind. (*Pause about 3 seconds*) Allow yourself to be curious about what the emotions and urges feel like—including any related sensations in your body. (*Pause about 3–5 seconds*)

(continued)

166

This is your chance to experience your emotions and urges on purpose. Emotions and urges won't make your head explode, even if they feel like they will. Urges don't predict the future. You can have emotions and urges without acting on them. You can ride them out—even though it's hard. (*Pause about 3 seconds*) This is your chance to step outside of automatic pilot and choose to experience whatever it is that you are experiencing. You might notice your emotions changing a little bit now that you're purposely aware of them—or you might not. (*Pause*) Be aware of what it's like to take your power back by purposely experiencing your emotions and urges—and riding them out. (*Pause for 5–7 seconds. Give one prompt to bring the client's mind back to emotions and urges.*)

Now S for sensations. Gently shift your attention to focus primarily on your physical sensations. (*Slight pause*) Do a quick mental scan of your body. If any area of your body feels tight or tense or heavy, imagine that your breath goes to that area when you inhale—and then surrounds and fills the area. When you exhale, some of the tightness may or may not leave with the breath. There is no right or wrong way to feel. (*Pause about 5 seconds*) If you notice your mind wandering, just give yourself credit for noticing, and bring it back to your breath. When you inhale, again imagine the breath going to any area that feels tight, tense, or heavy. And when you exhale, some of that tightness may or may not leave with the breath. Either way is fine. (*Pause about 3–5 seconds*)

Now allow yourself to be aware of T—your thoughts. Most of the time we act on thoughts as if they were facts, but your brain generates thoughts based on what you somehow learned to believe in the past. Thoughts don't necessarily equal facts. Thoughts don't predict the future. You can have a thought and let it pass without acting on it. (*Slight pause*) Gently shift your awareness to the thoughts that pass through your mind as you visualize yourself doing the BEST B. Then label each thought as "That's just a thought." You said you were having thoughts like (*list one relevant thought that the client reported*). Remind yourself: "That's just a thought." Thoughts don't predict the future. (*Slight pause*) You might be thinking (*another relevant thought*). Label it: "That's just a thought." (*Slight pause*) Maybe you're thinking, "I need to [target behavior] to get through this situation." That's just a thought. (*Pause about 3 seconds*) Notice your thoughts passing through your mind like clouds passing across the sky. Clouds come and go, but the sky remains the sky—just like thoughts come and go, but your mind remains your mind. (*Pause for about 3 seconds*) I'm going to be quiet a moment, as you just notice the thoughts that pass in and out of your mind. Just observe them . . . and notice that they're thoughts. (*Pause for about 5–7 seconds. Give one prompt to bring the client's mind back to thoughts.*)

Now that you've focused your attention on your emotions and urges, your sensations, and your thoughts, gently bring your attention back to your breath. Allow yourself to be aware of the sensations in your chest and stomach as you breathe in and breathe out. (*Pause*) Remind yourself of your commitment to work to be the kind of person you want to be. (*Slight pause*) Make a commitment to yourself to do whatever it takes to ride out the urges without acting on them—so that you keep moving toward that destination—a life that's more like the kind of life you want where you're more like the kind of person you want to be. Really picture yourself making that commitment—and be aware of what that feels like. (*Pause about 5 seconds*) Now, your urges and emotions may or may not have changed during the BEST B. Where are your urges now on a scale of 0–100? (*Pause, then continue matter of factly.*) That's fine. And where is your discomfort or distress? (*Pause*) That's fine, too. Now focus on a couple more breaths: the physical sensations as you breathe in and out. (*Pause*)

(continued)

And now, imagine that you're still in that situation, and you've finished the BEST B. Instead of acting on the urge, instead of letting the urges and the emotions control you, you decide to act in a way that fits the kind of person you want to be. Make a decision about what you will do instead of acting on the urges. Maybe you'll leave the situation. Maybe you'll do something from the Coping Toolbox. Maybe you'll get rid of any high-risk cues. (*Feel free to customize based on what you know about the client.*) Maybe you'll choose something else. But whatever you do, make sure it's something that keeps you moving toward the life that you want—toward the destination. (*Slight pause*) Do you have a plan? (*If not, provide suggestions.*) Now picture yourself taking that action. It's really hard at first to change your reactions. But do your best to fully imagine yourself making a choice about how you react—so you're not controlled by urges or emotions or other people. Really picture yourself taking that action. (*Pause for about 3 seconds*) And be aware of what it feels like as you do it. (*Pause*) Really be aware about how you feel about yourself. (*Pause*)

Have you pictured yourself taking action? (*Pause*) Good. This is hard mental work. I appreciate your doing this. (*Slight pause*) Now, start to bring your attention back into the room. One: Be aware of your breath as you inhale and exhale. (*Slight pause*) Two: Be aware of the feelings of your body against the chair and your feet against the floor. (*Slight pause*) Three: Be aware of the various sounds in and around the room. (*Slight pause*) And whenever you're ready, allow your eyes to open. And you might want to stretch a little. (*Pause and turn toward the client.*) What was that like for you?

H-C1

High-Risk Situations That May Cue Urges (Example)

Day	Situation	Physical Sensations	Emotions	Thoughts	BEST B? Y/N	How Did You Respond?	Positive Consequences	Negative Consequences
Wed.	Had argument with friend.	Tightness in stomach, racing heart.	Anger, anxiety, urges.	I can't stand her. I'll show her. I'll do [target behavior].	Yes	Left the situation and took a walk. Sang to my favorite music.	I felt happy that I didn't let urges control me.	Took a while for the anger to decrease.
Thurs.	Someone criticized me.	Emptiness in chest and stomach, heaviness.	Shame, hopelessness, urges.	I never do anything right. I can't stand this feeling.	Yes	Called a friend and talked. Then did home practice.	Felt good about myself afterward.	It was tough for a while, but no real negative consequence.
Fri.	Dinner with family.	Tightness in chest.	Bored, guilt, frustration.	I'm bored. I feel guilty that I want to leave. I need something to kill time.	Yes	Told family I needed to leave after dinner. Went to support group afterward.	Got through dinner with family without doing anything to feel guilty about.	Dinner was a little boring.
Sat.	At home alone all evening.	Tired.	Bored, lonely.	The time is crawling. I deserve to have some fun.	Yes	Did stuff from the Coping Toolbox (worked out, played with my dog) and then went to bed early.	When I woke up the next day, I was so happy I hadn't [done the target behavior].	I was bored for a while.
Tue.	Person I met said he/she didn't want to go out with me.	Tightness, lump in throat.	Shame, anger, sadness, hopeless.	Nobody will ever want me. There's something wrong with me. I need to get rid of this feeling.	No	Did an audio practice and took a hot shower.	Saved myself from feeling even worse later.	Had to feel my sadness in the short term.
Wed.	Got some good news.	Nothing big.	Happy. A little restless.	I want to celebrate. I deserve to have fun.	Yes	Texted the news to a friend. Met for coffee.	Felt grateful and proud that I acted in a way that fit my values.	Felt a little disappointed I couldn't let loose.

High-Risk Situations That May Cue Urges: Worksheet

Complete this sheet when you notice yourself starting to feel increased urges. Do your best to complete it as soon as you notice yourself experiencing the urges. However, if you can't complete it at that time, then please complete it afterward—no matter how you respond to the urges.

Day	Situation	Physical Sensations	Emotions	Thoughts	BEST B? Y/N	How Did You Respond?	Positive Consequences	Negative Consequences

Tracking Sheet, Week C

Please write the day and what you did each day in the appropriate column.

Day	Audio: Five Times	BEST B: At Least Once Daily Where? When?	Comments (Optional)
Wed.	Color Body Scan	1. While waiting for coffee, kitchen 2. On couch, evening	I felt a little nervous about doing the BEST B, but I think I'm starting to get used to it.

Home Practice Summary: High-Risk Situations

1. **Practice the audio at least five times.**

   Do your best to **practice the audio at least five times** before our next meeting. Remember that there is no right or wrong way to feel when practicing. Whatever you feel is fine. Just notice it— and do your best not to judge or try to change what you are feeling. Allow yourself to be curious about whatever you are experiencing. Just keep practicing, and we'll talk about it next week. Be sure to fill in the Tracking Sheet to record your practice.

2. **Do the BEST B at least once a day. (See *H-B2*: *BEST B*.) You're also encouraged to do a second BEST B each day while doing other activities.**

   Be sure to fill in the Tracking Sheet to record your practice.

3. **Complete *H-C2: High-Risk Situations Worksheet*** when experiencing increased urges.

4. **Complete the Tracking Sheet and the Daily Log each day.**

   Fill out the Tracking Sheet and the Daily Log each day. This helps us both keep track of what works best for you, what gets in your way, and how you are feeling throughout the week.

Note: When you fill out the Tracking Sheet and the Daily Log, please do your best to be honest. You will not be judged in any way about how much or little you have practiced, how strong or weak your urges are, or what behaviors you have or haven't engaged in during the week. The more honest you are on these forms, the more I can tailor your treatment to meet your needs. This will allow me to be more effective in helping you get closer to the kind of life you want to live. Also, please write any comments you have or anything that comes up during practice so we can talk about it at the next meeting.

MMT Session D (Fourth or Fifth Session)
Mindful Exposure, Part II:
Further Intentional Experiencing of Higher-Intensity Emotions/Urges

- Greet the client and review the previous week (15–20 minutes).
  - Assess client's experiences, home practice, and target behavior.
  - Actively reflect/validate/affirm throughout.
- Conduct mindful exposure, Part II (20–25 minutes).
  - Visualization of exposure to urges and uncomfortable emotions
  - Extended BEST B and alternative reaction:
    - Include visualization of reaction that is inconsistent with urges and consistent with the kind of person the client wants to be.
    - Provide suggestions *when needed.*
    - Briefly process the experience.
    - Assign home practice: *H-D1: High-Risk Situations Worksheet.*
- Wrap up session, check emotions/urges, and plan for upcoming week (5 minutes).
- Home practice: guided audio (five times), BEST B (at least once daily), Daily Log, *High-Risk Situations Worksheet (H-D1).*

Needed for session (all therapist sheets and handouts for this session are at the end of the Session D guidelines):

- Exposure/BEST B (TS-D1)
- High-Risk Situations Worksheet (H-D1)
- Tracking Sheet (H-D2)
- Practice Summary (H-D3)
- Daily Log (Use the version you downloaded and customized.)

SESSION D (FOURTH OR FIFTH SESSION)

The purpose of this session is to further the exposure and planning begun in Session C.

Greet the Client and Review the Previous Week
(15–20 Minutes)

Follow the protocol of the previous weeks.

- Review the Daily Log.
- Review Tracking Sheet (audio and BEST B).
- Briefly review *H-D1: High-Risk Situations Worksheet.* Affirm any (1) completion of the worksheet, (2) reports of doing the BEST B, and (3) urges that were followed by adaptive coping. Validate the difficulty of doing the BEST B (in the face of high urges) and choosing adaptive coping instead of habitual behavior.
- If needed, address difficulties with home practice (Strategy 4C, Chapter 5, pp. 67–71), create a shaping plan (Strategy 5, Chapter 5, pp. 71–78), and/or conduct a functional analysis of target behavior (Chapter 6, pp. 84–86).

    If the client did not complete *H-D1: High-Risk Situations Worksheet* and reported engaging in the target behavior the previous week, ask about the incidence of the target behavior and write the client's responses on the worksheet. Tell the client that you are not judging or criticizing, and that you understand how hard it can be to think and write about lapses. If the client did not complete the worksheet and did not engage in the target behavior, ask about a time during the week the client experienced urges, and write those responses in the relevant worksheet columns. Encourage the client to complete the sheet in the upcoming week, at least a few times, when she experiences urges.

Introduce and Discuss Session Topic: Mindful Exposure, Part II
(20–25 Minutes)

This session is largely a repeat of the previous session. Its purpose is to give the client the chance to either (1) plan and prepare for an additional high-risk situation, or (2) further plan and prepare for the original situation if you both believe further work is needed. Regardless, the exercise will provide additional exposure to urges/emotions without the client engaging in habitual reactions.

Conduct Visualization of Exposure to Urges and Uncomfortable Emotions: Extended BEST B and Alternative Reaction

Explain the reason for repeating the practice and then decide whether to repeat the previous situation or choose a new one. If the latter, ask the client to think of (1) an upcoming situation likely to cue urges and/or (2) a recent situation in which she engaged in the target behavior (especially if a similar situation is likely to occur soon). In the previous session, the client was advised not to choose a situation that felt intensely distressing. Unless your clinical judgment screams otherwise, you are encouraged not to give the client that advice this time. If the situation is one that is likely to happen, it can be helpful for the client to "practice" by experiencing it in session. This approach also shows the client that intense emotions are not dangerous experiences that need to be avoided. (You may continue to advise the client not to choose a past situation that was traumatic if you think she might choose such a situation.)

The template for eliciting information and conducting the first part of the visualization is the same as it was in the previous session: Find out what the situation is, who is involved, where the client will be, what the client thinks she may feel and think about the situation, and so on. Ask the client to sit up with feet on the floor and allow her eyes to close. Turn your chair around.

Lead the Client through TS-D1: Exposure Visualization and BEST B

After the visualization, ask what it was like for the client. Validate the difficulty in changing conditioned reactions, and also focus on processing (1) reported dissatisfaction with previous ways of reacting and (2) reported desire to change her reactions and/or confidence that she can do so. Problem solve any trouble the client may have had identifying adaptive methods of coping.

- Ask the client to rate her urges and discomfort/distress. Most of the time, they will be lower than the highest point in the exercise and near the level they were before the exercise. If so, point out how much urges can fluctuate even in a few minutes—but also stress that it would have been OK if the urges remained high, since having urges doesn't mean that a person has to act on them.

- If the client continues to report high urges and discomfort/distress, validate/reflect while staying matter-of-fact. You want to communicate that urges and negative emotions are not dangerous in and of themselves. Use a caring but calm tone to plan what the client will do to get through the rest of the day to decrease the chance he will act on the urges.

- Sometimes clients do not experience increases in urges during the exercise. Similarly, some clients say they have trouble visualizing. In these cases, normalize the experience and assure the client that the exercise still "worked."

Assign H-D1: High-Risk Situations Worksheet *for Another Week*

Briefly review the directions and answer any questions. Because you don't have a new practice to introduce, you may have more time flexibility than you had for the previous exposure session.

Check Emotions/Urges, Wrap Up Session, and Plan for Upcoming Week (5–10 Minutes)

● If you are conducting this session in the fourth week of treatment and the client has not yet been given a new audio, give her *Audio #2: Body Movement* as long as she has practiced the Color Body Scan at least once the previous week. Ask the client to do this new practice on at least 2 days, and then choose either of the practices the other 3 days.

● If the client is practicing much less than the assigned rate, use shaping and other strategies. Choose the semi-flex session for the next session and focus on motivation and commitment.

● Remind the client about the home practice: audio practice 5 days, BEST B at least once a day (with encouragement to do another when experiencing urges), and *H-D1: High-Risk Situations Worksheet* when the client experiences urges and/or engages in the target behavior. Get a commitment that the client will do her best to refrain from the target behavior and/or decrease the target behavior by an agreed-upon amount.

Exposure Visualization and BEST B: Therapist Script Template

A final script cannot be provided, since the visualization should (obviously) be specific to the client's situation. Instead, a (fairly muddled) script template appears below. Direct instructions to the therapist are in parentheses and italic. The underlined portions should be customized to fit the client. The portions that are not underlined can be said largely verbatim (if you choose). Please become familiar enough with the template that you can customize it as you lead the visualization. Start by asking clients to rate their urges to engage in the target behavior on a scale of 0–100. Also ask for levels of discomfort or distress (0–100). Then segue to the template.

Allow your eyes to close if you haven't already. I'm going to count from three to one to help you focus. Three, be aware of the various sounds in and around the room. (*Slight pause*) Two, be aware of the feelings of your feet against the floor and your body against the chair. (*Slight pause*) One, be aware of the physical sensations in your chest and stomach as you breathe in and breathe out. (*Slight pause*) Now, imagine that you're in the situation you just told me about. (*Provide a few details about the situation.*) Really visualize yourself in the situation. Do your best to really picture your surroundings. (*Pause*) (**Skip the rest of this paragraph if the client is alone in the chosen situation.**) Picture the person [people] who is [are] with you. Do your best to see that person [those people] in your mind. Imagine what they are saying to you. Really hear what they are saying—and then imagine how you respond.

Be aware of what you are doing—whether you are sitting or standing, and what is actually happening in the situation. (*Pause*) Tell me what's going on in the situation right now. (*Pause for answer. Reflect what the client said and lead the client a little further in imagining what is being said and/ or done. Give cues based on what you know. Then continue.*) What are you feeling as this happens? (*Pause for answer*) So you're feeling (*list relevant emotion*) and (*list relevant emotion*). Maybe you're also feeling (*list potentially relevant emotions*)? (*Reflect response*) Also be aware of your thoughts. You might be thinking things like (*provide potentially relevant thoughts, such as "I'll feel better after [target behavior]" or "Just this one more time"*). What are you thinking? (*Pause*) So you're having thoughts like (*list relevant thoughts*). What else are you thinking? (*Pause for answer*) OK, so you're feeling (*relevant emotion*) and (*relevant emotion*), and you're thinking (*relevant thought*) and (*relevant thought*).

What are your physical sensations? Do you feel tight or tense anywhere? Or perhaps any heaviness or burning? Or maybe pressure or emptiness? (*Pause for answer*) OK, what other sensations are you feeling? So you're feeling (*relevant emotion*), you're having thoughts that (*relevant thoughts*), and you're feeling (*relevant sensations*). (*If there is another person involved, ask what the other person does and how the client responds during all of this time.*) Now be aware of your urges. Be aware of urges to [target behavior]. Some people say that the urges feel almost like a magnet pulling them to act. What do the urges feel like for you? (*Pause*) What sort of thoughts are you having about the urges? (*Pause*) What sort of emotions and physical sensations are you having? (*Pause*) So your urges feel (*reflect the client's description*), and you're having thoughts that (*reflect thoughts*), and you're feeling (*reflect emotions*). Where are your urges right now on a scale of 0–100? (*Pause*) OK. Where is your discomfort or distress on a scale of 0–100? (*Pause*) OK. Now I'm going to be quiet a few moments to let you continue imagining

(continued)

yourself in the situation. Really imagine what's going on: what you do; what you feel; what it's like to feel the urges rising. If your mind starts to wander, just bring it back to the situation. (*Pause for about 15 seconds—with a prompt reminding the client to focus on the situation sometime in the middle. Then continue.*)

So you're (*describe the situation*). What emotions are you feeling now? (*Pause*) (*Repeat the emotions the client reports.*) What sensations are you feeling? (*Pause*) You're feeling (*list emotions*), and you're having physical sensations of (*list sensations*). In fact, these emotions and sensations might be growing even more intense. You're also having urges. Where are your urges now on a scale of 0 to 100? (*Pause*) You're in this situation, and you're having urges at (*number*), and you keep thinking about [target behavior]. (*Pause a few seconds*) What are you thinking now? (*Pause*) So you're feeling (*list emotions*) and you're thinking (*list thoughts*). (*Pause*) Now I'm going to be quiet again. Continue picturing yourself in the situation and being aware of what's happening. Really imagine what you're doing, what you're feeling, and what the urges are like. (*Pause for about 15 seconds, with a reminder prompt in the middle.*)

EXTENDED BEST B

(*Calm voice*) Continue being aware of the situation and your urges. (**If the client is alone in the situation, skip to the next paragraph.**) Now, I'd like you to imagine finding a way to leave the situation for a moment. Maybe you say that you need to step out to answer a text or return a call. Maybe you say that you need to go to the bathroom. Maybe you find another reason to leave. Whatever the reason, picture yourself leaving the situation for a moment to get some privacy. (*Pause*)

(**Skip to this paragraph if the client is alone.**) Now, instead of acting on autopilot and letting the urges control you, imagine taking a moment to do the BEST B. Picture where you are, and then picture yourself deciding to do a BEST B before making any decision about what to do. (*If the client is alone, ask him or her to move to another room or another part of the room if possible.*) I'm going to guide you through a long BEST B now. Do your best to picture yourself doing the BEST B in the situation—while also being aware of what you're experiencing now as you picture yourself. Does that make sense? (*If the client says no, talk through what you are asking.*) Remember: The purpose is not to try to change your emotions or urges. They may change, they may not. The purpose is just to experience whatever you experience—and to practice riding out the urges so you can stop feeling controlled by them.

First, B for the breath. Focus on your breathing for a few breaths; allow yourself to be aware of the physical sensations in your chest and stomach as you breathe in and breathe out. (*Pause for about 4 breaths*)

Next, E—emotions and urges. Gently bring your attention to your emotions and urges. Purposely experience what you're feeling. (*Pause about 3 seconds*) Allow yourself to be open to all of your emotions—without trying to control them. (*Pause about 2 seconds*) Mentally label the emotions and urges. (*Suggest emotions the client has mentioned.*) That is (*relevant emotion*). That is (*relevant emotion*). That is (*relevant emotion*). That's an urge. (*Pause*) You don't have to label every emotion you might be experiencing. Just be aware of the first few that come to mind. (*Pause about 3 seconds*) Allow yourself to be curious about what the emotions and urges feel like—including any related sensations in your body. (*Pause about 3–5 seconds*)

(continued)

178

This is your chance to experience your emotions and urges on purpose. Emotions and urges won't make your head explode, even if they feel like they will. Urges don't predict the future. You can have emotions and urges without acting on them. You can ride them out—even though it's hard. (*Pause about 3 seconds*) This is your chance to step outside of automatic pilot and choose to experience whatever it is that you are experiencing. You might notice your emotions changing a little bit now that you're purposely aware of them—or you might not. (*Pause*) Be aware of what it's like to take your power back by purposely experiencing your emotions and urges—and riding them out. (*Pause for 5–7 seconds. Give one prompt to bring the client's mind back to emotions and urges.*)

Now S for sensations. Gently shift your attention to focus primarily on your physical sensations. (*Slight pause*) Do a quick mental scan of your body. If any area of your body feels tight or tense or heavy, imagine that your breath goes to that area when you inhale—and then surrounds and fills the area. When you exhale, some of the tightness may or may not leave with the breath. There is no right or wrong way to feel. (*Pause about 5 seconds*) If you notice your mind wandering, just give yourself credit for noticing, and bring it back to your breath. When you inhale, again imagine the breath going to any area that feels tight, tense, or heavy. And when you exhale, some of that tightness may or may not leave with the breath. Either way is fine. (*Pause about 3–5 seconds*)

Now allow yourself to be aware of T—your thoughts. Most of the time we act on thoughts as if they were facts, but your brain generates thoughts based on what you somehow learned to believe in the past. Thoughts don't necessarily equal facts. Thoughts don't predict the future. You can have a thought and let it pass without acting on it. (*Slight pause*) Gently shift your awareness to the thoughts that pass through your mind as you visualize yourself doing the BEST B. Then label each thought as "That's just a thought." You said you were having thoughts like (*list one relevant thought that the client reported*). Remind yourself: "That's just a thought." Thoughts don't predict the future. (*Slight pause*) You might be thinking (*another relevant thought*). Label it: "That's just a thought." (*Slight pause*) Maybe you're thinking, "I need to [target behavior] to get through this situation." That's just a thought. (*Pause about 3 seconds*) Notice your thoughts passing through your mind like clouds passing across the sky. Clouds come and go, but the sky remains the sky—just like thoughts come and go, but your mind remains your mind. (*Pause for about 3 seconds*) I'm going to be quiet a moment, as you just notice the thoughts that pass in and out of your mind. Just observe them . . . and notice that they're thoughts. (*Pause for about 5–7 seconds. Give one prompt to bring the client's mind back to thoughts.*)

Now that you've focused your attention on your emotions and urges, your sensations, and your thoughts, gently bring your attention back to your breath. Allow yourself to be aware of the sensations in your chest and stomach as you breathe in and breathe out. (*Pause*) Remind yourself of your commitment to work to be the kind of person you want to be. (*Slight pause*) Make a commitment to yourself to do whatever it takes to ride out the urges without acting on them—so that you keep moving toward that destination—a life that's more like the kind of life you want where you're more like the kind of person you want to be. Really picture yourself making that commitment—and be aware of what that feels like. (*Pause about 5 seconds*) Now, your urges and emotions may or may not have changed during the BEST B. Where are your urges now on a scale of 0–100? (*Pause, then continue matter of factly.*) That's fine. And where is your discomfort or distress? (*Pause*) That's fine, too. Now focus on a couple more breaths: the physical sensations as you breathe in and out. (*Pause*)

(continued)

179

And now, imagine that you're still in that situation, and you've finished the BEST B. Instead of acting on the urge, instead of letting the urges and the emotions control you, you decide to act in a way that fits the kind of person you want to be. Make a decision about what you will do instead of acting on the urges. Maybe you'll leave the situation. Maybe you'll do something from the Coping Toolbox. Maybe you'll get rid of any high-risk cues. (*Feel free to customize based on what you know about the client.*) Maybe you'll choose something else. But whatever you do, make sure it's something that keeps you moving toward the life that you want—toward the destination. (*Slight pause*) Do you have a plan? (*If not, provide suggestions.*) Now picture yourself taking that action. It's really hard at first to change your reactions. But do your best to fully imagine yourself making a choice about how you react—so you're not controlled by urges or emotions or other people. Really picture yourself taking that action. (*Pause for about 3 seconds*) And be aware of what it feels like as you do it. (*Pause*) Really be aware about how you feel about yourself. (*Pause*)

Have you pictured yourself taking action? (*Pause*) Good. This is hard mental work. I appreciate your doing this. (*Slight pause*) Now, start to bring your attention back into the room. One: Be aware of your breath as you inhale and exhale. (*Slight pause*) Two: Be aware of the feelings of your body against the chair and your feet against the floor. (*Slight pause*) Three: Be aware of the various sounds in and around the room. (*Slight pause*) And whenever you're ready, allow your eyes to open. And you might want to stretch a little. (*Pause and turn toward the client.*) What was that like for you?

High-Risk Situations That May Cue Urges: Worksheet

Complete this sheet when you notice yourself starting to feel increased urges. Do your best to complete it as soon as you notice yourself experiencing the urges. However, if you can't complete it at that time, then please complete it afterward—no matter how you respond to the urges.

Day	Situation	Physical Sensations	Emotions	Thoughts	BEST B? Y/N	How Did You Respond?	Positive Consequences	Negative Consequences

Tracking Sheet, Week D

Please write the day and what you did each day in the appropriate column.

Day	Audio: Five Times	BEST B: Once Daily Where? When?	Comments (Optional)
Wed.	Color Body Scan	1. While waiting for coffee, kitchen 2. On couch, evening	I'm starting to get used to doing a BEST B when I notice urges.

Home Practice Summary: High-Risk Situations

1. **Practice the audio at least five times.**

   Do your best to **practice the audio at least five times** before our next meeting. Remember that there is no right or wrong way to feel when practicing. Whatever you feel is fine. Just notice it— and do your best not to judge or try to change what you are feeling. Allow yourself to be curious about whatever you are experiencing. Just keep practicing, and we'll talk about it next week. Be sure to fill in the Tracking Sheet to record your practice.

2. **Do the BEST B at least once a day. (See *H-B2*: *BEST B*.) You're also encouraged to do a second BEST B each day while doing other activities.**

   Be sure to fill in the Tracking Sheet to record your practice.

3. **Complete *H-D1: High-Risk Situations Worksheet*** when experiencing increased urges.

4. **Complete the Tracking Sheet and the Daily Log each day.**

   Fill out the Tracking Sheet and the Daily Log each day. This helps us both keep track of what works best for you, what gets in your way, and how you are feeling throughout the week.

Note: When you fill out the Tracking Sheet and the Daily Log, please do your best to be honest. You will not be judged in any way about how much or little you have practiced, how strong or weak your urges are, or what behaviors you have or haven't engaged in during the week. The more honest you are on these forms, the more I can tailor your treatment to meet your needs. This will allow me to be more effective in helping you get closer to the kind of life you want to live. Also, please write any comments you have or anything that comes up during practice so we can talk about it at the next meeting.

MMT Semi-Flex Session (Usually Fourth or Fifth Session)
Likely Will Occur as One of the First Five Sessions

The clinician chooses the topic of focus for the middle portion of this session and also determines which week (usually within the first five sessions) the semi-flex session would be the most useful.

- Review the week (the client's experiences, home practice, target behavior; 15–20 minutes).
- Focus on the topic you believe needs additional work (10–15 minutes), which may include:
    - Issues with motivation, commitment, and/or rapport;
    - Problems with home practice, attendance, and/or decreasing the target behavior;
    - Further (repeated) explanation on how the mindfulness practice "works";
    - Specific topics relevant to the client's particular target behavior; and/or
    - Other topics that you and the client agree would be helpful to address.
    - Be sure to leave 20 minutes for the Mirror Exercise and the session wrap up.
- Conduct the Mirror Exercise (15 minutes).
    - Guided visualization to enhance motivation and commitment
- Remind the client about home practice and wrap up session (5 minutes).
- Home practice: guided audio (five times), BEST B (at least once daily), Daily Log, *High-Risk Situations Worksheet (H-SF1)*

Needed for session (all therapist sheets and handouts for this session are at the end of the Semi-Flex Session guidelines):

- Mirror Exercise (TS-SF1)
- High-Risk Situations Worksheet (H-SF1)
- Tracking Sheet (H-SF2)
- Practice Summary (H-SF3)
- Daily Log (Use customized version.)

SEMI-FLEX SESSION
(USUALLY FOURTH OR FIFTH SESSION, BUT MAY BE THE THIRD SESSION IF NECESSARY)

Flex sessions allow the therapist to choose the session topic(s) based on client needs. Although the therapist chooses the primary topic(s) of the session, all flex sessions maintain the template of beginning by reviewing the previous week and ending by reminding the client about home practice (and providing the client with the Tracking Sheet and Daily Log).

The first five weeks of MMT include four fixed-topic sessions and one semi-flex session. (The session is only a *semi*-flex, as therapists are instructed to focus on a guided visualization in a portion of the session. Thus, only 10–15 minutes of the session are flexible.)

The 16-week version of MMT also includes one additional flex session, and the 20-week version includes three additional flex sessions (explained further in Chapter 12). You may use the flex sessions at any time during treatment. If the treatment is not time-limited, you may use as many flex sessions as deemed necessary; however, it is recommended that you not use multiple flex sessions in a row, as you would risk the client's becoming bored by home practice that never changes and losing motivation after not being exposed to new material.

The semi-flex session usually occurs during the fourth or fifth week of treatment, although you may conduct it earlier if needed to address issues of motivation and engagement.

Greet the Client and Review the Previous Week (15–20 Minutes)

Follow the protocol of the previous weeks.

- Review the Daily Log.
- Review the Tracking Sheet (audio and BEST B).
- Briefly review *H-D1: High-Risk Situations Worksheet.*
- If necessary, address any difficulties with home practice (Strategy 4C, Chapter 5, pp. 67–71), create a shaping plan to increase practice or days of abstinence from the target behavior (Strategy 5, Chapter 5, pp. 71–78), and/or conduct a functional analysis of instances of target behavior (Chapter 6, pp. 84–86).

If the client did not complete *H-D1: High-Risk Situations Worksheet* and reported engaging in the target behavior the previous week, ask about the incidents of target behavior and write the client's responses in the relevant worksheet columns.

Focus on the Topic You Believe Needs Additional Work (10–15 Minutes)

- Topics that are often relevant to clients in treatment for target behavior include (1) addressing issues with motivation, commitment, and/or the therapy relationship; (2) additional work on shaping to increase the home practice or decrease the target behavior; (3) further (and repeated) explanation on how the mindfulness practice works; (4) a focus on issues relevant to the client's specific target behavior; and/or (5) other areas you believe would be helpful to address.

- For ideas, instructions, and examples of methods of focusing on these topics, see
  - "Strong Focus on the Therapeutic Relationship," (Chapter 3, Strategy 1), or
  - "Strong Focus on Client Values" (Chapter 4, Strategy 2, pp. 42–50), or
  - "Strong Focus on Helping the Client Understand Self, Behavior, and Treatment" (Chapter 4, Strategy 3, pp. 50–59), or
  - Relevant "Questions, Obstacles, and General Issues" in Chapter 6.
- Examples of topics that are customized for specific target behaviors include (1) nutrition, overall food consumption, body image, or exercise for clients with eating-related behavior; (2) safety issues such as needle sharing, unsafe sex, or other behaviors that may be relevant to the client's target behavior; and/or (3) decreasing access to items that are part of the target behavior (e.g., not keeping drugs, alcohol, porn, binge-cueing food, computer games, or other related objects around the home).
- Keep track of time. The Mirror Exercise will take the full 15 minutes, plus you will need time to wrap up.

Introduce the Mirror Exercise (15 Minutes)

This exercise is a guided visualization to help clients realize the consequences of repeatedly telling themselves that they will stop the target behavior and start doing the home practice/ attending treatment "tomorrow." The previous sentence purposely does not use the word *procrastinate*, because many clients do not perceive themselves as procrastinating when they decide to do the home practice or stop the behavior "tomorrow." Instead, they often believe they will somehow be more motivated or have less difficulty in the future. (One client once expressed a fairly universal sentiment when he said he always thought his "future self" would be more together than his "current self.") Clients may also repeatedly convince themselves they just need to have "one last day" or "one last weekend" of fun before giving up the behavior.

You are encouraged to record yourself conducting the exercise so that the client can have a copy to play at home when needed. A generic version (*Audio #3: Mirror*) may also be downloaded from the publisher's website (see the box at the end of the table of contents), but a customized version is more effective. It is OK if you stumble on words, lose your place, or stutter. The purpose is not to create a flawless, professional-sounding recording. The purpose is to allow the client to practice an exercise that can potentially increase motivation and improve outcome. Although you will usually conduct the Mirror Exercise within the first 5 weeks of treatment, the audio is not shared with the client until Week 5 or 6 to give the client more opportunities to practice the more standard mindfulness practices (the Color Body Scan, Audio #1, and Body Movement, Audio #2).

Although *TS-SF1: Mirror Exercise* is introduced during the semi-flex session, it can be conducted again, when needed, to increase motivated action. The first time that you conduct the Mirror Exercise, explain that this visualization is conducted for every client as a reminder of the importance of doing the work of the program. This setup decreases the chance that the client will feel defensive or criticized when you lead him through a visualization of not succeeding in treatment. You do not want the client to think you are suggesting that he will not succeed. You can discuss possible consequences of continued noncompliance after the exercise, as long as you stress that the client still has time to start practicing and/or working toward stopping the target behavior. Stress that you still fully believe that the client can be successful in moving past the target behavior and toward the destination.

Note: The template for *TS-SF1: Mirror Exercise* requires substantial customization. You are encouraged to download the template from the publisher's website (see the box at the end of the table of contents) and modify it before reading it for the client. The template should be customized to fit the client's (1) specific target behavior, (2) history of attendance and home practice completion, (3) level of target behavior at the time of reading the script, and (4) core life values. For example, if the client usually completes most of the home practice but still engages in the target behavior, you would focus the first portion of the exercise on the target behavior but not the home practice. If the client is not doing the practice, you will focus the first portion on never getting around to doing the home practice—which means that the client never learns the skills necessary to stop the behavior or remain abstinent over the long term.

Here's an example regarding values: If a client cares a lot about her relationship with her child, you can have the client imagine what kind of mother she would be and what the child might think of her as he gets older and sees how much the target behavior controls her life. If the client is pressured into treatment by her job, you can include a focus on imagining what her career would be like if she continues to engage in the behavior—and what kind of job she might have in 5 years as a result. If the client is mandated to treatment by the courts, she might be incarcerated 6 months from now—and then have the trauma of the incarceration *and* the record of the incarceration 5 years from now. Since she will still be at risk of engaging in the target behavior once her incarceration ends, she also will have the fear of getting arrested again.

The script can also be customized to fit the therapeutic setting (e.g., private practice, mandated program). The portions of the script most likely to be customized are <u>underlined</u>.

Tell the client you are going to lead her in a visualization. Ask her to sit with both feet on the floor and hands in her lap or on the chair/couch. Turn your chair around. Lead the client in *TS-SF1: Mirror Exercise*.

After guiding the client through the visualization, ask which response the client chose and what the exercise was like for her. Stress that you would not have judged the client if she had chosen the first path, although you hoped she would choose the second. Reflect and validate the difficulty of choosing the second path. Affirm the client for her choice.

Wrap Up and Plan for Upcoming Week (5 Minutes)

Remind the client about the home practice: guided audio five times, daily BEST B (with encouragement to do a second BEST B with eyes open during routine activity), Daily Log, and *H-SF1: High-Risk Situations Worksheet*.

Mirror Exercise: Therapist Script Template

A final script cannot be provided, since the visualization is (obviously) specific to the client's situation. Instead, a (muddled) script template appears below. Direct instructions to the therapist are in parentheses and italic. The underlined portions should be customized to fit the client. The portions that are not underlined or in parentheses can be said largely verbatim (if you choose). Please become familiar enough with the template that you can customize it as you lead the visualization. Alternatively, you can download it from the publisher's website (see the box at the end of the table of contents) and modify it before reading it to the client (which is recommended, at least the first one or two times you conduct the exercise for a client).

For clients with eating or body issues, you can stress that the mirror is a small mirror that only shows the face. If the client expresses difficulty with even imagining looking into a small mirror, you can say that the client is standing in front of her/his sink getting ready in the morning—and just leave out the mirror reference. Stay consistent throughout the script.

Allow your eyes to close if you haven't already. I'm going to count from three to one to help you focus. Three: Be aware of the various sounds. (*Slight pause*) Two: Be aware of the feelings of your body against whatever it is touching. (*Slight pause*) One: Focus on your breathing as you breathe in and breathe out. (*Slight pause*) During this exercise, your mind will wander, and that's fine. When you get distracted, just notice it and then bring your attention back to the visualization.

Imagine that you're standing in front of your bathroom mirror or whatever mirror you stand in front of to get ready in the morning. You're getting ready for your day, and it's 6 months from now. (*Note: Tailor the timeframe to fit the length of the program, if applicable.*)

<u>You're no longer in this treatment program [or] You're still in treatment, but you're no longer working on decreasing [target behavior].</u> As you stand in front of the mirror 6 months from now, you think back on the current time.

(***For clients who always complete home practice, skip to paragraph #5. For the following paragraphs, modify the level of home practice completion based on the client.***) During your first few weeks of treatment, <u>you may have done the home practice a little</u> . . . but then you would start to feel unmotivated . . . or something else would get in the way. So you'd miss home practices. <u>And maybe you'd even miss a session here and there.</u> You did try to start doing the home practice regularly . . . but a lot of days you'd feel like you were just too busy . . . or maybe you were just not feeling motivated. And you'd think, "I'm having a rough day. I'll start doing the home practice tomorrow." Or you'd think, "I've already missed a few days of practice this week, so I'll wait until next week so I can get a fresh start." So you'd put it off a few more days. And then a few days later, you'd think, "Just this one more day without the practice won't hurt. I'll have more time tomorrow." (*Pause*) And that just kept happening. Day after day. (*Pause*) You always thought in the back of your mind you'd get yourself to start doing the practice at some point. But little by little, weeks started going by without your ever doing the practice regularly or really getting involved in the treatment. And <u>even though you may have been able to decrease the</u>

(continued)

[target behavior] a little at first, you never fully learned ways to cope that were necessary to deal with your urges and move closer to the life you want.

(*PARAGRAPH #5: For clients not engaging in their target behavior, skip to paragraph #6.*) You did really work to stop [target behavior] . . . and you may have had times when you went a while without [target behavior] now and then. But sooner or later, you'd have at least 1 day when you felt bored, or bad about yourself, or out of sorts. And you'd have high urges. And you'd think, "I'm having a rough day. Just this once won't hurt. I'll stop [target behavior] tomorrow." Or maybe you'd think, "I'll do the [target behavior] for the rest of this week to get it out of my system—and start working on it next week when I feel more motivated." And then the next week, you'd think, "Just this once more time won't hurt. I'll stop [target behavior] tomorrow or next week." (*Pause*) And that just kept happening. Week after week. (*Pause*)

(*PARAGRAPH #6: Pick whichever is a possibility.*) And eventually you got discouraged about not making enough progress, and you just quit therapy [or] you got discouraged about not making enough progress, and you and your therapist decided to quit working on [target behavior] [or] you finished the treatment program without ever really doing the practice and getting the benefits of the treatment.

So you're standing in front of a mirror 6 months from now. Six months have gone by, and [target behavior] has returned [if applicable] and is not much better than it was when you started treatment. (*For clients pressured into treatment, focus on consequences of continuing the behavior. The client may have been fired from a job, dumped by a partner, had probation extended, sent to jail, dropped out of school, etc.*)

Just be aware, when you look in the mirror, of how you feel about yourself—knowing that you're still controlled by your urges and the target behavior. (*Modify next sentence to fit things important to the client. Pause briefly between every item.*) Be aware of how you feel about your life . . . about your future. (*Pause*) What is your health like? What about your relationships? (*Perhaps mention relationships with children and/or other specific important people.*) How is your career/school? (*Pause*) Really be aware of how you feel about what's going on with your life. As you stand in front of the mirror, think back to 6 months before, when you were still telling yourself that you'd start regularly doing the home practice or that you'd stop the [target behavior] the next day or next week. (*Slight pause*) Really be aware of how you feel about yourself as you realize that 6 months have gone by. (*Longer pause*)

And now I'd like you to imagine that you're standing in front of the mirror a year from now. A whole year has gone by. You're no longer in this treatment, but every once in a while, you've tried to stop or decrease [target behavior]. But it's so much effort, especially when you're feeling stressed and you're no longer in treatment to help you. So you've never been able to stick with it. A lot of things are similar to the way they were before starting the program: the [target behavior], feeling hopeless about being able to change, the feeling of being controlled by urges and emotions. As you get ready to start your day, be aware of realizing that a whole year has gone by, and you're just as controlled by [target behavior] as you were before you started treatment. (*Pause*) We don't know what all will be happening in your life, but be aware of some of the potential consequences of continuing to engage in [target behavior] for another whole year. (*Customize. Slight pause after every question.*) How do you feel about your life? (*Slight pause*) What are your relationships like? (*Slight pause*) How does [target behavior] affect your

(continued)

relationships? (*Slight pause; mention specific relationships if applicable.*) <u>What is your health like?</u> (*Slight pause*) <u>What about your career/school?</u> (*Slight pause*) As you stand in front of the mirror getting ready for your day, how do you feel—knowing that you're going to have to get through yet another day of the same ol', same ol'? How do you feel about the future? (*Slight pause*) How do you feel about yourself? (*Longer pause*)

And now imagine that 5 years have gone by. You're 5 years older; 5 more years of your life have passed. (*If the client has children or close family members, remind her/him that these family members are 5 years older as well.*) You're standing in front of a mirror in the morning after 5 more years of [target behavior]. There have been various times you've tried to stop [target behavior], but then it's always been, "Well, something stressful is going on, so I'm really going to stop [target behavior] tomorrow . . . or in a week or two." Then later you've tried to stop again for a while, but there were always high urges, and you'd think, "I'll get started working on this in another couple of weeks." And somehow 5 whole years have gone by. (*Slight pause*) You're still doing [target behavior] as much as before you started this treatment—probably even more by this time. (*Slight pause*) As you get ready for your day, be aware of what your life is like. (*Pause now and after each topic.*) Be aware of what your relationships are like. (*Slight pause*) (*If the person has a child, focus her/his relationship with the child.*) <u>Your child/children is/ are 5 years older. How do you feel about each other?</u> (*Slight pause*) <u>What kind of child/children is/are she/he/they?</u> (*Slight pause*) <u>How is the child's emotional functioning?</u> (*Slight pause*) <u>What does your child think of you now that they understand how controlled you are by the [target behavior]?</u> (*Slight pause*) <u>What is your health like?</u> (*Slight pause*) <u>How are your finances?</u> <u>What is your career like?</u> [or] <u>Were you able to finish school, or did [target behavior] get in the way of that?</u>

Five more years have gone by, and you're realizing that this is probably what you can expect for the rest of your life. This is pretty much how the rest of your life will be—feeling controlled by your urges to [target behavior]. (*Pause*) How do you feel about yourself and your life? (*Pause*) How do you feel about starting your day knowing that the rest of your life is probably going to be like this? (*Pause*) Really be aware of what it feels like. (*Longer pause*)

And now, keeping your eyes closed, I'd like you to let that image go and shake out your body just a little bit. (*Pause*)

Now imagine again that you're standing in front of the same mirror, and it's 6 months from now. But this time, imagine that you were able to get involved with the treatment. You weren't perfect—but on average, you did get on track with the home practice. And even though you thought your head would explode at times, you were able to stop/greatly reduce [target behavior]. You had days that felt bleh, you had days that felt stressful, and you had times of high urges. But you kept doing the home practice even when you were busy and didn't feel like doing it, and you did whatever you had to do to get through more and more days without [target behavior]. And now you haven't [target behavior] in a few months. You still have urges, but the urges don't totally control you. You're not fully where you want to be, but you notice a difference.

We don't know all the specifics of what your life will be like in 6 months, but be aware of how you might feel knowing that you no longer feel controlled by [target behavior]. Be aware of how your relationships might be. (*Slight pause*) <u>How your work/school/free time feels these days.</u> (*Slight pause*) How do you feel about yourself? (*Slight pause*) Your life? (*Slight pause*) Your future? (*Pause*)

(continued)

And now imagine that it's a year from today. You're standing in front of a mirror about to start your day. And you're still free of being controlled by [target behavior] (*say the following underlined portion only if you know it is what the clients wants*) and perhaps you're doing the [target behavior] in moderation. You still have urges sometimes, but you don't feel controlled by urges or negative emotions. You still practice some of the exercises, and you still have to be careful around some cues, but you don't lose control like you used to. You've taken back your power; your urges no longer have power over you. Be aware of how your relationships may have changed. (*Slight pause*) And what other people think of you now that you've shown you can get past [target behavior]. (*Slight pause*) Be aware of your feelings about yourself. (*Slight pause*) Your life. (*Slight pause*) Your future. (*Pause*)

And now imagine that it's 5 years from today. You still may have urges every now and then, and you still do the practice, but you have no problem with [target behavior]. You feel like your life is your life, as opposed to someone else having the remote control. Yes, you have difficult days, but you're able to get through them without doing things that leave you suffering from negative consequences. As you stand in front of the mirror, be aware of how different your relationships are now. With your loved ones . . . and perhaps new relationships. How do you feel about yourself? How do you feel about yourself as a mother/father/partner/friend/daughter/son? How do you feel about your life? (*Pause*) How do you feel about your future? (*Pause*) Be aware of knowing what it feels like to have taken back your power, and to know you're really free from being controlled by the target behavior. (*Pause*)

Now, I'd like you to really think about those two different paths you can take. Ask yourself which one you would rather live. That sounds like a rhetorical question, but it's not. The second path will take much more work and be a lot harder than the first one in the short term. Some people don't think it's worth the effort. So I'd like you to decide: Is it worth it? Knowing how hard it is to do the home practice and how difficult it will be for a while to go without the [target behavior]—is it worth it? Make a choice right now; choose which version is the life you want to live. (*Pause*) Because not making a choice—not making a commitment—is really choosing the first version—where life goes by, little by little, without any change. (*Pause*) So I'd like you to make a commitment to yourself about which life you choose. And commit to doing whatever it takes to have that life. (*Pause for about 3 seconds*) Be aware of what it feels like to make that commitment to yourself. (*Pause for about 3 seconds*) And know that either decision is hard. The first in the long term because of the things you'll have to deal with as consequences. The second in the short term because of giving up [target behavior] and doing practices that can feel burdensome. But make that commitment, regardless of the difficulty. (*Slight pause*) Know that what you're doing is very tough. It takes a lot of effort to be here and to go through these exercises, and I commend you on what you're doing. (*Pause*)

Now, start to bring your attention back to this room as I count from three to one. (*Slight pause*) Three: Be aware of your breathing. Two: Be aware of the feelings of your body against whatever it is touching. One: Be aware of the various sounds. Whenever you're ready, you can open your eyes and stretch a little bit. (*Pause. Turn chair around and face the client.*) What was that like for you? (*Pause*) Which one did you choose?

High-Risk Situations That May Cue Urges: Worksheet

Complete this sheet when you notice yourself starting to feel increased urges. Do your best to complete it as soon as you notice yourself experiencing the urges. However, if you can't complete it at that time, then please complete it afterward—no matter how you respond to the urges.

Day	Situation	Physical Sensations	Emotions	Thoughts	BEST B? Y/N	How Did You Respond?	Positive Consequences	Negative Consequences

Tracking Sheet, Semi-Flex Session

Please write the day and what you did each day in the appropriate column.

Day	Audio: Five Times	BEST B: Once Daily Where? When?	Comments (Optional)
Wed.	Color Body Scan	1. In bed, morning 2. In park, after lunch	I sometimes get antsy during the audio, but I keep doing it anyway.

Home Practice Summary: High-Risk Situations

1. **Practice the audio at least five times.**

   Do your best to **practice the audio at least five times** before our next meeting. Remember that there is no right or wrong way to feel when practicing. Whatever you feel is fine. Just notice it— and do your best not to judge or try to change what you are feeling. Allow yourself to be curious about whatever you are experiencing. Just keep practicing, and we'll talk about it next week. Be sure to fill in the Tracking Sheet to record your practice.

2. **Do the BEST B at least once a day. (See *H-B2*: *BEST B.*) You're also encouraged to do a second BEST B each day while doing other activities.**

   Be sure to fill in the Tracking Sheet to record your practice.

3. **Complete *H-SF1: High-Risk Situations Worksheet* when experiencing increased urges.**

4. **Complete the Tracking Sheet and the Daily Log each day.**

   Fill out the Tracking Sheet and the Daily Log each day. This helps us both keep track of what works best for you, what gets in your way, and how you are feeling throughout the week.

Note: When you fill out the Tracking Sheet and the Daily Log, please do your best to be honest. You will not be judged in any way about how much or little you have practiced, how strong or weak your urges are, or what behaviors you have or haven't engaged in during the week. The more honest you are on these forms, the more I can tailor your treatment to meet your needs. This will allow me to be more effective in helping you get closer to the kind of life you want to live. Also, please write any comments you have or anything that comes up during practice so we can talk about it at the next meeting.

CHAPTER 9

Mindful Emotion Regulation Module

MMT Session E
Identifying, Scheduling, and Participating in Activities That Are Pleasant and/or Fulfilling

- Review the week (the client's experiences, home practice, target behavior; 15–20 minutes).
- Engage in mindfulness practice: Focus on Object (5–6 minutes).
- Discuss the importance of mindfully participating in activities that are pleasant and/or fulfilling (15–20 minutes).
  - Complete *H-E1: Pleasant and/or Fulfilling Activities.*
    - ◆ Work with client to identify possible pleasant and/or fulfilling activities.
    - ◆ Client chooses from activities on worksheet and may also generate additional activities.
  - Discuss/normalize potential avoidance urges and negative emotions that may occur prior to (or even during) pleasant/fulfilling activities.
  - Assign new home practice: the *Pleasant/Fulfilling Activity* column on the Tracking Sheet.
- Wrap up and plan for the upcoming week (5 minutes).
- Home practice: guided audio (five times), BEST B (at least once daily), *Pleasant/Fulfilling Activities (H-E1*; once daily), Daily Log.

Needed for session (all therapist sheets and handouts for this session are at the end of the Session E guidelines):

- Mindfulness: Focus on Object (TS-E1)
- Pleasant/Fulfilling Activities (H-E1)
- Tracking Sheet (H-E2)
- Practice Summary (H-E3)
- Daily Log

SESSION E

....

This session focuses on identifying and planning pleasant and/or fulfilling activities. Clients will record these activities throughout the rest of treatment.

Greet the Client and Review the Previous Week (15–20 Minutes)

See the instructions for home practice review at the end of the relevant session.

Engage in Mindfulness Practice: *TS-E1: Focus on Object* (5–6 Minutes)

Tell the client you are going to transition to the new topic by leading him in a mindfulness practice. Ask him to sit with his hands on his lap, and turn your chair or body around so you are not looking at him. Hand him the object and set a timer (or watch a clock) to conduct the practice for 4 minutes. Afterward, ask the client what his experience was like. Do your best not to spend more than a minute or two on processing, or you will not have time to adequately cover the rest of the session material. Encourage the client to practice this exercise on his own.

Introduce the New Topic: Discuss the Importance of Mindfully Participating in Activities That Are Pleasant and/or Fulfilling (15–20 Minutes)

- Explain that since the client is giving up target behavior(s) that brought pleasure as well as relief, it is important that he find other ways to bring pleasure and/or fulfillment into his life. Because the client has likely grown accustomed to finding pleasure from the target behavior, making time to engage in other potentially pleasurable activities may not feel natural to him.

- You will also need to explain that positive and negative emotions are not segregated. Avoiding or suppressing negative emotions will eventually decrease the ability to experience positive emotions as well. Because of the client's likely history of working to "turn off" negative emotions and/or urges (e.g., the boiling pot metaphor), he may currently have trouble feeling positive emotions as strongly and/or as easily as he once did.

- Thus, clients can benefit from mindfully engaging in activities that have the potential to be enjoyable and/or fulfilling. Such activities can retrain the client's brain to once again experience pleasure and fulfillment from activities other than the target behavior.

- If the client says he would rather focus on stopping the target behavior than spending time on pleasure or fulfillment, explain that adding pleasurable/fulfilling activities is helpful in stopping the behavior and preventing relapse. Individuals tend to have greater difficulty stopping dysregulated behavior and higher chances of relapse if their lives have few pleasurable and fulfilling activities.

Complete H-E1: Pleasant/Fulfilling Activities, *Page 1*

Read the instructions on the first page aloud to the client:

Write down some activities, people, places, and situations that you enjoy; that help you feel confident; and/or that help you feel like you're living according to what you value—but that don't involve behaviors you would regret later. These can be things from the past, things from the present, or things you'd like to add to your life in the future.

Ask the client to write down the first few answers that come to mind—and to then take the sheet home to continue adding items as he thinks of them. Briefly review the client's answers, but do not spend much time on this portion. The purpose is mainly to "jump-start" the client into thinking about activities, people, etc., that may add pleasure and fulfillment to life.

The Client Will Choose from Activities on the List and May Also Generate Additional Activities

- Hand the client the second page and tell him that the list includes activities that many people find pleasurable and/or fulfilling. Ask the client to:
  - Read the list and put a checkmark by anything he has done in the last few months (regardless of whether he felt any pleasure at the time).
  - Read the list a second time and put a checkmark by anything he might be willing to do at some point in the future.
    - Tell the client that this is not a commitment.
    - If you are pressed for time, you can just have the client read through the list once and mark any anything he has recently done and/or would be willing to do.
  - Encourage the client to choose some items specifically relevant to his target behavior, if applicable (e.g., some form of exercise or meal plan for eating issues) or to use the blank lines to add such items. He can also use the blank lines to add anything else he might enjoy.
  - If a client is lacking in social support, suggest considering at least one or two activities that involve building on strengthening social connections.
- Briefly review the list with the client, commenting, affirming, and asking about chosen items.

Assign the Home Practice: Do One Pleasant or Fulfilling Activity per Day and Record It in the Pleasant/Fulfilling Activity Column on the Tracking Sheet

- Explain that the activities can be pursuits that the client (1) currently enjoys, (2) has enjoyed in the past, (3) might potentially enjoy, and/or (4) might not enjoy in the moment, but might feel good about himself afterward and/or feel like he's living a life more consistent with his values. Examples of a fulfilling activity might be doing a favor for a friend, working out, building a skill, volunteering, taking a class, etc.
- The daily activity can be from the worksheet, or it can be anything else the client finds pleasant or fulfilling.
- Stress that the activity can take a substantial amount of time (e.g., going to an amusement park, attending a workshop), but it can also take 5 minutes (e.g., drinking a favorite flavor of

coffee, walking a block out of the way to go through a park, reading for pleasure, listening to a favorite song).

- Encourage the client to add at least a few activities not normally in his standard routine, but tell him that he can also count more routine activities, as long as those activities are potentially pleasurable or fulfilling. The difference is that he is instructed to *be mindful of what he is feeling* during at least some portion of the activity—instead of just engaging in the activity automatically without much awareness.

- **Ask the client to plan one activity that he commits to doing this week but that he might not do during an average week.** Write it on the Tracking Sheet. The activity does not have to be particularly significant or time-consuming; it just needs to be something that (1) he does not do regularly, and that (2) he knows he will be able to do this week. Write that activity on top of the *Pleasant Activity* column on the Tracking Sheet. That activity will count as one of his daily activities for the week.

  - Help the client pick an activity that he *knows* he will do. The key factor is that he actually engages in the activity—as opposed to committing to something that might sound interesting but not following through.

  - Ask when and how he will engage in the activity; make sure he has the time and resources. Consider asking the client to set an alarm on his phone as a reminder.

- **Important: Warn the client that he might not actually enjoy the "pleasurable" activities at first.** Such experiences are normal, and you do not want the client to judge himself or feel like he is failing.

  - The client may be so accustomed to engaging in the target behavior for pleasure, and so distant from some of his emotions from years of putting the lid on the boiling pot, that he might initially have trouble experiencing pleasure from any other activities—even when he tries to do so.

  - He may also be conditioned to believe that he doesn't *deserve* to feel pleasure or spend time on himself.

- Assure the client that engaging in the activities is beneficial even if he does not experience pleasure or fulfillment. Such an experience does not mean that anything is wrong with him, nor does it mean that he will not be able to experience pleasure in the future. By taking time to do things specifically planned to bring pleasure/fulfillment, he is retraining his brain to believe that he *deserves* to feel pleasure. He is building emotional muscles to start feeling pleasure from activities other than the target behavior. Encourage him to continue to engage in the activities even if he does not enjoy them at first.

- **Normalize urges to avoid. Advise the client to engage in the activities even when he feels urges to avoid doing so.** Prepare the client for potential anxiety, guilt, and/or urges to procrastinate. Validate his reactions, while also encouraging him to engage in a planned activity for *at least a few minutes* each day in order to retrain his brain.

- Sometimes the clients will complain that you are assigning too much home practice. Feel free to point out the humor in the fact that the client is *complaining* about being told to do things he enjoys.

Wrap Up and Plan for Upcoming Week (5 Minutes)

Remind the client about the rest of the home practice: guided audio (five times), BEST B (at least once daily, with encouragement to do more BEST Bs with eyes open during routine activities), Pleasant/Fulfilling Activity (once daily), Daily Log.

Review the Home Practice the Week after Assigning Pleasant/Fulfilling Activities

Although you will be reviewing the home practice in the week following this session, you have the option of arranging the sessions' order to fit the client's needs. Thus, since the next session for your client might not be the next session listed in this manual, the instructions for reviewing the home practice after assigning Pleasant/Fulfilling Activities are provided here:

- Review the Daily Log, the Tracking Sheet, and the previous week as you normally would.
- If the client has not engaged in a pleasant or fulfilling activity at least 4 days, assess and address the obstacles, and then use shaping (see Strategy 5, Chapter 5, pp. 71–78).
  - Remind him that activities can be very brief (eating an apple, watching a YouTube video [if Internet use is not a target behavior], sending a text, listening to a song, etc.).
  - Remind the client that activities do not always have to take extra time. He can also count some activities he already does, as long as he is mindful of his experiences during the activities. (However, encourage the client to choose at least one or two activities each week that he might not normally schedule—at least for a few weeks.)
  - Asking the client to read through the list again (in session) and choose additional potential activities can often be helpful.
- If the client listed the same activity almost every day, affirm his completion of the assignment; then gently encourage him to find additional activities on at least a day or two each week. (He can still continue to engage in the original activity.)
- Sometimes clients feel distressed because they do not experience pleasure when engaging in the activities. Assess this possibility. Normalize and then remind the client of the explanations you gave when assigning the practice.
- When checking Pleasant/Fulfilling Activities in subsequent weeks, you may also suggest activities that are particularly relevant for the client's target behavior (e.g., healthy eating) or that address an area in the client's life that needs more focus (e.g., building social support for a client who is isolated). Use your clinical judgment.
- Although daily activities are assigned, maintenance of four or more per week is acceptable. The key is to find a schedule the client can maintain. Once you find a schedule, you may change the assigned number in the Practice Summary and Tracking Sheet each week.

Mindfulness: Focus on an Object—Therapist Template

Choose a common object (e.g., leaf, rock, coin). Give the object to the client and begin:

Three: Be aware of sounds. (*Pause*) Two: Be aware of the feelings of your feet against the floor, body against the chair. (*Pause*) One: Be aware of your breath. (*Pause*) During this practice, I will provide some prompts and ask some questions. You do not need to answer the questions aloud.

The following is a template. After a few breaths, lead the client through variations on the following instructions. Pause for a few seconds between each instruction/question. Allow 4–5 minutes for the exercise.

- Focus on the sensations of holding the object in your hand. Be aware of any weight of the object. . . . Does it feel warm or cool? . . . Can you tell if it's rough or smooth?
- Open your eyes and study the object. Allow yourself to *really see* it. Notice the details you might normally miss. . . . Allow yourself to be curious. Notice the shape . . . the edges . . . the colors . . . the pattern. . . . Do your best to let go of judgments.
- Do your best to find some sort of beauty in the object.
- Now move the object around in your hands. Turn it over . . . rub the edges . . . bring it closer to your eyes or farther away.
- Notice how the light falls on the object. Does the color change at all?
- Is the object's surface rough or smooth? How does it feel to rub against your hand or fingers?
- Now I'm going to pause for a while to let you really look at the object. When you notice your mind wandering, just bring it back to your breath—and then back to the object. *[Give prompts to gently bring mind back to object every 10 seconds.]*

A point to make afterward: The client sees that object regularly—but probably rarely really sees it. Sometimes we get so caught up in life that we forget to be curious about what's around us. We lose touch with the beauty. Encourage the client to look for the beauty in the upcoming week.

Pleasant and/or Fulfilling Activities

Write down a few people, activities, and situations that you enjoy, that help you feel confident, and/or that help you feel like you're living according to what you value. Only pick things that don't involve behaviors you would regret later. You can pick things from the past, things from the present, or things you'd like to add to your life in the future.

Person, activity, or situation	How do you usually feel?

(continued)

POSSIBLE ACTIVITIES

____ Spending more time with certain people (Who?)

____ Going to a park (e.g., walking a trail, sitting on a bench and reading, sitting on the grass and meditating, watching dogs play, watching people, sitting on a swing)

____ Creating something:
- Photography
- Creative writing
- Journaling
- Painting
- Sewing, knitting, crotcheting, needlepoint
- Drawing
- Arranging flowers
- Fixing something
- Redecorating a room
- Building something (with tools)
- Building something from a kit

____ Joining a club, a group on Meetup (*www.meetup.com*), or some other organization

____ Taking a class (for credit or for fun)

____ Working out (yoga, running, aerobics, weights) on your own, at a gym, or with DVD/online class

____ Working to become a better (parent, sibling, friend, partner, daughter/son). What would you do?

____ Making a plan to eat healthier and working to stick to it (making a meal plan, buying the food, etc.)

____ Keeping in touch (email, phone calls, texts, and/or letters) with someone important to you

____ Going certain places you enjoy (What place or places?)

____ Doing anything from the Coping Toolbox

____ Volunteering (ex: serving food to the homeless for 2 hours, answering phones at a nonprofit, visiting a nursing home, walking shelter animals, sorting donations)

____ Going to an art gallery, another kind of gallery, or some kind of museum

____ Taking a walk or hike (down a street with fun stores, on a hiking trail, in quiet neighborhood)

____ Planting/tending a garden, doing yardwork, or adding plants to your home

____ Cooking or baking something (for yourself or others; only if this isn't a cue for a target behavior)

____ Spending time by a lake, a river, at the beach, or in the country

____ Playing a sport on a team or casually with friends, or practicing on your own

____ Going to church, synagogue, mosque, or another place of worship, or going to a meditation center

____ Going to a movie or streaming a movie (only if this isn't a cue for a target behavior)

____ Spending time with someone important to you—or making a new friend (What would you do?)

____ Eating a type of food you love (only if this isn't a cue for a target behavior)

____ Going to a library/bookstore, downloading a book you'd like read, and/or reading a book you own

____ Working toward getting a job or a job you like better (What would you do?)

____ Dancing in a class, by yourself at home, or at a club (only if this isn't a cue for target behavior)

____ Going to support group meetings

____ Listening to (and maybe singing with) your favorite songs and/or downloading or streaming a song you like

____ Doing something to take care of yourself (getting a haircut, massage, manicure, etc.)

____ Taking a day trip out of town

____ Driving/walking and listening to the radio, to songs you've downloaded, or to a podcast

____ Going to a free or ticketed concert, lecture, film, or other event

____ Add your own _____

____ Add your own _____

____ Add your own _____

Put a checkmark by anything you've done recently. Now read through the list again and put a checkmark by anything you might like to do. (This doesn't mean that you have to do the things.)

Tracking Sheet

Please write the day and what you did each day in the appropriate column.

Day	Audio: Five Times	BEST B: At Least Once Daily Where? When?	Pleasant/Fulfilling Activity	Comments (Optional)

Home Practice Summary: Pleasant/Fulfilling Activities

1. **Do one audio practice at least 5 days this week.**

   Be sure to fill in the Tracking Sheet to record your practice.

2. **Do the BEST B at least once a day. (You're also encouraged to do a second BEST B each day while doing other activities).**

   Be sure to fill in the Tracking Sheet to record your practice.

3. **Do at least one Pleasant and/or Fulfilling Activity each day. (See H-E1 for suggestions.)**

   One activity should be the activity that you chose for this week. The others can be anything you want to do. Be sure to fill in the Tracking Sheet to record your practice.

4. **Complete the Tracking Sheet and Daily Log each day.**

   Fill out the Tracking Sheet and Daily Log each day. This helps us both keep track of what works best for you, what gets in your way, and how you are feeling throughout the week.

Note: When you fill out the Tracking Sheet and the Daily Log, please do your best to be honest. You will not be judged about how much or little you have practiced, how strong or weak your urges are, or what behaviors you have or haven't engaged in during the week. The more honest you are on these forms, the more I can tailor your treatment to meet your needs. This will allow me to be more effective in helping you get closer to the kind of life you want to live. Also, please write any comments you have or anything that comes up during practice so we can talk about it at the next meeting.

MMT Session F
Urge Roadblocks

- Review the week (the client's experiences, home practice, target behavior; 15–20 minutes).
- Engage in mindfulness practice: People through the Room (5–6 minutes).
- Introduce new topic: urge roadblocks (15–20 minutes).
  - Briefly review peaks-and-valleys example and discuss recent urges:
    - Introduce the concept of *urge roadblocks*. Urge roadblocks help the client continue to move toward a more valued life instead of acting on urges—even during peak periods of urges. *Note:* Roadblocks are against acting on urges, not against experiencing urges.
  - Read through and explain *H-F1: Urge Roadblocks:*
    - Once in general terms (although also focusing on the client's target behavior), and
    - Another time using one of the client's specific potentially high-risk situations.
  - Assign new home practice: *H-F1: Urge Roadblocks.*
- Wrap up and plan for upcoming week (5 minutes).
- Home practice: guided audio (five times), BEST B (at least once daily), Pleasant/Fulfilling Activity (once daily), *Urge Roadblocks (H-F1),* Daily Log.

Needed for session (all therapist sheets and handouts for this session are at the end of the Session F guidelines):

- Mindfulness: People/Room (TS-F1)
- Urge Roadblocks (H-F1)
- Tracking Sheet (H-F2)
- Practice Summary (H-F3)
- Daily Log

SESSION F

This session helps clients ride out urges by purposely "blocking" (or at least decreasing) opportunities to act on the urges. Some urge roadblocks can be planned and implemented even before high urges occur; others need to be implemented once urges begin to rise.

Greet the Client and Review the Previous Week (15–20 Minutes)

See the instructions for home practice review at the end of the relevant session.

Engage in Mindfulness Practice: *TS-F1: People through the Room* (5–6 Minutes)

Tell the client that you are going to transition to the new topic by leading her in a mindfulness practice. Ask her to sit up with her hands on her lap, and turn your chair or body around so you are not looking at her. Conduct the practice by reading *TS-F1: People through the Room*.

Introduce New Topic: Urge Roadblocks (20 minutes)

The general concept of urge roadblocks may have already been mentioned for some target behaviors (e.g., not having alcohol in the home for clients in treatment for alcohol use); however, this session includes a more detailed focus on urge roadblocks in a variety of contexts.

Remind the Client of the Peaks-and-Valleys Example

Briefly remind the client of the peaks-and-valleys example (Session B): Urges rise and fall like waves. If a client rides out the peak urge instead of acting on it, the urge will eventually subside on its own. Once a client rides out enough peak urges without acting on them, the overall peaks will eventually decrease in intensity and frequency. But every time the client acts on an urge, the urges are reinforced, and the peaks are more likely to remain high. (Demonstrate with your hands. For example, move your hands to show urges rising—staying high while the client rides out the urges—and then slowly decreasing on their own, as in Figure 8.2 from Session B (p. 150). Demonstrate how the urges eventually decrease dramatically, as in Figure 8.3 (p. 150).

Relate the peaks-and-valleys explanation to any recent episodes of urges the client has experienced. If the client rode through the urges without acting on them, affirm the effort and tell the client that she is making progress toward decreasing those urges. Tell her the new lesson will provide ways to continue getting through urges without acting on them, even when urges are at their highest. If she acted on the urges, validate her effort, and stress that today's topic will provide more ways to ride out future urges. If the client reports no urges, remind her that urges will likely return, and stress the importance of planning so as not to be taken by surprise.

Introduce the Concept of Urge Roadblocks

Urge roadblocks are planned actions that make it harder to act on an urge when the urge is at its peak. Thus, urge roadblocks help the client ride out high urges and move toward a valued life by "blocking" (or at least impairing) opportunities to act on the urges.

- Urge roadblocks should be used when the client starts to feel a high urge and/or when the client finds her resolve to ride out an urge starting to waver.

- Urge roadblocks can also be set up in advance when a client knows she will likely experience a high-risk situation (e.g., an evening with no plans or a visit by family).

- Finally, setting up urge roadblocks can be imperative when the client is still working to stop the behavior or is newly abstinent, even if the client is *not* experiencing urges at the moment.

  - Examples (dependent on the behavior) include not having alcohol/drugs or binge-cueing food around the home; closing or cutting up credit cards; closing accounts for online gaming; deleting and blocking the numbers of drug dealers or an ex that the client compulsively texts; etc.

This topic was mentioned in the first session; however, some clients have difficulty believing they need to take actions that they may feel are extreme. This session provides you with structured handouts and additional time to further address and generalize the issue.

Be sure to stress that the roadblocks are against acting on urges—not against *experiencing* urges. Remind the client that urges will decrease on their own, but that sometimes she may need a little help "blocking" herself from acting on the urges while they are at their peak—especially until she builds her emotional muscles.

Read through and Explain H-F1: Urge Roadblocks

- Read through and explain the handout once in general terms (while also focusing on the client's target behavior).

- Talk through the handout a second time using one of the client's potentially high-risk situations as an example.

  - The handout is largely self-explanatory. Feel free to delete any behaviors that you are sure are not relevant to the client.

  - Due to the large number of potential dysregulated behaviors, the handout does not contain every possible target behavior. If the client's target behavior is not listed, you are encouraged to add it to the list prior to printing the handout.

- Work with the client to decide which specific actions will most likely work for her.

  - Choose from the list of suggestions, or create roadblocks that fit the client that might not appear on the list.

Assign New Home Practice: H-F1: Urge Roadblocks

Instruct the client to set up an urge roadblock and complete the sheet at least one time this week. Also encourage her to set up urge roadblocks even when not recording her actions on the worksheet. (She may record these instances in the "Comments (Optional)" column on the Tracking Sheet, although she is also free not to do so.)

Wrap Up and Plan for Upcoming Week (5 Minutes)

Remind the client about the rest of the home practice: guided audio (five times), BEST B (at least once daily, with encouragement to do a second BEST B with eyes open during routine activities), Pleasant/Fulfilling Activity (once daily), *H-F1: Urge Roadblocks,* Daily Log. If you have not yet conducted Session E, then just cross out the column labeled *Pleasant/Fulfilling Activity* and tell the client that she has a preview of a future session.

Review the Home Practice the Week after Assigning Urge Roadblocks

Although you will be reviewing the home practice in the week following this session, you have the option of arranging the session order to fit the client's needs. Thus, since the next session for your client might not be the next session listed in this manual, the instructions for reviewing the home practice after assigning *H-F1: Urge Roadblocks* are provided here:

- Review the Daily Log, the Tracking Sheet, and the previous week as you normally would.
- If the client did not complete the *Urge Roadblocks* assignment, assess and address the obstacles. Briefly review the handout based on the client's target behavior, and reassign *H-F1: Urge Roadblocks* for the upcoming week (along with the new assignment).
  - If the client says she did not have any urges the previous week, remind her that urges will likely return, and she can use it then.

Mindfulness: People through the Room—Therapist Script

Set a timer (or watch a clock) to conduct the practice for 4 minutes. Start with the standard MMT mindfulness setup of counting from three to one.

Imagine you're in a long room with a door on either end. It's a bare room except for a chair or two in the middle. There's nothing threatening. You don't need to worry about what it looks like or why you're there. That's not important. As you sit or stand there, the door to the right opens, and in walks someone you like or love a lot—whom you haven't seen in a while. (*Slight pause*) Imagine that the person walks through the doorway and comes toward you. (*Slight pause*) Be aware of your reactions. (*Slight pause*) Be aware of the emotions you feel as the person walks up to you. What are your physical sensations? Do you have any impulses to do anything or move in any way? Just be aware of your reactions. (*Pause*) After a while, the person has to go. The person says "goodbye" and then walks to the other door and leaves the room. (*Slight pause*)

And then the first door opens again. This time, someone you *don't* like walks through the doorway. It might be someone whose actions have led to pain for you or people you care about—or someone you just do not like. (*Slight pause*) Be aware of your reactions as you see *that* person walking toward you. (*Slight pause*) Be aware of the emotions that you are feeling. Do you have any impulses to do anything or move in any way? Notice any physical sensations. (*Slight pause*) Just be aware of your reaction. (*Pause*) After a while, that person also walks to the other door and then leaves the room. (*Slight pause*) Now, I'm going to be quiet for a while, and I'd like you to imagine various people coming in the room, staying for a moment, and then walking out the other door. Bring in some people you feel very positive about, some people you don't really like, and some people you don't care strongly about one way or another. And just be aware of your reactions. Your emotions. Your impulses. Your physical sensations. And when you notice your mind wandering, just gently bring it back to the exercise.

[*Every 15–20 seconds, prompt the client to bring her attention back to the exercise when her mind wanders. Proceed to the following script approximately 30 seconds before you want the exercise to end.*] If there's someone in the room with you now, allow that person to leave. (*Slight pause*) Now there's time for one more person. You get to choose who you want. It can be someone who has already been in the room or someone new. That person comes into the room and walks over to you. Just allow yourself to be aware of your reactions. (*Pause 5–7 seconds*) Then that person has to leave, and the person walks over to the door—and out of the room. (*Pause*) Now, whenever you're ready, allow your attention to come back into the room. (*Slight pause*) And whenever you're ready, allow your eyes to open. What was that like for you?

Talking Points

- What were the client's reactions?

- Did the client notice feeling different emotions, impulses, and/or sensations for different people? (Most clients do, at least a little. For the first person, many clients report feeling positive emotions, impulses

(continued)

to walk toward the person, and urges to smile. For the second, clients often report urges to turn away, ignore the person, or hide.)

- Ask the client to notice the fact that her reactions changed over such a short period of time.

- When we feel emotions and have reactions to situations, it can be easy to think that we'll feel that way forever. But the client's emotions and reactions changed over the course of a 4-minute practice—in reaction to people she was only imagining! This exercise shows how strongly our minds can affect our emotions and overall reactions.

Setting Up Urge Roadblocks

(If Those Urges Don't Fit Your Values)

1. Ask yourself:

   A. What is my urge at this moment? (Write it down.)

   B. What emotion or emotions am I feeling? (Possible examples: bored, angry, stressed, sad, frustrated, empty, anxious, ashamed, lonely, numb, etc.)

   C. Would acting on the urge have long-term consequences that are more positive than negative?
   ____ Yes ____ No

   D. Would acting on the urge fit my values for the kind of person I want to be? ____ Yes ____ No

   If the answers to C and D are both "Yes," then feel free to stop this exercise. Otherwise, do your best to SET UP URGE ROADBLOCKS by continuing this exercise.

2. *Stop* and engage in a short BEST B. Make a commitment to react mindfully by continuing to complete this form instead of acting on the urge.

   • Did you do the BEST B? ____ Yes _____ No

3. Set up urge roadblocks, which can be anything that makes it harder to act on the urge while it is at its peak. (See the following pages for some examples.) What are you going to do?

4. What did you end up doing?

5. Do you feel better or worse about yourself than you would have if you had acted on the urge? Explain:

6. Wait until the following day. Write the answer to number 5 again in the space below:

(continued)

Examples of Urge Roadblocks

Important: You are *not* telling yourself not to feel the emotion or urge. *You are setting up roadblocks to make it harder to act on the urge.* The urges will eventually become weaker on their own. You are just helping yourself ride out the strongest part of the urge without acting on it and without doing anything to cause yourself negative consequences later. You are helping yourself live a life that fits your values—to take back your power so that you're no longer controlled by urges.

If the urge is to . . .

Drink alcohol/ use drugs	Do something that makes it difficult or impossible to drink or use drugs at that moment. Make plans with a non-user; call someone and ask them to come over or take you somewhere; go to an area where drugs/alcohol are not available (movie theater, museum, gym, certain parks, place of worship, etc.); call a friend; go to a 12-step meeting or other support group; get as far away from alcohol or drugs as you can. Say "no" to any invitations to parties or bars. Ask your friends in advance to never invite you to do anything that involves alcohol or drugs. Do an audio or do other home practice—especially something from the Coping Toolbox. *If you have alcohol or drugs in your home, throw them away in an outside dumpster, flush them down the commode, or give them to someone who doesn't live with you! Now!*
Binge eat/ overeat	Do something that makes it difficult or impossible to binge or overeat at that moment. Make plans with someone to do something that doesn't involve food; call someone and ask them to come over or take you somewhere; go someplace where food is not easily available (a museum, gym, park, meditation center, place of worship, etc.); call a friend; throw yourself into an activity that doesn't involve food. Avoid grocery stores or other places you often buy food for binges. Say "no" to any invitations to restaurants that are likely to cue binges (such as restaurants with free chips or bread, or restaurants with certain cues). Set an alarm for the next time you can eat a meal or snack—and work to wait until the alarm goes off to eat your next serving. Do an audio or do other home practice—especially something from the Coping Toolbox. *If you have any food in your home that you often use for binges and that doesn't belong to other people, throw it away in an outside dumpster, flush it down the commode, or give it away. Now!*
Attack someone verbally or physically	Do something that makes it difficult or impossible to attack the person at that moment. Get away from the person for at least a little while; leave the room or the building; end the call or stop texting. Focus on your breathing and think of the long-term *consequences of acting on your urge.* Ask yourself if you want to give the person power over you (power to get you to do something you will regret later). Another option: After separating yourself from the person, focus on your breathing and think about the difficulties and suffering the person has in his or her life; let yourself feel pity for the person. Do an audio or do other home practice—especially something from the Coping Toolbox.
Avoid a situation that's important to you	Tell yourself "I will not let this situation force me off the road toward my destination. I will not avoid!" Mindfully force yourself to participate in the situation. Break the situation down into tiny steps and just do one small step of it. If applicable, text someone and ask them to go with you. Or text/email someone to confirm that you will turn in the project by a certain time or see them at the meeting/gathering/dinner. Basically, do something that leaves another person expecting you to participate in the activity or complete the project. Focus on your breathing; do your home practice. Use the Coping Toolbox.
Play computer games or surf the Internet	Do something that makes it difficult or impossible to spend time surfing the Internet or playing computer games. Go somewhere without your laptop, tablet, smartphone, or gaming console. (Consider investing in a flip phone if necessary for times when you need to be away from your

(continued)

	smartphone.) For Internet surfing or games that require the Internet, temporarily disconnect your mode of accessing the Internet by giving your devices (including your smartphone if necessary) to a housemate or neighbor during high urges. Alternatively, disconnect your wifi and disconnect your other devices from your cell service, and only use the Internet when you're at a desktop computer in a room with other people. For games that have already been downloaded, consider deleting the games or giving away the DVDs (even temporarily).
	Slightly lower roadblock: Set an alarm for the next time you can use the Internet—and work to wait until the alarm goes off before logging on. Decide in advance how long you will allow yourself to stay logged on, and set an alarm for that amount of time. (In other words, you might set one alarm for 60 minutes and one alarm for 80 minutes. The first tells you that you can use the Internet; the second tells you it's time to stop using the Internet.) Do an audio or do other home practice—especially something from the Coping Toolbox.
Shop online	See above for Internet surfing. In addition, close your online accounts in stores. Close any accounts you use for online payment. Cancel or suspend credit cards. Do an audio or other home practice—especially something from the Coping Toolbox.
Shop in stores	Do something that makes it difficult or impossible to shop at the moment. Cancel or suspend credit cards. When you go out, only take enough cash for exactly what you need to buy. Avoid stores that are cues for you (such as clothing stores, department stores, or electronics stores). Do an audio or do other home practice—especially something from the Coping Toolbox.
Pornography/ sex	See above for Internet surfing. In addition, cancel any accounts/subscriptions to porn sites. Make plans with someone with whom you would not watch porn. Go to an area where porn is not available (museum, gym, a park, a place of worship, a mainstream movie theater). Stay away from pickup type bars or clubs. Delete accounts to online dating/sex sites. Install parental control software. Go to a support group meeting. Do an audio or do other home practice—especially something from the Coping Toolbox.
Gambling	For online gambling, see above for Internet surfing and online shopping. In addition, close any gambling-related accounts, and close any accounts used for online payments. Also avoid casinos, poker games, or other places that provide opportunities to gamble. Make plans with someone who does not gamble. Say "no" to any invitations to casinos, poker games, or activities that could be cues. Ask your friends in advance to not ask you to do anything that involves gambling. Do an audio or do other home practice—especially something from the Coping Toolbox.
Hibernate at home/sleep all day	Make yourself get up and do *something*. Take a walk or engage in some other physical activity. Go to a store, a museum, a movie, a park, a coffee shop, or other places with people around—even if it's just for a few minutes. Just get on the bus and ride for a while or just drive for a while. (You can promise yourself that you'll come home and hibernate afterward, if that will help.) Call or email someone and ask if they want to meet for lunch/coffee or just come over. Do your home practice. Use your Coping Toolbox.
	Note: There's nothing wrong with hibernating now and then. You only need to use urge roadblocks if hibernating would be inconsistent with your values and impede your progress to the life you want.
Pull hair/pick skin	Put on thick gloves or mittens. Slick your hair back with hair gel (and put it in a bun if it's long enough).
	Slightly lower roadblocks: Draw/doodle, wash dishes in the sink, knit, crochet, play with yarn, mold clay, squeeze a stress ball, or do other tasks to keep your hands busy. Do an audio or do other home practice—especially something from the Coping Toolbox.
Add your own:	

Tracking Sheet

Please write the day and what you did each day in the appropriate column.

Day	Audio: Five Times	BEST B: At Least Once Daily Where? When?	Pleasant/Fulfilling Activity	Comments (Optional)

Home Practice Summary: Urge Roadblocks

1. **Do one audio practice at least 5 days this week.**

   Be sure to fill in the Tracking Sheet to record your practice.

2. **Do the BEST B at least once a day. (You're also encouraged to do a second BEST B each day while doing other activities.)**

   Be sure to fill in the Tracking Sheet to record your practice.

3. **Do one Pleasant/Fulfilling Activity each day.**

   Be sure to fill in the Tracking Sheet to record your practice.

4. **Complete *H-F1: Setting Up Urge Roadblocks* at least once.**

5. **Complete the Tracking Sheet and the Daily Log each day.**

   Fill out the Tracking Sheet and Daily Log each day. This helps us both keep track of what works best for you, what gets in your way, and how you are feeling throughout the week.

Note: When you fill out the Tracking Sheet and the Daily Log, please do your best to be honest. You will not be judged about how much or little you have practiced, how strong or weak your urges are, or what behaviors you have or haven't engaged in during the week. The more honest you are on these forms, the more I can tailor your treatment to meet your needs. This will allow me to be more effective in helping you get closer to the kind of life you want to live. Also, please write any comments you have or anything that comes up during practice so we can talk about it at the next meeting.

MMT Session G
Freeing Yourself from Being Controlled by Your Thoughts

- Review the week (the client's experiences, home practice, target behavior; 15–20 minutes).
- Engage in mindfulness practice: Thoughts (5 minutes).
- Introduce new topic: freedom from being controlled by thoughts (15–20 minutes).
  - ◾ Discuss automatic thoughts.
  - ◾ Explain *H-G1: Common High-Risk Thoughts*.
  - ◾ Ask the client to circle the thoughts he has experienced before engaging in the target behavior.
  - ◾ Explain and discuss the diagram of thoughts and reactions in *H-G2: Path to Make a U-Turn versus Path toward the Person You Want to Be*.
  - ◾ Assign home practice: *H-G3: Thought Tracking*.
  - ◾ Wrap up and plan for upcoming week (5 minutes).
  - ◾ Home practice: guided audio (five times), BEST B (at least once daily), Pleasant/Fulfilling Activity (once daily), *Thought Tracking (H-G3)*, Daily Log.

Needed for session (all therapist sheets and handouts for this session are at the end of the Session G guidelines):

- Mindfulness: Thoughts (TS-G1)
- Common High-Risk Thoughts (H-G1)
- Path to Make a U-Turn (H-G2)
- Thought Tracking (H-G3)
- Tracking Sheet (H-G4)
- Practice Summary (H-G5)
- Daily Log

SESSION G

Clients frequently react to thoughts as though thoughts were facts, often unaware that they have the option of responding otherwise. This session helps clients become aware of high-risk thoughts and begin to learn adaptive ways of reacting to those thoughts.

Greet the Client and Review the Previous Week (15–20 minutes)

See the instructions for home practice review at the end of the relevant session.

Engage in Mindfulness Practice: *TS-G1: Mindfulness: Thoughts—Therapist Script* (5 Minutes)

See previous weeks for setup of the mindfulness practice.

Introduce New Topic: Thoughts (20–25 Minutes)

Discuss automatic thoughts. Remind the client that our brains spew out thoughts based on what we were taught to believe in the past—regardless of whether or not those thoughts fit the present circumstances. (Customize the following to fit what you know about the client.)

- *If you were wearing blue-tinted glasses, everything around you would look at least a little blue—regardless of what color the objects really are. That object* (point to a blue object) *would look bluer than that object* (point to a white object), *but almost everything would have at least a little tint of blue to it.*

- *Sometimes your beliefs are the same way. The things you learned to believe in the past color the way you interpret situations now—regardless of the facts of the situation.*

- *For example: If someone learned to believe that he is stupid, he'll tend to automatically interpret information to fit the belief that he's stupid. If that person didn't do well on one test, he might think, "That's proof that I'm stupid"—even if he made good grades on every other test. Instead of thinking that maybe he just didn't study enough for this test, he might automatically believe that he is stupid, because that's what he's accustomed to believing. And he may take actions that fit those beliefs.*

- *Unfortunately, at some point you have learned that the target behavior was the best way to cope with negative emotions and other cues. You've gotten so accustomed to using the target behavior as a way to cope that your brain might not believe you can use any other coping mechanisms. So whenever you try to stop the target behavior, your brain will spew out thoughts to try to convince you to use the behavior again.*

- *These thoughts may be things like, "The urges are too high; I can't take it anymore. I have to engage in the target behavior today." Or maybe, "I'll just do the target behavior one more time, and then I'll make a fresh start tomorrow." Or maybe things about yourself, like, "I fail at everything; I know I'll fail at this, too."*

● *In the past, you've acted on those thoughts as though they were facts that predicted the future. But that has kept you stuck. What I'd like you to do now is to:*

   1. *Work to be aware of your thoughts,*

   2. *Remind yourself that thoughts don't necessarily equal facts or predict the future, and*

   3. *Make an effort to choose how you react to your thoughts—instead of letting your thoughts have control over you.*

Important: The purpose of this lesson is not to try to decide whether or not each thought is true. The purpose is to learn that thoughts don't necessarily equal facts or predict the future—so that the client has a choice whether or not to act on the thoughts.

Explain/Discuss H-G1: Common High-Risk Thoughts

Read the instructions aloud. Tell the client that the thoughts on the sheet are common to people who struggle with the target behavior. **Note:** The generic term *target behavior* is underlined when included in the sheet. You are encouraged to replace the generic term with the client's specific target behavior before printing.

Ask the Client to Read through the Thoughts and Circle the Numeral by Each of the Thoughts the Client Has Ever Experienced before Engaging in the Target Behavior

After the client circles the numerals by the relevant thoughts, ask him to add any additional thoughts that have cued lapses but are not already listed. Once the client has circled and added thoughts, explain that these thoughts are high-risk thoughts that have controlled him in the past. All thoughts on the list are common thoughts that have controlled other people who've struggled with the target behavior. However, by learning to recognize these thoughts as they're occurring and then *make a choice about whether or not to act on these thoughts,* the client can take back his power and choose to act in a way that fits his values. Like urges, the high-risk thoughts will eventually become less frequent and less intense as the client continues to ride them out without acting on them.

Explain and Discuss H-G2: Path to Make a U-Turn

Choose a recent situation in which the client engaged in the target behavior, and briefly talk through the lower path of the diagram. (Remind the client that you are neither judging nor criticizing.) Then talk through how the client might respond to similar situations in the future by taking the upper path. Discuss the thoughts the client may experience (based on past experiences), and then discuss new ways the client might respond to thoughts that will keep him moving toward the kind of person he wants to be. *Note:* Depending on the order in which you conduct the sessions, the client may not have been exposed to some of the MMT strategies listed on the handout. Focus on the ones the client has learned and tell him that he will learn the rest in the upcoming weeks.

The main point of the diagram is to give clients a visual picture of how their reactions to thoughts determine their paths—either toward or away from the people they want to be. Stress that the choice is difficult (to say the least), but that by being aware of their thoughts and choosing to free themselves from being controlled by those thoughts, they are building their muscles and decreasing the amount of power their thoughts have over them. In other words, making the choice to act in a way that fits their values will get easier over time.

It's critical to stress that clients are not instructed to try to ignore their thoughts or to suppress their thoughts. Doing so would just lead to stronger, more pressing thoughts. Instead, clients are instructed to work to become aware of thoughts and then make a choice on how they want to act. Here are the key phrases:

- Thoughts are just thoughts.
- Thoughts don't necessarily equal facts.
- Thoughts don't predict the future.
- (Most important): You can have a thought without acting on it.

Assign Home Practice: H-G3: Thought Tracking

H-G3: Thought Tracking is similar to a previous assignment (*H-D1: High-Risk Situations Worksheet*). The difference is that this assignment places more focus on thoughts, without including positive and negative consequences. Instruct the client to pay particular attention to his thoughts this week, and to be aware of thoughts that match those listed as *Common High-Risk Thoughts (H-G1)*. Instruct him to write down his thoughts whenever he has urges or even notices high-risk thoughts without urges. Encourage him to do a BEST B whenever he notices high-risk thoughts; however, he is instructed to complete the sheet whether or not he does a BEST B.

Wrap Up and Plan for Upcoming Week (5 Minutes)

Remind the client about the rest of the home practice: guided audio (five times), BEST B (at least once daily, with encouragement to do a second BEST B with eyes open during routine activities), Pleasant/Fulfilling Activity (once daily), *H-G3: Thought Tracking*, Daily Log.

Review the Home Practice the Week after Assigning *H-G3: Thought Tracking*

Although you will review the home practice in the week following this session, you have the option of modifying the session order. Thus, the instructions for reviewing home practice the week after the Thought Tracking assignment are provided here.

- Review the Daily Log, the Tracking Sheet, and the previous week.
- Review *H-G3: Thought Tracking.* Affirm (1) any completion of the sheet, (2) any reports of using the BEST B, and (3) any urges that were followed by adaptive coping. Ask about the client's experience of being aware of his thoughts and his reactions to those thoughts.

- If the client did not complete *H-G3: Thought Tracking*, assess and address the obstacles. Reassign the sheet for the upcoming week, along with the new assignment. Ask if the client has potentially high-risk situations in the upcoming week, and encourage the client to complete the sheet during that time.
  - If the client engaged in the target behavior during the week, ask about thoughts and other antecedents to the behavior. Write responses in the relevant columns.
  - If the client did not engage in the target behavior, ask about a time during the week when the client experienced urges, and write responses in the relevant columns.

Mindfulness: Thoughts—Therapist Script

Ask the client to close his or her eyes or to focus on a spot in front of him/her.

Three: Be aware of the sounds. (*Slight pause*) Two: Be aware of the feelings of your body against the chair and your feet against the floor. (*Slight pause*) One: Be aware of your breathing—the physical sensations in your chest and stomach as you inhale and exhale. (*Slight pause*) Now, we've started most practices by taking a moment to be aware of the sensations of breathing. I'd you like to stay with the breath for a moment, but instead of focusing on the sensations in your chest and stomach, just allow yourself to notice *whatever aspect of the breath* you happen to notice. Maybe your attention will be drawn to the sensations in *just* your chest or *just* your stomach. (*Pause*) Maybe you'll notice the sensations in your nostrils or in your throat as the breath passes in and out. (*Pause about 3 seconds*) Your attention may also go to the *sounds* of your breathing as you inhale and exhale. (*Slight pause*) Maybe the sounds are so soft that you can barely hear them—or perhaps you can't hear them at all, but instead just have more of a *sense* that they're there. (*Pause about 3 seconds*) Instead of sounds, maybe your attention will be drawn to the rhythm or pattern of your breathing. (*Pause about 3 seconds*) Just notice as various aspects of your breathing move in and out of your awareness. (*Pause about 5 seconds*) If you notice your mind wandering, just gently bring it back to your breathing. (*Pause about 10 seconds*)

Now, broaden your attention to the sounds around you. (*Pause*) Notice that some sounds may seem close (*Pause*) and some may seem further away. (*Pause for about 3 seconds*) Some sounds may seem loud (*Pause for about 3 seconds*) and some may seem much softer. (*Pause for about 3–5 seconds*)

And now, allow your awareness of sounds to fade to the background, and gently open your awareness to the thoughts passing through your mind. (*Slight pause*) You might notice thoughts about [target behavior]—or thoughts about this practice. (*Slight pause*) You might notice thoughts about the past or the future . . . or thoughts of happiness . . . or thoughts of worry. (*Pause about 3 seconds*) Just allow the thoughts to move through your mind like clouds moving through the sky. (*Pause about 3 seconds*) Thoughts come and go, but your mind remains your mind, just like the sky remains the sky. (*Pause about 5 seconds*) Allow yourself to be curious. Instead of being controlled by your thoughts, you can notice them as they move into your mind . . . stay a few moments . . . and then eventually fade. (*Pause about 10 seconds*) Now let yourself be curious about what comes next. Ask yourself, "What thought will pass through my mind next?" And then observe the answer. (*Pause about 5 seconds*) Once you've observed the answer, you can continue watching thoughts pass through your mind, or whenever you're ready, you can ask yourself again, "What thought will pass through my mind next?" And observe the answer. (*Pause about 5 seconds*) When you notice your mind wandering, give yourself credit for noticing, and then gently bring your mind back to noticing your thoughts. (*Pause about 5 seconds*) Remember, you are not your thoughts. Your mind is like the sky, and the thoughts are just moving across it. You can have a thought without acting on it. (*Pause about 5 seconds*) Now, when you're ready, allow your attention to come back into the room. And when you're ready, allow your eyes to open.

Common High-Risk Thoughts
(*Freeing Yourself from Being Controlled by Your Thoughts*)

Your brain automatically spews out thoughts based on what it has learned to believe in the past—regardless of whether those thoughts are true in the present. The following thoughts can be cues for lapses—*but only if you automatically see them as facts and act on them.* By being aware of your thoughts and realizing that *thoughts are just thoughts,* you can choose not to act on them (even though it's really hard at first). Once you practice enough times, you can gain freedom from being controlled by your thoughts.

Remember: Thoughts are just thoughts. Thoughts don't predict the future. You can have a thought without acting on it.

Circle the thoughts you've had before [target behavior(s)]:

1. These feelings or urges are unbearable. I can't stand them anymore. I have to act on them.
    a. (Variation:) I'm so bored or numb; I need to act on the urges in order to feel something.
2. The urges are so strong that I'm going to act on them sooner or later anyway—so I might as well do it now and get it over with (so I can start fresh tomorrow).
3. I deserve some fun in my life, so I *deserve* to [target behavior].
4. With everything bad that has happened to me, I deserve to [target behavior] so I can get some relief.
5. I'm just going to do it this one time (or these next few days). I'll stop tomorrow (or next week).
6. One more time won't make a difference.
7. I'm so mad! I'll show him/her—I'll just [target behavior]!
8. [Target behavior] doesn't count as much if you're with friends and they're doing it too. It's only polite to do it with them.
9. My health or life is so bad anyway that [target behavior] probably won't make it any worse.
10. Life has been unfair enough to me already. I shouldn't have to be the one to make the effort. I shouldn't have to make the effort to do the home practice.
11. It doesn't matter if I [target behavior] and then others get upset with me. I already have so many problems in my life—a little more won't make that much difference.
12. I fail at everything anyway, so I might as well just act on the urges.
13. I'm not strong enough to live without acting on my urges.
14. I'm not feeling motivated, so I'll probably have more success if I [target behavior] the rest of the day and then start fresh tomorrow when I'm motivated.
15. It doesn't count as much if nobody else knows I did it.
16. [Target behavior] is the only thing I have that's just mine. I need to do it right now.
17. I need [target behavior] to help me relax.

Add other thoughts you've had before [target behavior(s)]:

18. _____
19. _____
20. _____

Path to Make a U-Turn
versus Path toward the Person You Want to Be

Think of a past situation in which you reacted in a way that had negative consequences for you. Think about the cue, the initial thoughts that followed, and the occurrences along each step of the path you took. Now think of a possible risky situation in the future. Think about how a different response to the thoughts could change the path you follow.

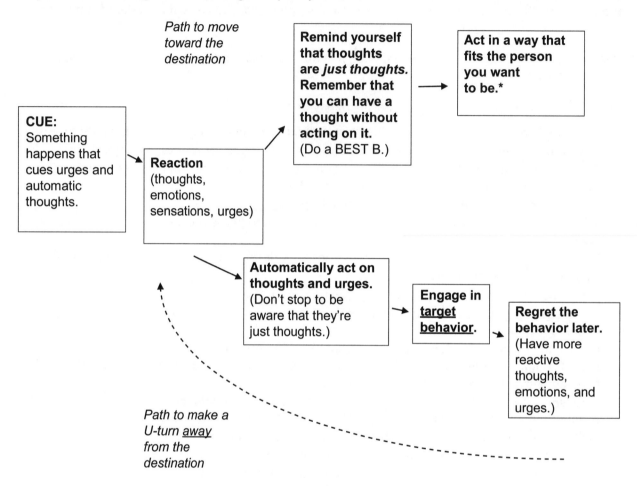

*This might include the BEST B, Coping Toolbox (maybe several things from the Toolbox), Pleasant/Fulfilling Activities, Step toward Goal, Urge Roadblocks, OFFER, Freeing Yourself from Control and Gaining Power (Acceptance Exercises), one of the audio practices, reminding yourself about your commitments, or anything else you do that keeps you from engaging in the behavior.

Thought Tracking: U-Turn versus Moving toward the Person You Want to Be

Complete this sheet whenever you notice yourself experiencing increased urges and/or if you're experiencing high-risk thoughts. Do your best to complete it as soon as you notice yourself experiencing the urges and/or thoughts. However, if you can't complete it at that time, then please complete it afterward—no matter how you responded. Pay particular attention to your thoughts.

Day	Situation	Thoughts	Emotions	Physical Sensations	BEST B Y/N	What Did You Do?

Tracking Sheet

Please write the day and what you did each day in the appropriate column.

Day	Audio: Five Times	BEST B: At Least Once Daily Where? When?	Pleasant/Fulfilling Activity	Comments (Optional)

Home Practice Summary: Thoughts

1. **Do one audio practice at least 5 days this week.**

   Be sure to fill in the Tracking Sheet to record your practice.

2. **Do the BEST B at least once a day. (You're also encouraged to do a second BEST B each day while doing other activities.)**

   Be sure to fill in the Tracking Sheet to record your practice.

3. **One Pleasant/Fulfilling Activity each day.**

   Be sure to fill in the Tracking Sheet to record your practice.

4. **Complete *H-G3: Thought Tracking* when appropriate.**

5. **Complete the Tracking Sheet and Daily Log each day.**

   Fill out the Tracking Sheet and Daily Log each day. This helps us both keep track of what works best for you, what gets in your way, and how you are feeling throughout the week.

Note: When you fill out the Tracking Sheet and the Daily Log, please do your best to be honest. You will not be judged about how much or little you have practiced, how strong or weak your urges are, or what behaviors you have or haven't engaged in during the week. The more honest you are on these forms, the more I can tailor your treatment to meet your needs. This will allow me to be more effective in helping you get closer to the kind of life you want to live. Also, please write any comments you have or anything that comes up during practice so we can talk about it at the next meeting.

MMT Session H
Identifying, Breaking Down, and Moving toward Goals

- Review the week (the client's experiences, home practice, target behavior; 15–20 minutes).
- Engage in mindfulness practice: Counting Breath (5–6 minutes).
- Introduce new topic: goals (15–20 minutes).
  - Discuss importance and potential difficulty of setting and moving toward goals.
  - Review *H-H1: Breaking Down Goals (Examples)*.
  - Identify one or more goals the client would like to work to achieve.
  - Choose one goal that is feasible (achievable within a few weeks at most) and can be broken into small steps.
  - Complete *H-H2: Breaking Down Goals* for the identified goal.
  - Assign home practice: Complete at least one step on the *Goals* worksheet. (Each step may count as one Pleasant/Fulfilling Activity.)
  - Discuss/normalize potential avoidance urges and negative emotions.
- Wrap up and plan for upcoming week (5 minutes).
- Review home practice: guided audio (five times), BEST B (at least once daily), Pleasant/Fulfilling Activity (once daily), one step toward goal (created in session on *H-H2*), Daily Log.

Needed for session (all therapist sheets and handouts for this session are at the end of the Session H guidelines):

- Mindfulness: Counting Breath (TS-H1)
- Breaking Down Goals (Examples) (H-H1)
- Breaking Down Goals (H-H2)
- Tracking Sheet (H-H3)
- Practice Summary (H-H4)
- Daily Log

SESSION H

This session works to help the client identify and start taking steps toward a valued goal.

Greet the Client and Review the Previous Week (15–20 Minutes)

See the instructions for home practice review at the end of the relevant session.

Engage in Mindfulness Practice: *TS-H1: Mindfulness: Counting Breath* (5–6 Minutes)

See previous weeks for setup of the mindfulness practice.

Introduce New Topic: Identifying, Breaking Down, and Moving toward Goals (15–20 Minutes)

Making progress toward a valued goal can add pleasure and/or a feeling of fulfillment to the client's life, while also providing a sense of confidence for further activities. In addition, once the client masters the skill of identifying and taking steps toward one goal, she can use these skills for moving toward additional goals that may also seem overwhelming.

Discuss Importance and Potential Difficulty of Setting and Moving toward Goals

Most people have things they want to do that they just never get around to doing. It's common for years to go by while a person tells herself she will take action at some point, without ever taking the action. One problem is that people often see the goal as one big endeavor that may seem overwhelming to begin. (This is especially relevant for clients who are working to give up a target behavior and so are more likely to feel overwhelmed in general.) Instead, goals are easier to move toward if they are broken into very small (perhaps tiny) steps.

Review H-H1: Breaking Down Goals *(Examples)*

The examples on the handout may seem like "small" goals (volunteering, cleaning the kitchen); however, they illustrate that almost any multistep activity can sometimes seem overwhelming. Read through the examples with the client and explain how the goals were broken into steps. In the first example (volunteering), the person committed to completing at least one step a week. Point out that although the goal took several weeks to complete, the person had been wanting to volunteer for years but had never gotten around to doing so. Thus, spending a few weeks taking steps toward the goal allowed the client to arrive much faster than if she had continued to procrastinate, as she had in the past.

In the second example, the person completed a step every other day. Again, although her kitchen was not guest-ready for more than a week, she had been telling herself that she "should" clean her kitchen for several weeks without doing so. (In fact, the kitchen became messier during this time.) If your client dismisses some steps as "too small," stress that it is more important for the goal setter to take small steps and keep moving forward than it is to set larger steps but then stop because of not having time or feeling overwhelmed.

Identify One or More Goals the Client Would Like to Attain

Identify one or more potential goals, and then choose one that is feasible (achievable within several weeks at most), that has at least some value to the client, and that can be broken down into small steps. The goal does not have to be a lofty, life-changing goal! Although you can discuss various possibilities, the chosen goal needs to be achievable within the timeframe of the client's treatment, if possible. Another option would be to break a larger goal into subparts and work to complete one subpart during the time the client is in treatment. For example, one client ultimately wanted to get a job that better fit her skills, but she had never applied for a job that required a résumé. Thus, she set the goal of finding/attending a half-day course at a local community center on creating a résumé. That goal was then broken into small steps. Once she completed that goal, she set another goal of applying for at least four jobs. And so on.

Offer the client examples of possible goals. Encourage the client to choose a goal that feels as though it would add pleasure to her life, feel valuable to her, and/or address an obstacle to her moving forward. Possibilities in addition to cleaning, creating a résumé, and volunteering include the following: taking a class (for credit or no credit), starting (or resuming) a hobby, taking up a sport, joining a community sports team, attending a Meetup group, attending a support group (12-step or otherwise), starting a window garden, joining and attending a gym, writing/sending an email to an estranged friend or family member, scheduling and attending a doctor's appointment, renewing a lapsed registration for a car (which involves getting the car inspected), etc.

You may also suggest goals that are relevant to the client's specific target behavior and/or that address areas in need of focus (e.g., consulting a nutritionist, gaining social support). However, the decision about which goal to pursue should ultimately be up to the client.

If the client has trouble coming up with any goals (which happens rarely), continue to offer potential suggestions until the client chooses one. Offer any of the examples provided in this text, and feel free to generate your own suggestions based on what you know about the client's life. If you run out of ideas, another possibility is to choose one of the pleasant activities the client mentioned in a previous session but has not yet done. Do your best not to let the session end without choosing a goal and breaking it into steps.

Work with Client to Complete H-H2: Breaking Down Goals for the Chosen Goal

The key is to break down the goal into the smallest steps possible. If you are going to err, err on the side of making the steps too small and easy to achieve. It is much better to choose steps that seem "too small" and have the client actually take those steps than it is to risk the client not taking steps to which she committed. Remember: Many people who struggle with dysregulated behavior have a history of feeling like failures, so working to achieve any goal often brings up intense anxiety and/or urges to procrastinate. By making each step as small and easy as possible, you increase the chance that the client will take the steps despite anxiety and avoidance urges. See *H-H1: Breaking Down Goals (Examples)* as well as the examples that follow.

- *Taking a class* (for fun, not for credit). Steps included (1) choosing a topic that interested the person, (2) searching for classes online, (3) narrowing potential classes based on cost, (4) narrowing further based on times/days, (5) choosing a class, (6) signing up for the class, (7) preparing any necessary materials, (8) planning the travel route, and (9) attending the class.

- *Starting a hobby.* One person wanted to begin knitting again after stopping for several years; however, she had been having trouble getting herself to start again. Her plan included (1) deciding what she wanted to knit, (2) finding her knitting needles in a box in the overhead closet, (3) searching the Internet to find the type and colors of yarn she wanted, (4) ordering the yarn, (5) putting the yarn and needles on the coffee table so she would have them available when she watched TV, and (6) starting to knit. (This client had a tendency to search the Internet for hours before deciding on products, so Step 3 included a caveat that the search could only last an hour before she had to choose.)

- *Going to a Meetup meeting.* Steps involved (1) looking online to get an idea of Meetup groups in the area that fit the client's interests, (2) going online again and choosing five (or fewer) groups with upcoming meetings, (3) creating a Meetup profile (which can be just a username and email), (4) "joining" at least three of the five groups (which meant just pushing the "join" button and the client would now receive notices of upcoming meetings), (5) choosing one of the upcoming meetings to attend and RSVP-ing "yes," (6) planning travel route, and (7) attending the meeting for at least 30 minutes.

> Clients sometimes write several random steps without building on any of them. Be sure that each step builds on the previous step to lead to the goal. Example: A client who wanted to start working out broke down her goal into these steps: (1) Check to see what yoga studios are located near me, (2) buy a workout DVD, and (3) start walking instead of driving. Notice that she did not write what she would do after she found yoga studios, what steps she would take to find the particular DVD, how she would get herself to practice the DVD workout, or how she would make time to walk instead of drive. She then rewrote the list, adding steps until they resulted in the goal: "(1) Check yoga studios near me, (2) choose a studio based on type of yoga, (3) check for classes that fit my schedule, (4) find yoga pants online (no more than 45 minutes), (5) order yoga pants, (6) sign up for a class, (7) attend class," etc.

Assign Home Practice: One Step toward the Goal

Ask the client to commit to completing at least one step that she listed on *H-H2: Breaking Down Goals.* The client may complete more than one step if she chooses to do so, but encourage her to *commit* to only one step. (Again, it is better for the client to undercommit and complete more tasks than planned than for her to overcommit and become accustomed to not keeping commitments.) Once the client has completed the steps she committed to do for a week or two, you can increase the number of steps the next week—if *(and only if) the client requests to do so.* Even so, continue to err on the side of *under*committing.

Each step the client completes may count as one Pleasant/Fulfilling Activity on the *H-H3 Tracking Sheet.* Thus, on a day the client completes a step toward a goal, she will write that step on the Tracking Sheet, and as a consequence, does not "have to" engage in an additional Pleasant/Fulfilling Activity. (However, she is free to engage in such activity if she would like!)

Discuss/Normalize Potential Avoidance Urges and Negative Emotions That May Occur Prior to Completing Steps toward Goals

Tell the client that she may experience strong urges to procrastinate whenever she thinks about completing one of the planned steps. Prepare her for potential anxiety or other uncomfortable emotions she may experience when actually choosing to complete a task. Explain that such feelings are normal, and troubleshoot how she can get herself to take the step even if experiencing urges to procrastinate. Work with her to plan a time when she might complete the first task. *Note:* The first two steps should be especially simple and easy to achieve. In that way, clients will be able to build at least a little self-efficacy by successfully completing some tasks in the early stages of moving toward the goal.)

Wrap Up and Plan for Upcoming Week (5 Minutes)

Remind the client about the rest of the home practice: guided audio (five times), BEST B (at least once daily, with encouragement to do a second BEST B with eyes open during routine activities), Pleasant/Fulfilling Activity (once daily), at least one step listed in *H-H2: Breaking Down Goals* (which counts as a Pleasant/Fulfilling Activity), Daily Log.

Review the Home Practice the Week after Assigning *H-H2: Breaking Down Goals*

Home practice will be reviewed in the week following the above session.

- Review the Daily Log and Tracking Sheet as you normally would.
- If the client has not engaged in at least one step toward the goal, address the obstacles, and then use shaping (see Strategy 5, Chapter 5, pp. 71–78).
  - As long as the client reports wanting to continue to work on the chosen goal, reassign the same step for the upcoming week (along with new home practice). Troubleshoot.
  - If the client reports wanting to change goals and you believe the change is adaptive, quickly work to break the new goal into steps and assign at least one step for the upcoming week.
- If the client completed at least one step, ask if she's willing to commit to doing at least one more step in the upcoming week. Work with her to plan specifics, if needed. Continue to track her steps toward the goal in the upcoming weeks. (You're encouraged to make a note on the *MMT Session Chart (TS-2)* to remind yourself to check each week.)

Mindfulness: Counting Breath—Therapist Script

Set a timer for 4 minutes. Prior to starting timer, instruct the client:

Sit up as straight as is comfortable for you, with both hands in your lap, and allow your eyes to close. Three: Be aware of sounds. (*Slight pause*) Two: Be aware of the feelings of your feet against the floor, your body against the chair. (*Slight pause*) One: Be aware of your breath—the physical sensations as you inhale and exhale. (*Slight pause*)

For this practice, I'd like you to continue focusing your attention on the physical sensations of your breath. Then when I tell you to start counting, I'd like you to mentally count each time you inhale. In other words, inhaling the first time will be *1*, and then you'll exhale. Inhaling the second time will be *2*, and then you'll exhale. Keep counting each inhale until you get to *10*. Once you get to *10*, start over at *1*. And then keep repeating. When your mind wanders, just notice—and gently bring your attention back to the physical sensations of breathing—with the counting starting at *1* again. If you're like most people, you might have times when you suddenly notice that you've gone past *10* and are continuing to count upward. When that happens, just notice, bring your attention to the sensations of your breath, and then start counting from *1* again. If you find that you are judging yourself, just do your best to let go of the judgment and bring your attention back to your breath. (*Slight pause*) Now, whenever you're ready, start counting your inhales—being aware of the physical sensations of your breath as you do so. [*Give prompts every 45–60 seconds for the client to bring her or his attention back to the breath when noticing the mind wandering.*]

After the practice, ask the client what it was like for her or him. Normalize difficulties.

Breaking Down Goals (Examples)

EXAMPLE 1: Volunteer

Choose one goal you would like to start working toward. Make sure it's feasible.

Overall goal: Start volunteering up to 3 hours per week.

First start with a one-time volunteer commitment to get used to it.

Break into steps toward completion.

1. Search for volunteer centers on the Internet; write down or bookmark addresses.
2. Look through opportunities at one center (more if first center doesn't have any that fit).
3. Choose two or three opportunities that interest me. I will choose simple opportunities to start out.
4. Complete online form to apply for one of the positions.
5. Read their reply email, which will ask me for more information or tell me the position is filled.
6. Return email with additional information (if needed), or return to Step 4 for another position.
7. Confirm a time to volunteer for the position.
8. Make sure I have clean clothes ready.
9. Check directions/transportation schedule and plan route.
10. Show up for volunteer job.

EXAMPLE 2: Clean kitchen so I can have my friends visit

Choose one goal you would like to start working toward. Make sure it's feasible.

Overall goal: Clean my kitchen so I can have my friends visit.

It doesn't have to be perfect—just clean enough that I feel comfortable letting other people visit.

Break into steps toward completion.

1. Throw out the old food in the refrigerator, and then take out the trash.
2. Wipe up the spills in the refrigerator.
3. Remove everything from the sink and wash the sink with cleaning solution.
4. Wash the dishes.
5. Put dishes away.
6. Put away anything else on the counter that doesn't belong there.
7. Clean the counters and stove with cleaning solution.
8. Vacuum or sweep kitchen floor.

Commit to taking at least one step this week. Each step you take toward your goal counts as one of your Pleasant/Fulfilling Activities on your Tracking Sheet.

(*Note: The person in the second example ultimately chose to take one step every other day, for a total of four steps in the first week. But there is no pressure to commit to that many.*)

Breaking Down Goals

Choose one goal you can begin taking steps toward immediately. Make sure it's feasible.

_____

_____

Break into steps toward completion.

_____

_____

_____

_____

_____

_____

_____

_____

_____

_____

_____

_____

_____

Commit to taking at least one step this week. Each step you take toward your goal counts as one of your Pleasant/Fulfilling Activities on your Tracking Sheet.

Tracking Sheet

Please write the day and what you did each day in the appropriate column.

Day	Audio: Five Times	BEST B: At Least Once Daily Where? When?	Pleasant/Fulfilling Activity	Comments (Optional)

Home Practice Summary: Goals

1. **Do an audio practice at least 5 days this week.**

   Be sure to fill in the Tracking Sheet to record your practice.

2. **Do the BEST B at least once a day. (You're also encouraged to do a second BEST B each day while doing other activities.)**

   Be sure to fill in the Tracking Sheet to record your practice.

3. **Do one Pleasant/Fulfilling Activity or take one step toward a goal each day. (See H-H2.)**

   From now on, any step toward a goal can be counted as your daily Pleasant/Fulfilling Activity. Be sure to fill in the Tracking Sheet to record your practice.

4. **Do your best to do at least one step toward the goal you chose in session.**

   Record it under Pleasant/Fulfilling Activity.

5. **Complete the Tracking Sheet and the Daily Log each day.**

   Fill out the Tracking Sheet and the Daily Log each day. This helps us both keep track of what works best for you, what gets in your way, and how you are feeling throughout the week.

Note: When you fill out the Tracking Sheet and the Daily Log, please do your best to be honest. You will not be judged about how much or little you have practiced, how strong or weak your urges are, or what behaviors you have or haven't engaged in during the week. The more honest you are on these forms, the more I can tailor your treatment to meet your needs. This will allow me to be more effective in helping you get closer to the kind of life you want to live. Also, please write any comments you have or anything that comes up during practice so we can talk about it at the next meeting.

CHAPTER 10

Mindful Communication/ Relationships Module

MMT Session I
Saying No: OFFER Mindful Refusal Skills

- Review the week (the client's experiences, home practice, target behavior; 15–20 minutes).
- Introduce new topic: mindful refusal skills (20–25 minutes).
  - Identify a situation in which the client may need to use mindful refusal skills. If necessary, choose a past situation that might occur again.
  - Work to identify a concrete reason for refusing to engage in the target behavior.
  - Explain the OFFER acronym for mindful refusal skills.
  - Help the client become mindful of the other person's perspective.
  - Work with the client to write an informal "script" using OFFER format.
  - Conduct informal role play: The client plays him/herself, and the therapist plays the person encouraging the target behavior. Provide affirmations and constructive suggestions for improvement.
  - Assign new home practice: Engage in OFFER once this week if possible (*H-I2: Saying No: OFFER*).
- Wrap up and plan for upcoming week (5 minutes).
- Home practice: guided audio (five times), BEST B (at least once daily), Pleasant/Fulfilling Activity (once daily), *H-I2: Saying No: OFFER,* and Daily Log.

Needed for session (all therapist sheets and handouts for this session are at the end of the Session I guidelines):

- Saying No: OFFER Example (H-I1)
- Saying No: OFFER (H-I2; two copies)
- Tracking Sheet (H-I3)
- Practice Summary (H-I4)
- Daily Log

SESSION I

Clients often have trouble refusing offers to engage in the dysregulated behavior. The purpose of this session is to help clients become more effective in refusing such offers, while also decreasing the chance of harming the client's relationship with the person offering.

Greet the Client and Review Previous Week (15–20 Minutes)

See the instructions for home practice review at the end of the relevant session.

Introduce New Topic: Mindful Refusal Skills (20–25 Minutes)

First, validate the difficulty of saying "no" when others encourage the client to engage in the target behavior or to become involved in situations that will likely lead to the behavior. Clients often report feeling guilty (as though they were letting the other person down), ashamed (as though they were admitting a flaw), anxious (about harming the relationship), and a host of other unpleasant reactions when attempting to refuse such encouragements. In addition, refusals are often (at least initially) met with stronger attempts from others to persuade the client to engage in the behavior.

Second, work with the client to identify any upcoming situations in which he might be encouraged to engage in the target behavior. Encourage him to avoid those situations, if possible, at least for the first several weeks of treatment. (For example, a client working to stop drinking would avoid going with friends to bars or parties that serve alcohol.) Also encourage him to avoid people who tend to pressure him into engaging in the behavior—such as bookies, dealers, or even certain friends and family members—if at all possible. Avoiding such situations for at least a few weeks gives the client a chance to build emotional muscles—to increase the chance that he can successfully refuse offers to engage in the target behavior in the future.

Finally, since clients often do not have the option of avoiding people who might encourage their target behavior, clients can also benefit from learning mindful refusal skills.

> Most dysregulated behaviors are encouraged by other people to some extent. However, although refusal skills are relevant for most dysregulated behaviors, they may not be relevant to all such behaviors. If, after a discussion with your client, you decide that refusal skills are not relevant, feel free to jump to Session J, which you may choose to conduct twice. (Many clients need 2 weeks of OFFER communication practice.)

Identify a Situation in Which the Client May Need to Use Mindful Refusal Skills in the Near Future

Situations (depending on the behavior) may include:

- Being asked to go out for a drink (or to a meal where others will be drinking).
- Being encouraged to participate in an online game.
- Being offered extra helpings of food, or being persuaded to take home extra food.
- Being offered drugs or alcohol.

- Being asked to go to a casino, bet in fantasy football, join a poker game, or go to the track.
- Being asked to go shopping with someone or buy items for an event.
- Being approached for sex, invited to go to a pickup-type bar, or contacted online.
- Being asked to go outside and smoke with someone.

If the client cannot think of a situation, offer prompts based on what you know about him. Sometimes the situation is a direct offer, and sometimes the situation is less obvious (being asked to go to a work party—which the client knows often involves alcohol or poker games). If you and the client still cannot generate a situation that will likely occur in the near future, ask the client to choose a past situation that might occur again.

Work to Identify a Concrete Reason for Refusing to Engage in the Target Behavior

Sometimes clients can successfully refuse to engage in their target behavior just by telling others that they have stopped the behavior (without giving a specific reason for doing so). If a client wants to take such a course of action, he should be encouraged to do so. However, many clients have extreme difficulty refusing offers unless they can provide a reason or "excuse" for their refusal. This difficulty often becomes even stronger if others persist in pressuring them to engage in the behavior. Thus, helping the client identify a specific reason for refusing can help him successfully refuse in the first place, while also helping him continue to refuse, even if others repeatedly pressure him. It can also decrease the chance that the client will become sidetracked if the other person uses multiple arguments to persuade him to engage in the target behavior.

Reasons should have long-term relevance—*at least* 6 months in duration. (Once the 6 months are drawing near an end, the client will likely be more comfortable continuing to refuse without a specific reason.) Of course, the client can always say that the behavior was interfering with his life and that he is therefore working to stop it. But if the client is not comfortable sharing such personal information, other potential excuses include (but are not limited to):

- I'm working to be healthier, so I've promised myself I won't [drink, eat dessert, eat second helpings, do drugs] for at least 6 or 12 months.
- My doctor advised me not to engage in [target behavior] for at least 6 months due to a health issues [high blood pressure, recurrent illness, blood sugar, unspecified].
- My partner [or friend] and I made commitments to each other to stop [target behavior] and work to be healthier for the next 6 months. We promised each other we'd help keep each other on track, and I don't want to break my promise.
- I've been gaining weight or I want to lose weight [or] I've noticed my clothes are all tight lately, so I'm going to give up [taking food home, eating sweets, eating second helpings, drinking] for the next 6 months. [If the other person says that one drink/sweet/extra helping won't hurt, the client can say that he knows himself well enough to know that he won't just stop at one; if the person says the client can take food home to take to the office the next day, the client can say that he knows he will eat at least some if he takes it home.]
- [For mandated clients] I got a ticket/I've been arrested [for target behavior], and if I'm caught doing the behavior any time in the next x months, I will [go to jail, be on longer probation, be charged a bigger fine]. I have to stop the behavior until this legal issue gets cleared up. [Note:

The person does not have to say that he deserved to be arrested. Many mandated clients report that the arrest was unfair; however, the consequences remain the same.]

- The [target behavior: computer gaming/gambling/drinking/drug use/sexual activity] is interfering with my relationship. I promised my partner I won't engage in the behavior for at least *x* months. I don't want to jeopardize my relationship or lie to my partner.
- My job is conducting random drug screens. I could get fired if I used drugs.
- I've noticed that the behavior is taking too much of my time. I need to stop for x months so I can spend more time focusing on [work/partner/other central thing in client's life].
- My work [or relationship] has suffered since I've been engaging in [target behavior] so late at night. I know once I start, I'm not going to be able to stop in time to go to sleep earlier. So I'm taking a 6-month break. I can't risk losing my job [or relationship].
- My parents [or partner] said that they will not let me continue to live at home unless I stop the [target behavior]. So I have to stop for at least [number] months until things settle down.
- The behavior is keeping me from spending quality time with my kids. I'm going to stop so I can be a better parent.
- I've been spending too much money on [target behavior]. I need to save money for [something essential]. [Or] I've already used up a lot of my savings. [Or] My credit card debt is too high. I'm going to stop the behavior for at least 6 months until I get back on track.

The following reasons are *not* effective, because they are only relevant for a short amount of time (which will encourage the other person to ask again later) and/or they can be easily solved.

- Feeling sick
- Needing to get up early the next day (unless the client needs to get up early every day)
- Not having money at the moment (as the encourager can just offer to cover for the client that one time)

Explain the OFFER Acronym for Mindful Refusal Skills

OFFER MINDFUL REFUSAL

- O = *Other* (Express what the other person might be feeling or going through.)
- F = *Facts* (Tell the facts of the situation—not opinions or judgments.)
- F = *Tell your Feelings and/or the Consequences* of the situation for you. (Be nonjudgmental as you tell how you feel and/or what the consequences are for you. Be specific.)
- E = *Explain* (Explain that you are refusing. Be clear. Ask that the person not to try to persuade you again.)
- R = *Reward* (Let the person know how respecting your request can be beneficial to her/him—even if it's just that you'll appreciate the person.)

If the person persists, stress that the issue is important to you. Say that if the person cares about you, he/she will not keep trying to persuade you to do something that has negative consequences for you.

Introduce the OFFER by going through *H-I1: Saying No: OFFER Example.* Explain that the OFFER provides a way for the client to decline to engage in target behavior, even when pressured, while also:

- Increasing the chance that the client will be successful in staying abstinent,
- Decreasing the chance that the other person will be upset, and
- Increasing the chance that the other person will respect the client's wishes.

However, stress that the OFFER is not magic. Some people will get upset or ignore the client's refusal regardless of how well the client communicates. The OFFER just decreases the chance that that will happen.

Work with the Client to Write an Informal "Script" Using H-I2: Saying No: OFFER

After you have walked the client through the examples, create an OFFER (*H-I2*) for the situation the client chose earlier. Before composing an OFFER, the client is instructed to:

1. *Choose a reason you are willing to give the other person for saying "no."*
2. *Think about what the other person is going through at that moment—and why the person might want you to engage in the behavior. Do your best to be nonjudgmental.*

Point 1: Review the reason the client has identified for refusing to engage in the target behavior. *Point 2:* Have the client take a moment to be mindful about what the other person may be experiencing. Explain that if the client works to understand and express the perspective of the other person, the other person is less likely to feel upset/defensive and more likely to listen to the client's perspective. Stress the need to be nonjudgmental—because the more the client can understand the *other person's* perspective, the more effective the client will be in conducting the OFFER. Being nonjudgmental does not mean the client agrees with the other person or approves of the person's behavior; instead, it means the client works to understand the other person's point of view. Explain that the client can be mindful of the other person's perspective while also choosing to live according to his own values.

After Points 1 and 2, ask the client for a response to each prompt of the OFFER acronym, and write his replies on the sheet. If the client's answers are judgmental, too general, or in other ways don't fit the prompts, gently validate/affirm while also suggesting modifications. Write the answers in a conversational, unstilted tone. Key elements of the OFFER include:

- *Facts:*
  - Avoid generalizations such as *always* or *never.* If the client says, "I always lose money when I gamble," the other person might bring up a time when the client gambled but didn't lose money—which would take the conversation on a tangent.
  - Be nonjudgmental by *focusing on facts.* If the client says, "Engaging in [target behavior] is wasting my time," the other person might feel defensive and argue with the client's judgments. A more effective option would be: "I've been spending hours a day on [target behavior], and I haven't had time to study as much as I need to do."

- *Feelings/consequences:* Don't blame the other person. Instead of "You make me feel bad about myself when I do that," the more effective option would be, "I feel bad about myself when I do that."
- *Explain:* Be firm, clear, and specific. Saying, "I think I should probably stop [target behavior] or "I need to stop [target behavior] for a while" implies that the client is open to being persuaded otherwise.
- *Reward:* Although the reward can be specific (e.g., going with the other person to a place that doesn't involve the target behavior), it often involves less concrete things like appreciating the other person, feeling like the other person is a good friend, etc.

Additional key points:

- If the other person continues to try to persuade the client after he has used the OFFER, the client should continue to emphasize that he will not engage in the behavior. **Important:** Tell the client to say that if the other person is a true friend and/or cares about the client, the other person won't want the client to do anything that causes negative consequences.
- If the other person tries to move the conversation off-topic, which often includes accusations about inconsistencies in the client's past, the client is advised to stick to refusing to engage in [target behavior] and not get caught up in tangents.
- The other person may accuse the client of not being a good friend, of rejecting the other person, of thinking he/she is better than the other person, of letting the other person down, etc. In these cases, the client is advised to briefly respond to the person's point, but quickly return to the main points: the consequences to the client and the client's refusal.
  - *I don't think I'm better than you, and I'm not rejecting you. I'd like to get together to do something that doesn't involve [target behavior]. But I'm not going to [target behavior], because [insert consequences for the client]. If you really care about me, please quit trying to get me to do something that will hurt me.*

Another example:

> OTHER PERSON: You said that [target behavior] takes so much of your time that you're not the kind of parent you want to be for your daughter. Well, I have a kid, too, and I spend that much time on [target behavior]. So you're saying you don't think I'm a good parent.
>
> CLIENT: I'm not saying that at all. Maybe you have better time management than I do. I don't know. All I'm talking about is *my* time and *my* daughter—not about your parenting. I'm not going to [target behavior] anymore. Please quit asking me.

Note: Sometimes the client may not have to use a full OFFER when refusing to engage in the target behavior. However, by preparing and practicing the full OFFER, the client will be familiar enough with what he wants to say that he can use the full OFFER if needed. By preparing and practicing the OFFER in advance, he is also gaining general experience with the OFFER template. The ultimate goal is for the client to be so accustomed to using the OFFER that he can automatically use it whenever he needs—without having to prepare beforehand.

Informal Role Play: The Therapist Plays the Person Encouraging the Target Behavior, and the Client Plays Him/Herself

If you are like most people, you dislike role plays. If your clients are like most people, they also dislike role plays. Thus, you may be tempted to skip the role play. You are strongly encouraged not to do so! Clients will often seem to understand OFFER but then become frazzled and get confused when they actually try to communicate the OFFER. (Trust us on this one.)

Before setting up the role play, read the client's OFFER aloud using a conversational tone. Then tell the client that you would like to do a role play with him to practice the OFFER, with you playing the person encouraging the client to engage in the behavior. Normalize the client's likely discomfort by saying that most people dislike doing role plays, and validate that the role play will feel awkward and artificial. However, explain that it can be helpful anyway.

Ask basic questions, such as where the client will be sitting or standing and what that person might say to encourage him to engage in the target behavior. Tell the client your character (you) will listen to the OFFER but then try to persuade him to engage in the behavior based on arguments people often use. Encourage him to continue to refuse and to ask your character to stop pressuring him.

- Start the role play by using the phrase the client said the encourager will use.
- Listen as the client goes through the OFFER. Do your best not to jump in and provide assistance if at all possible. In other words, stay in character!
- Once the client completes the OFFER, do your best to pressure him—which allows the client to practice responding to pressure. The client will sometimes later report feeling like the character you are playing must not care about his (the client's) needs, since the character continued to pressure him even though he reported negative consequences. Such a realization is helpful, as it can decrease the chance the client will be concerned about hurting the other person's feelings if such pressure occurs in "real life."

Possible (and common) arguments include:

- *Please. Just this once—for old time's sake. I'd do it for you.*
- *Come on. Just this one [drink/smoke/bet] won't make a difference.*
- *You think you're better than me now. You think you're too good for me.*
- *I've been there for you all this time, but now you're not there for me.*
- *You were more fun when you [underline]target behavior[/underline]. You're going to lose all of your friends.*
- *You don't need to worry about [health/weight/money/etc.]*
- *[For mandated clients] If you take this medicine [and/or] drink gallons of fluid [and/or] tape someone else's urine in a bag next to your body, the drugs won't show up in the urine test. [Important: That's not true. Urine tests can assess for adulterated urine, and the client will*

likely get in even more trouble. Also, a clinic employee almost always watches to make sure that clients don't substitute other urine for their own.] The client's response can include an explanation of the above, plus: *Do you really want me to risk going to jail [or losing my job]? It's not worth risking jail time [or getting fired].*

Add your own client response, based on what you know about the client's circumstances.

Provide Affirmation and Suggestions for Improvement

Find at least some aspects of the client's performance to affirm; then gently offer suggestions for improved performance. Also discuss various methods for responding based on potential reactions of the other person (or persons).

Assign the New Home Practice: H-12: Saying No: OFFER

Instruct the client to engage in at least one OFFER in the upcoming week. The simplest course would be to engage in the OFFER that was composed and practiced in session. Discuss how and when the client can engage in that OFFER. Instruct him to write a sentence or two on the back of the sheet after conducting the OFFER to describe how it went. In case that situation does not present itself this week, give the client a second (blank) *H-12: Saying No: OFFER* for composing another OFFER for a different circumstance.

Be sure to prepare the client for being nervous when conducting the OFFER. Assure him that it might not sound perfect, but as long as he sticks to his refusal, he will be getting practice. If nobody encourages the client to engage in the target behavior this week, ask the client to (1) think about the OFFER composed in session, and (2) compose another OFFER based on a circumstance that may occur in the future. However, encourage the client to actually do an OFFER if possible.

Wrap Up and Plan for Upcoming Week (5 Minutes)

Remind the client about the rest of the home practice: guided audio (five times), BEST B (at least once daily, with encouragement to do more BEST Bs during routine activities), Pleasant/ Fulfilling Activity (once daily), *H-12: Saying No: OFFER*, Daily Log.

Review the Home Practice
the Week after Assigning *H-12: Saying No: OFFER*

Home practice is reviewed in the week following the above session.

- Review the Daily Log, the Tracking Sheet, and the client's week as you normally would.
- If the client completed the OFFER and refrained from the target behavior, affirm the

success, validate the difficulty and effort, and ask about the experience. Briefly discuss times the client might use the OFFER in the future.

- If the client completed the OFFER but had trouble and/or engaged in the behavior anyway, affirm the client's effort to engage in the OFFER and assess what went wrong. Validate the client while also working to problem solve for future situations.
- If the client did not engage in the OFFER, assess the obstacles.
  - If the client truly did not have a chance to conduct an OFFER, discuss times in the future the OFFER might be used.
  - If the client had a chance but did not use the OFFER, further assess the obstacles and respond accordingly.
- Be sure to mention the OFFER in future sessions when you are aware of any potential need for mindful refusal skills.

Saying No: OFFER (Example]

Mindful Refusal Skills

Beforehand:

1. Choose a reason you are willing to give the other person for saying "no."

2. Also think about what the other person is going through at that moment—and why the other person might want you to engage in the behavior (in a nonjudgmental way).

1. **O = *OTHER*** (Express what the other person might be feeling or going through.)

   I understand that it's more fun to drink when a drinking buddy is with you, and I know we always have a good time when we go out.

   [Or]

   I know that you've put a lot of work into making that cake, and I can understand how you'd want to share it.

2. **F = *FACTS*** (Tell the facts of the situation—not opinions or judgments.)

   But I've made a commitment to be healthier, and I've given up drinking for the next 6 months.

   [Or]

   But my clothes have all been tight lately, and I've decided to give up sweets.

3. **F = *Tell your FEELINGS and/or the CONSEQUENCES* of the situation for you.** (Be nonjudgmental as you tell how you feel and what the consequences are for you.)

   This is really important to me, and I've already started feeling better since I've stopped drinking. I don't want to start feeling sluggish again like I did when I was drinking.

   [Or]

   This is really important to me, because I've been feeling bad about my weight, and I'll feel better about myself when I don't eat sweets.

4. **E = *EXPLAIN*** (Explain that you are refusing. Be clear. Ask the person not to try to persuade you again.)

   So even though I'd like to spend time with you, I'm not going to be going out drinking with you. And I'd appreciate it if you don't ask me to go drinking again.

   [Or]

   So I'm not going to have any of that cake. Please don't offer me any more dessert.

5. **R = *REWARD*** (Let the person know how respecting your request can be rewarding to him/her— even if it's just that you'll appreciate the person.)

   I really appreciate your understanding and support with this. Maybe later we can go to a movie or do something that doesn't involve alcohol.

   [Or]

   I appreciate your support with this. Thanks for understanding and being a good friend.

[If the person persists:] Seriously, this is very important to me. I know you're not the kind of friend who would want me to do something that causes me to feel unhealthy or that keeps me from feeling good about myself. So if you care about my health/how I feel about myself, please don't keep asking me.

Saying No: OFFER

Mindful Refusal Skills

Beforehand:

1. Choose a reason you are willing to give the other person for saying "no."

2. Also think about what the other person is going through at that moment—and why the other person might want you to engage in the behavior (in a nonjudgmental way).

1. **O = *OTHER*** (Express what the other person might be feeling or going through.)

_____

_____

2. **F = *FACTS*** (Tell the facts of the situation—not opinions or judgments.)

_____

_____

3. **F = *Tell your FEELINGS and/or the CONSEQUENCES* of the situation for you.** (Be nonjudgmental as you tell how you feel and what the consequences are for you.)

_____

_____

4. **E = *EXPLAIN*** (Explain that you are refusing. Be clear. Ask the person not to try to persuade you again.)

_____

_____

5. **R = *REWARD*** (Let the person know how respecting your request can be rewarding to him/her—even if it's just that you'll appreciate the person.)

_____

_____

If the person persists, point out that the issue is important to you. Say that if the person cares about you, he/she will not keep trying to persuade you to do something that has negative consequences for you.

Tracking Sheet

Please write the day and what you did each day in the appropriate column.

Day	Audio: Five Times	BEST B: At Least Once Daily Where? When?	Pleasant/Fulfilling Activity	Comments (Optional)

From *Treating Impulsive, Addictive, and Self-Destructive Behaviors: Mindfulness and Modification Therapy* by Peggilee Wupperman. Copyright © 2019 The Guilford Press. Permission to photocopy this material is granted to purchasers of the book for personal use or use with individual clients (see copyright page for details). Purchasers can download additional copies of this material (see the box at the end of the table of contents).

Home Practice Summary: Saying No: OFFER

1. **Do an audio practice at least 5 days this week.**

   Be sure to fill in the Tracking Sheet to record your practice.

2. **Do the BEST B at least once a day. (You're also encouraged to do a second BEST B each day while doing other activities.)**

   Be sure to fill in the Tracking Sheet to record your practice.

3. **Do one Pleasant/Fulfilling Activity or take one step toward a goal each day.**

   Be sure to fill in the Tracking Sheet to record your practice.

4. **Complete H-12: *Saying No: OFFER* at least once if at all possible.**

   You can conduct the OFFER planned in session, or you can conduct a new OFFER that you plan on your own.

5. **Complete the Tracking Sheet and the Daily Log each day.**

   Fill out the Tracking Sheet and the Daily Log each day. This helps us both keep track of what works best for you, what gets in your way, and how you are feeling throughout the week.

Note: When you fill out the Tracking Sheet and the Daily Log, please do your best to be honest. You will not be judged about how much or little you have practiced, how strong or weak your urges are, or what behaviors you have or haven't engaged in during the week. The more honest you are on these forms, the more I can tailor your treatment to meet your needs. This will allow me to be more effective in helping you get closer to the kind of life you want to live. Also, please write any comments you have or anything that comes up during practice so we can talk about it at the next meeting.

MMT Session J
Mindful Assertiveness Skills: OFFER

- Review the week (the client's experiences, home practice, target behavior; 15–20 minutes).
- Engage in mindfulness practice: May You Be exercise (7–8 minutes).
- Introduce new topic: mindful assertiveness (15–20 minutes).
  - Discuss: Many people have difficulty effectively asking for their needs to be met.
  - Explain the OFFER acronym for mindful assertiveness. Discuss importance of being aware of other person's perspective.
  - Identify an applicable situation for mindful assertiveness in the client's life.
  - Work with client to write an informal "script" using OFFER format (*H-J2*).
  - Conduct an informal role play: The client practices OFFER; the therapist plays the target person.
    - ◆ Provide affirmations and constructive suggestions for improvement.
  - Assign new home practice: Engage in OFFER once this week.
- Wrap up and plan for upcoming week (5 minutes).
- Review home practice: guided audio (five times), BEST B (at least once daily), Daily Pleasant/Fulfilling Activity (once daily), *H-J2: Assertiveness OFFER*, Daily Log.

Needed for session (all therapist sheets and handouts for this session are at the end of the Session J guidelines):

- Mindfulness: May You Be (TS-J1)
- Assertiveness OFFER Examples (H-J1)
- Assertiveness OFFER (H-J2; two copies)
- Tracking Sheet (H-J3)
- Practice Summary (H-J4)
- Daily Log

SESSION J

This session provides opportunities for clients to further practice and generalize the OFFER acronym for communication.

Greet the Client and Review the Previous Week (15–20 Minutes)

See the instructions for home practice review at the end of the relevant session.

Engage in Mindfulness Practice: *TS-J1: May You Be* (7–8 Minutes)

The "May You Be" practice is a modification of the Buddhist loving-kindness or *metta* meditation. The name was changed not to deny credit, but because some clients in pilot trials were skeptical about a practice that sounds like its sole purpose is to promote love and kindness toward others. Although increasing love and kindness may be a welcome secondary outcome of the practice, the primary purpose in MMT is to help clients gain freedom from feeling controlled by their reactions to others. *Note:* The practice takes 5–6 minutes to complete. Due to time constraints, you will need to limit the discussion after the practice in order to have time for the rest of the material in the session. (The guided audio #5 includes an extended version of the "May You Be" practice. You do not have to assign that audio at the same time you conduct the practice in session.)

Introduce New Topic: Mindful Assertiveness Skills (15–20 Minutes)

Mindful assertiveness may reduce resentment and relational discord that are often cues for dysregulated behavior. Use of these skills can increase the likelihood that (1) the client gets her needs met and (2) the other person continues to feel positively toward the client.

Discuss: Many People Have Difficulty Effectively Asking for Their Needs to Be Met and/or Asking Others to Change Their Behavior

If the client is like a lot of people, she might think that people in her life should somehow know when her (the client's) needs are not being met. She may believe that if other people care about her, they will *just know* when she is upset or needs help—so she should not *have* to ask for her needs to be met. She may (or may not) also believe that being assertive is selfish or impolite. Thus, she may remain silent instead of asserting herself. However, the reality is that other people are not mind readers, and most people are not aware that someone's needs are not being met unless the person tells them. By choosing not to express needs, the client runs the risk of several negative consequences:

1. If the client does not express her needs, it is unlikely that her needs will be met and unlikely that others will change the behavior that she finds upsetting.

2. The client will probably feel a building resentment and anger at the other person for not meeting her needs and/or for continuing with behavior she finds upsetting.

   ▪ Eventually, built-up resentment can start to feel uncomfortable and exhausting—like she is tied up in knots inside.

   ▪ In other words, the client is the one who suffers.

3. Once resentment grows, it can get so strong that the client may not be able to hold it in. The client may then express her resentment (a) in a way that is more intense than she would have liked, (b) in ways that do not directly address the original situation in which the client felt her needs were not met, and/or (c) by engaging in dysregulated behavior. (Resentment and anger are often cues for dysregulated behavior.)

   ▪ Such methods are unlikely to be effective in getting the client's needs met, and (again) the client is probably the one who will experience negative consequences.

   ▪ Consequences may include ruptures in relationships, feeling guilty or embarrassed by the strength of her reaction, or facing the consequences of the target behavior.

Thus, the client can likely benefit by learning how to express her needs effectively.

As you go through the above explanation, ask the client about her own experiences, and tailor the explanation to fit her answers. Tell the client that she is not expected to express her needs in every situation. Instead, by learning OFFER assertiveness skills, she will have more of a choice as to whether or not to express her needs.

Finally, in contrast to the above explanation, some clients *do* report expressing their needs strongly and regularly. However, these clients may not do so effectively. They may have never learned effective ways to assert themselves, their strong emotions may have gotten in the way of such communication, and/or they may have experienced other environmental factors that have impeded their efforts at effective assertiveness. The OFFER can be beneficial for these clients by helping them communicate in a way that increases the chance of their needs being met.

Explain the OFFER Acronym for Mindful Assertiveness

OFFER ASSERTIVENESS

- O = *Other* (Express what the other person might be feeling or going through.)
- F = *Facts* (Tell the facts of the situation—not opinions or judgments.)
- F = *Tell your Feelings and/or the Consequences* of the situation for you. (Be nonjudgmental as you tell how you feel and/or what the consequences are for you. Be specific.)
- E = *Explain* (Explain what you want/need. *Be specific.* Don't assume that the person already knows.)
- R = *Reward* (Let the person know how respecting your request can be beneficial to her/him—even if it's just that you'll appreciate the person.)

Of course, the OFFER for mindful assertiveness (H-J1) is almost identical to the OFFER for mindfully refusing target behavior (H-I1). The OFFER for assertiveness is introduced in a separate session because (1) the OFFER for assertiveness reflects a different focus, and (2) clients often need to be exposed to the OFFER for two sessions before they master it.

Introduce the OFFER for assertiveness by first going through *H-J1: Assertiveness OFFER Examples.* Explain that use of the OFFER does not guarantee that the client will always get her needs met; however, using the OFFER *does increase* the chance that (1) the client will get what she wants, and (2) the other person will feel positive toward the client and the relationship after the client makes the request.

H-J1: Assertiveness OFFER Examples also includes an example of saying "no" to a request, to show that the OFFER can be used to refuse requests other than just those related to dysregulated behavior. However, since the previous week's discussion focused on refusing to engage in dysregulated behavior, the current week's discussion should focus on assertive requesting if possible.

Identify an Applicable Situation for Mindful Assertiveness in the Client's Life

Ask the client to think of a situation in which she might ask someone for help, ask for a need to be met, or ask someone to change a behavior. Potential examples include asking someone to:

- Not engage in the target behavior in the client's home.
- Not leave items that are cues for the target behavior in the client's home.
- Help the client with certain tasks or projects.
- Text or call in advance when the person anticipates being late or needs to cancel.
- Give the client a raise or vacation time (boss).
- Not use certain language or call the client certain names.
- Pay for half of expenses on a night out or in daily life.
- Help take care of a pet or child.
- Set aside a certain amount of time to talk every day.
- Not play certain sexist or obscene songs when the client or client's child is around.
- Fix something in the apartment (landlord or maintenance person).
- Allow client to pay off debt in installments.
- Stop encouraging the client to engage in behavior that is against the client's values.

If the client cannot think of a situation in which to use the OFFER, suggest a situation that has recently occurred and might recur. Provide suggestions based on your knowledge of the client.

Work with the Client to Write an Informal "Script" Using H-J2: Assertiveness OFFER

After the client has chosen a situation, complete the Assertiveness OFFER worksheet (*H-J2*). Before composing an OFFER for mindful assertiveness, instruct the client to:

1. *Decide what you want out of the situation.*
2. *Think about what the other person is going through at that moment.*

The first point is often less obvious than it seems, since people can get so caught up in strong emotions that they lose sight of what they really want out of a situation. For example, perhaps a person values a friendship and looks forward to spending time with the friend. If that friend cancels plans at the last minute twice in a row, the person may feel hurt, disappointed, and angry—and may express those feelings by lashing out at the friend, which may drive the friend away. Although such a reaction may be understandable, it does the opposite of what the person ultimately wants, which is to be able to spend time with the friend. A more effective response would be to share the disappointment about not getting to see the friend after expecting to do so—and then ask the friend to call or text in advance if she needs to cancel again. Thus, deciding what one wants out of a situation can be crucial before asserting oneself.

The second point (i.e., think about what the other person is going through at that moment) may be even more critical in assertiveness than it is for mindful refusal skills. The importance should be stressed before composing the OFFER and again as the OFFER is composed:

> *By showing the other person that you care enough about her [him] to take time to think about what she [he] is going through, you decrease the chance the other person will feel defensive, increase the chance the person will listen to you, and increase the chance the person will feel positively toward you after the conversation.*

The final instruction prior to composing the OFFER: *Write down what you want out of the situation. Be specific.* Being specific reduces the chance of confusion or disagreement. If the person in the example had simply said that she wanted the partner to share more of the housework, the partner could do dishes one extra night and technically be complying with the request. Instead, the person wrote: "I want my partner to share more of the housework by doing dishes or cooking dinner each night."

Compose the OFFER by asking the client for a response to each prompt and recording her replies. If the client's answers are judgmental, are too general, or in other ways do not seem to be effective, gently validate/affirm while also suggesting modifications. Write the answers in a conversational tone—not a stilted tone. Key points:

- *Facts:*
  - Be specific: Avoid generalizations such as *always* or *never*. If the client says, "You're always late," the other person will likely think of a time when he or she was *not* late—which can derail the OFFER. Instead, tell the client to be specific. For example: "I had to wait at restaurants by myself for more than an hour the last two times I saw you." Also avoid vagueness or opinions. Saying "You don't do your share of work" is an opinion that could lead to an argument. Saying, "I had to close the shop every night for the last 10 days" is a specific fact that cannot be disputed.
  - Be nonjudgmental by *focusing on facts*. If the client says, "You selfishly hog the TV every night," the other person will likely feel defensive and be less likely to be open to the client's request. A more effective option would be to factually describe the situation: "I've been wanting to watch the shows I recorded, but I haven't gotten to use the TV any night for the past week."

- *Feelings/consequences:*
  - Don't downplay the feelings/consequences, but *also do not exaggerate.*
  - Don't blame the other person. Instead of "You were insensitive" or "You don't value my time," a more effective response would be, "When you're late and I don't hear from you, I get worried that something happened to you. So I have trouble focusing on my work, plus I'm tense and upset by the time you get here."
- *Explain what you want:* Again, be clear and specific. If the client says, "Will you please spend less time on your phone when we're eating dinner?," the other person could spend 59 minutes on the phone instead of 60 and technically be complying with the client's request. Instead, a more effective request would be: "Will you please not check your phone when we're eating dinner?"
- *Reward:* The reward can be specific (helping the person with something the person needs, engaging in an activity with the person), but it often involves less concrete things like appreciating the other person, feeling like the person is a good friend, being less irritable around the person and so improving the relationship, being better company, etc.

  Additional key points:

- The other person may bring up tangents that can derail the conversation. In these cases, the client is advised to continue to stick to the main point.
  - Ineffective example:

    OTHER PERSON: But you've been late before. You do many things that bother me.

    CLIENT: I was late that one time, but you've been late the last three times.

    OTHER PERSON: You were late more than once. And that time last spring you were an hour late.

    CLIENT: It wasn't a full hour. (*Notice that the point of the OFFER has been lost.*)
  - Effective example:

    OTHER PERSON: But you've been late before. You do many things that bother me.

    CLIENT: We can talk about those later if you'd like, but right now I'm just asking you to text me from now on if you're going to be late.

- If the other person tries to change the subject without saying whether she or he will comply with the client's request, tell the client to gently but firmly bring the topic back to the request.
- If the person refuses the client's request, the client has the option to compromise. Ask if there is any compromise she is willing to make—and then generate possible options. However, strongly urge the client not to compromise immediately. Encourage her to first work to get the other person to agree to her full request.

Informal Role Play: Client Practices OFFER; Therapist Plays the Target Person

Again, you are strongly encouraged to conduct a role play despite your potential urges to avoid it. Clients often gain marked understanding and effectiveness from practicing the script in session.

Before setting up the role play, read the OFFER you've written aloud using a conversational tone. Then say you'd like to do a role play with the client practicing the OFFER, with you playing the person the client chose earlier. Normalize that most people dislike role plays, and validate that the role play will probably feel awkward and artificial.

- Listen as the client goes through the OFFER. Do your best not to jump in and provide assistance if at all possible. (Stay in character.)
- Once the client completes the OFFER, briefly try to sidetrack her—by attempting to change the subject or arguing gently. This allows the client to practice sticking to the main point. (Be sure to warn the client in advance that you will be arguing with her as part of the role play.)

Provide Affirmations and Suggestions for Improvement

Affirm the client's performance and provide constructive feedback. Briefly discuss additional ways the other person might react—as well as ways the client might respond to such reactions.

Assign the New Home Practice: H-J2: Assertiveness OFFER

Instruct the client to engage in at least one OFFER during the upcoming week. The simplest course would be to engage in the OFFER composed and practiced in session. Plan how and when the client will engage in the OFFER. Instruct her to write a sentence or two on the back of the sheet after conducting the OFFER to describe how it went. Give the client a second (blank) *H-J2: Assertiveness OFFER* sheet in case she wants to conduct another OFFER during the week.

Troubleshoot how the client will cope with urges to avoid doing the OFFER, and prepare her for being nervous before and during the time she conducts the OFFER. Remind her that the OFFER is not magic, and that she may not get what she wants even if she does the OFFER perfectly. However, remind her that the OFFER *does increase* the chance that (1) she will get what she wants, and (2) the other person will continue to feel positively toward the client and the relationship.

> The OFFER owes extensive credit to the DEAR MAN assertiveness skills from DBT (Linehan, 1993b) and, to a lesser extent, to the basic assertive and refusal skills from CBT. Although MMT integrates strategies from these and other empirically supported therapies throughout the treatment, the OFFER is one of the skills that is most directly related to its sources of inspiration.

Wrap Up and Plan for Upcoming Week (5 Minutes)

Remind the client about the rest of the home practice: guided audio (five times), BEST B (at least once daily, with encouragement to do more BEST Bs during routine activities), Pleasant/Fulfilling Activity (once daily), one *H-J2: Assertiveness OFFER*, and Daily Log.

Review the Home Practice the Week after Assigning *H-J2: Assertiveness OFFER*

Home practice is reviewed in the week following the above session.

- Review the Daily Log and Tracking Sheet as you normally would.
- If the client completed the OFFER successfully, affirm the success, validate the difficulty and effort, and ask about the experience. Briefly discuss times the client might use the OFFER in the future.
- If the client completed the OFFER but did not get the desired response, assess whether the result might be due to the environment or to the client's use of the OFFER. Affirm the client for engaging in the OFFER and validate discouragement. Problem solve for future situations, and encourage the client to do another OFFER in the near future.
- If the client did not engage in the OFFER, assess the obstacles.
  - If the client truly did not have a chance to conduct an OFFER (i.e., the target person was out of town or did not return the client's request to talk), discuss times in the near future when the OFFER might be used.
  - If the client had a chance but did not use the OFFER, further assess the obstacles and respond accordingly.
- Be sure to mention the OFFER in future sessions when you are aware of any situations that might benefit from mindful assertiveness.

"May You Be" Mindfulness Meditation: Therapist Script

Sit with both feet on the floor, hands in your lap. Allow your eyes to close. Three: Be aware of the sounds. (*Very slight pause*) Two: Be aware of the feelings of your feet against the floor, body against the chair or couch. (*Very slight pause*) One: Be aware of the physical sensations as you breathe in and out. (*Very slight pause*)

Sometimes we all feel a little disconnected from the world—or we forget that other people have inner struggles—which can make them seem much more powerful and less vulnerable than they are. This exercise can help us realize that other people also have struggles and vulnerabilities—which can help us feel more connected to the world, while also helping to free ourselves from feeling controlled by our reactions to others' behavior.

Now, think of someone you love or like a lot. You don't have to feel 100% positive about the person. That's very rare. But pick someone you generally feel positive about and care about. (*Slight pause*) Do you have someone in mind?

Now I'm going to read a list of intentions. You can think of them as wishes for the person, or as prayers, or as positive thoughts—whatever fits for you. I'm going to say an intention and then pause for you to repeat the intention in your mind toward the person. You may or may not feel the words you are saying in your mind. Do your best not to judge yourself. Any way you feel or don't feel is fine.

Now do your best to picture the person you've chosen, and then mentally repeat each intention directed toward the person.

CORE INTENTIONS

Note: Pauses should be just long enough for the client to mentally repeat each statement.

- May you be safe from danger. (*Slight pause*)
- May you be free from illness. (*Slight pause*)
- May you be free from suffering. (*Slight pause*)
- May you be at peace. (*Slight pause*)

You may have really felt the intentions toward the person, or you may have felt nothing. Or you may have felt something different. Any way is fine.

[*Repeat the Core Intentions—the bulleted statements above—once again.*]

Now I'd like you to picture someone you don't know very well. Maybe a neighbor you rarely talk with, a coworker you see in passing, or a store clerk you see regularly. (*Slight pause*) Do you have anyone in mind?

(continued)

It's easy to forget that people have entire lives outside of what we know about them—that the person has loved; has had times of feeling lonely, scared, and rejected; and has had illnesses just like anyone else. So now do your best to picture that person, and then mentally repeat each intention directed toward that person. Whatever you feel *or don't feel* is fine.

[*Read the Core Intentions from first bullet point to last bullet point, and then repeat a second time.*]

Now, I'd like you to think of someone you dislike. It might be someone whose actions have led to pain for you or people you care about—or just someone you don't like. (*Slight pause*) Do you have anyone in mind? [*If the client cannot think of anyone, suggest picking someone from the news or a celebrity. But first encourage the client to pick someone he or she knows personally.*]

When we don't like someone, it's easy to forget that the person has experienced sadness, illness, fear, and rejection, just like anyone. Remember that these intentions are not that the person has great happiness or success. You're just sending the intentions that the person isn't harmed, isn't seriously ill, and doesn't suffer. Regardless, it's OK if you don't feel the intentions as you say them—or even if you feel anger. Do your best not to judge yourself. Now repeat each statement in your head, directed toward that person.

[*Read the Core Intentions from first bullet point to last bullet point, and then repeat a second time.*]

Finally, I'd like you to think of yourself. Some people like to picture themselves when they were young and more vulnerable, but if you do, know that you're sending the intentions to yourself as you are today. Other people like to picture themselves as their current age. And some people prefer to imagine the intention being sent inside—to their heart or core. Do whatever works for you. And just remember that it's OK if you have difficulty. Whatever you feel—or don't feel—is fine.

[*Read the Core Intentions from first bullet point to last bullet point, and then repeat a second time.*]

Now gently allow your attention to come back into the room. (*Slight pause*) And whenever you're ready, allow your eyes to open. (*Slight pause*) What was that like for you?

Note: This exercise is a little longer than most of the short mindfulness practices. It generally takes 5–6 minutes. Thus, be extra careful not to spend much time on processing, or you might not have time for the rest of the lesson. Points for processing:

* Many people have trouble feeling much of anything as they do the exercise. That's fine.
* Many people have an especially difficult time feeling the intentions for the person they don't know well, the person they dislike, and/or themselves. Normalize any difficulty the client experiences. Remind clients that their ease or difficulty in feeling intentions toward the people in the exercise has nothing to do with whether they are or are not caring people.
* Suggest that clients practice this exercise on their own when they are feeling disconnected, vulnerable, or frustrated with others.

Mindful Assertiveness: OFFER (Examples)

Example 1: Asking for What You Want/Need

Beforehand:

1. Decide what you want out of the situation.

2. Also think about what the other person is going through at that moment.

Write down what you want out of the situation. Be nonjudgmental and specific.

I want my partner to share more of the work at home.

[Needs to be more specific. See alternate version below.]

I want my partner to share more of the work by doing the dishes or cooking dinner each night.

1. **O = OTHER** (Express what the other person might be feeling or going through.)

   I know you're probably tired after your long day, but I'd like to talk with you.
   [Or]

   I realize that your job is really rough right now, and I'm sorry it's so stressful for you. I know you're tired, but I'd like to talk to you about something.

2. **F = FACTS** (Tell the facts of the situation—not judgments or opinions.)

   In the last 2 weeks, I've cooked dinner every night, and I've washed dishes every night except 2.
   (*Note:* Saying, "You don't do your share of the work" would not be effective!)

3. **F = Tell your FEELINGS and/or the CONSEQUENCES** of the situation for you. (Be nonjudgmental as you tell how you feel and/or what the consequences are for you.)

   I've been feeling really pressured—and I'm so tired by the end of dinner and dishes that I find myself feeling irritable and on edge.

4. **E = EXPLAIN** (Explain what you want in a nonjudgmental way. *Be specific.* Don't assume that the person already knows. *Tell the person.*)

   Since we both work full time, I'd like you to help out with the dishes or dinner. What if I cooked dinner and you did the dishes? Or if we switched off?

5. **R = REWARD** (Let the person know ways that working with you can be beneficial to her/him—even if it's just that you'll appreciate the person.)

   If you'd do this, I'd really appreciate it. Thank you for being such a caring partner.

You could also add specifics:

If you'd help with the dishes, I'd feel less pressured, and we'd probably enjoy each other's company more [or wouldn't argue as much].
[Or]

If you'd do this, I'd have more time in the evenings so we could watch TV together like we used to enjoy.

(continued)

Example 2: Saying "No" When Someone Asks You to Do Something You Don't Want to Do

1. **O = OTHER** (Express what the other person might be feeling or going through.)

   I know it can be really stressful to try to find a babysitter.

2. **F = FACTS** (Tell the facts of the situation—not opinions or judgments.)

   But I already have a lot of stuff I have to do this evening. If I take care of your son, I'll have to stay up very late
   to get everything done.

3. **F = Tell your FEELINGS and/or the CONSEQUENCES of the situation for you.** (Be nonjudgmental as you tell how you feel and what the consequences are for you.)

   And then I'll be really tired and feel out of sorts all day tomorrow.

4. **E = EXPLAIN** (Explain that you are refusing. Be clear.)

   So I'm going to have to say "no" for tonight.

5. **R = REWARD** (Let the person know how respecting your request can be beneficial to her/him—even if it's just that you'll appreciate the person.)

   I appreciate your being a good enough friend that you'll understand. And maybe I can help out some other time
   when I'm not as busy.

Mindful Assertiveness: OFFER

Beforehand:

1. Decide what you want out of the situation.

2. Also think about what the other person is going through at that moment.

Write down what you want out of the situation. Be nonjudgmental and specific.

_____

_____

1. **O = OTHER** (Express what the other person might be feeling or going through.)

_____

_____

2. **F = FACTS** (Tell the facts of the situation—not judgments or opinions.)

_____

_____

3. **F = _Tell your FEELINGS and/or the CONSEQUENCES_ of the situation for you.** (Be nonjudgmental as you tell how you feel and/or what the consequences are for you.)

_____

_____

4. **E = EXPLAIN** (Explain what you want in a nonjudgmental way. _Be specific._ Don't assume that the person already knows. _Tell the person._)

_____

_____

5. **R = REWARD** (Let the person know ways that working with you can be beneficial to her/him— even if it's just that you'll appreciate the person.)

_____

_____

If the person refuses, work to be nonjudgmental while (1) pointing out that the issue is important to you, and (2) telling him/her that you appreciate the person for listening. If the person agrees to your request, be sure to thank him/her!

Tracking Sheet

Please write the day and what you did each day in the appropriate column.

Day	Audio: Five Times	BEST B: At Least Once Daily Where? When?	Pleasant/Fulfilling Activity	Comments (Optional)

Home Practice Summary: OFFER Assertiveness

1. **Do an audio practice at least 5 days this week.**

   Be sure to fill in the Tracking Sheet to record your practice.

2. **Do the BEST B at least once a day. (You're also encouraged to do a second BEST B each day while doing other activities).**

   You may also choose to do a "May You Be" on your own (without the audio), in place of a BEST B, for a couple of days. Be sure to fill in the Tracking Sheet to record your practice.

3. **Do one Pleasant/Fulfilling Activity or take one step toward a goal each day.**

   Be sure to fill in the Tracking Sheet to record your practice.

4. **Complete *H-J2: Mindful Assertiveness: OFFER* at least once if possible.**

   You can conduct the OFFER planned in session, or you can conduct a new OFFER that you plan on your own.

5. **Complete the Tracking Sheet and the Daily Log each day.**

   Fill out the Tracking Sheet and the Daily Log each day. This helps us both keep track of what works best for you, what gets in your way, and how you are feeling throughout the week.

Note: When you fill out the Tracking Sheet and the Daily Log, please do your best to be honest. You will not be judged about how much or little you have practiced, how strong or weak your urges are, or what behaviors you have or haven't engaged in during the week. The more honest you are on these forms, the more I can tailor your treatment to meet your needs. This will allow me to be more effective in helping you get closer to the kind of life you want to live. Also, please write any comments you have or anything that comes up during practice so we can talk about it at the next meeting.

CHAPTER 11

Acceptance/Empathy Module

MMT Session K
Freeing Yourself from Being Controlled and Taking Back Your Power, Part I: Acceptance and Tolerance

- Review the week (the client's experiences, home practice, and target behavior (15–20 minutes).
- Introduce new topic: accepting situations that can't immediately be changed (20–25 minutes).
  - Explain introduction from *H-K1: Freeing Yourself from Being Controlled: Acceptance.*
  - Discuss power of choosing to accept/tolerate; provide examples.
    - Accepting does not mean approving or liking.
    - Accepting does not mean giving up; one can still work for change.
  - Identify a situation that the client is having difficulty accepting and tolerating.
  - Explain exercises from *H-K1: Freeing Yourself . . . Acceptance.*
  - Conduct mindfulness practice: exercises from *H-K1.*
  - Discuss the client's experience with the exercises and offer feedback.
  - Assign home practice: Do the acceptance/tolerance exercises from *H-K1: Freeing Yourself . . . Acceptance.* (Can replace one BEST B per day.)
- Wrap up and plan for upcoming week (5 minutes).
- Home practice: guided audio (five times), BEST B (at least once daily), Pleasant/Fulfilling Activity (once daily), acceptance/tolerance exercises from *H-K1: Freeing Yourself . . . Acceptance* (can replace BEST B), Daily Log.

Needed for session (all therapist sheets and handouts for this session are at the end of the Session K guidelines):

- Freeing Yourself . . . Acceptance (H-K1; two copies)
- Tracking Sheet (H-K2)
- Practice Summary (H-K3)
- Daily Log

SESSION K

When a person has difficulty accepting and tolerating things that cannot be changed, the person may react to such things with distress and with urges to engage in target behavior. This session focuses on helping clients begin learning to accept and tolerate things that cannot be changed.

Greet the Client and Review the Previous Week (15–20 Minutes)

See the instructions for home practice review at the end of the relevant session.

Introduce New Topic: Accepting Situations That Can't Immediately Be Changed (20–25 Minutes)

Hand the client *H-K1: Freeing Yourself from Being Controlled: Acceptance (Taking Back Your Power)* and read the introduction:

> *When you refuse to accept and tolerate something you can't immediately change (a situation, actions of another person, etc.), you give that thing power over you. You let that thing have at least a little control over your emotions and/or actions. That thing has the power to (1) lead you to do things that hurt you in the long run [example: target behavior], and/or (2) get you so upset that you feel tied up in knots and ruminate about the thing. Either way, you are the one who suffers. This practice is about freeing yourself from being controlled and taking back your power by choosing to accept and tolerate the thing instead of letting it control your reactions.*
>
> > *Important: Accepting and tolerating something does not mean that you approve. Accepting is a way to free yourself from being controlled and to ease your own distress. You are not necessarily saying that you accept that the thing will stay the same forever, but you're accepting and tolerating that it is that way now. You might even work to change the thing, but you accept that it's the way it is now.*

Discuss the Importance of Accepting and Tolerating

Key points to discuss after reading the introduction to the worksheet include the following.

- [Ask the client:] Have you ever been so upset about something that seemed unfair that you walked around feeling tied up in knots inside? That can really wear you down after a while. Maybe you even had trouble sleeping because you were worrying about the thing or arguing about it with someone in your head. Over time, that can be exhausting. And when you feel like that, *you* are the one who suffers.

- [Emphasize the following:] By choosing to accept and tolerate something, you are not saying that you approve, and you are not "giving up." You may still hope that the thing changes—and you may still even work for change—but you are accepting that the thing is the way it is *right now*.

• For example, someone may hate the fact that some people in the world don't have enough to eat while other people are millionaires. He may do volunteer work for organizations that work to end world hunger. However, no matter how much he volunteers, he can't end all world hunger right at this moment. He could react by becoming so angry about the unfairness in the world that he becomes tied up in knots and has trouble sleeping—but that won't help anyone who is hungry. That will only cause *him* to suffer. Instead, he takes back his power by choosing to accept that hunger exists in the world. That doesn't mean he likes the fact or that he will stop working to end world hunger. It just means that he will work to accept the fact so that he doesn't suffer needlessly.

• Sometimes it's hard to choose to accept something that seems very upsetting, because it feels like accepting it means you're saying that the thing isn't a big deal and that you shouldn't be upset by it. But that's not the case. You can still be upset and think it's a big deal while also accepting and tolerating that the thing is happening at the moment. Accepting doesn't mean that you won't be angry or sad or worried. It means you're just choosing to decrease the thing's ability to control you and cause you even more misery.

Discuss the Power of Choosing to Accept Something That Can't Be Changed and Provide an Example (from Your Own Life, If Possible)

After discussing the above points, provide the client with an example of a time when someone did not accept a situation and suffered needlessly. A brief example from your own life (not too personal, of course) can be especially helpful, as it can decrease the chance that the client will feel judged or ashamed when discussing his own problems with acceptance. The following is a true example from an MMT therapist.

> When I moved across country, one of my best friends rode with me. We had 3 days to travel several hundred miles, so we were in a hurry. But when we got only a few blocks from the old apartment, the rental truck broke down. The repair person from the truck company didn't show up for over an hour, and then he kept leaving on lengthy trips to get additional parts. We were stranded in the 100-degree heat for several hours before the truck was fixed.
>
> After a few hours, my friend and I were invited to wait in the air-conditioned home of someone my friend knew in the neighborhood. I was so upset about the situation that instead I spent the time on my phone complaining to anyone I could reach at various offices of the truck rental company. I wanted to be told that that they'd get another repair person to us immediately, that they'd replace the truck with a new one, and that they'd immediately refund my money. Instead, they said that no other repair person was available, no other truck was available, and company rules did not allow refunds until the truck reached the destination. But I felt I was being treated so unfairly that I couldn't let it go. I just kept demanding to talk to supervisors and being put on hold for extended periods—only to be told again there was nothing anyone could do. The result? I didn't get anything I demanded. Instead, I became exhausted by pacing in the heat, I got a painful sunburn, and

I missed getting to spend time with my friend. I also felt tied up in knots because I was so upset. If I had just worked to accept and tolerate the situation once I realized it couldn't be changed, I could have saved myself some misery, and I might even have gotten some pleasure from the afternoon. But instead, I just needlessly increased my own suffering.

Note: The story happened many years ago, before the woman began practicing mindful acceptance. Let's assume she would handle the situation more effectively now.

Identify a Situation the Client Is Having Difficulty Accepting and Tolerating

If the client cannot think of a situation, you can offer suggestions based on what you know about the client—but be sure he chooses a situation that he *wants* to work to accept. Encourage the client to choose a situation that is minor to medium in intensity, as the client will likely need to build his mental muscles before choosing extremely distressing situations. Work with the client to describe the facts of the situation without judgment, and then write the description of the situation on *H-K1: Freeing Yourself from Being Controlled: Acceptance. Note:* Sometimes clients will find themselves needing to accept that the fact that they still have urges to engage in the target behavior; however, for the first round of practice, you are encouraged to find another situation if possible.

Explain Exercises in H-K1: Freeing Yourself from Being Controlled: Acceptance

Once the client has chosen something that has power over his reactions, explain that the bulleted exercises on H-K1 can help him gain freedom from feeling controlled. Briefly talk through the exercise on the sheet. [As always, replace *target behavior* with the client's specific behavior(s) before printing.] Most of the bulleted options are largely self-explanatory, but others include further explanation.

- *Purposely was aware of emotions/urges, sensations, and thoughts ["EST" of BEST B]. Did a quick mental body scan and breathed in to any tense areas. Allowed tension to release with the breath. Repeated until at least some tension was released.* [This does not need to take as long as a BEST B. The primary focus is the release of tension.]
- *Reminded myself that I can have emotions, urges, sensations, and thoughts without their controlling me.*
- *Breathed and thought, "It is as it is" on each inbreath and each outbreath.*
  - Mention that this bulleted point is rated as the most effective by a large number of clients. Explain that the client can use this point to get some emotional distance from the situation. Urge him to practice this bullet point even when he does not have the time or ability to close his eyes and engage in the practice for the full 3–5 minutes (e.g., when driving in traffic, when sitting in a meeting, at lunch with others).
- *Thought about the facts that had nothing to do with me that led to the situation as it is now. Worked to understand how these facts combined to lead up to the current situation. (This doesn't mean that it's OK that it happened or that I approve; it just means I want to free myself*

from being controlled by it.) This also helps remind me that things aren't always entirely about me, even when they affect me.

- Mention to the client that it can be easy to take things personally when upset; however, taking things personally tends to increase a person's distress. Taking things personally is also often the result of one's brain spewing out thoughts based on what one was taught to believe—as opposed to what might actually be occurring: that is, the facts.
  - ◆ Example 1: If you're running late to work and get caught in a traffic jam, it can be easy to think, "Bad things always happen to me. Of course traffic is bad on the day I'm running late!" Instead, look at the facts that have little or nothing to do with you. Two cars had a fender-bender, an occurrence that happens regularly and has nothing to do with you. Because hundreds of extra people are on the roads this time of day, the combination of the wreck and the extra traffic mean there's no way anything other than a traffic jam could have happened. The traffic jam also had nothing to do with you or the fact that you're late. (You still won't be happy that you're late, but accepting the traffic jam and your lateness may help you ease your distress.)
  - ◆ Example 2: You might be disappointed and irritated that your partner rarely gives you compliments. But if your partner was raised in a family that didn't give compliments (or perhaps the parent of the partner's identified gender did not give compliments), then it makes sense that your partner may have trouble remembering to compliment you. Perhaps it has more to do with your partner and your partner's experiences than it has to do with you, personally. You may still be disappointed, and you may want to work with your partner to improve communication, but perhaps you can accept that your partner has trouble giving compliments at this time.

- *[If the thoughts involve a person:] Thought about or imagined other things in the person's life that he/she might be concerned, sad, scared, and/or insecure about. This does not mean that I approve of the person's behavior or that I like the person—but just that I can feel sympathy for her/him as a human being.*
  - When you think of another person as all-confident and capable, it can be easy to feel weak and vulnerable by comparison. In other words, it can be easy to give that person the power to get you tied up in knots or do things that can have negative consequences for you. But by thinking of the vulnerabilities and struggles of another person, you can gain sympathy and perhaps even a little pity for that person. This can allow you to gain back your power—instead of letting that person's behavior have power over you. Thus, you can decrease the chance that you'll react in ways that have negative consequences for you.
  - Note: Saying that the person's behavior has power over you does not mean that the person chose to have power over you or that the person even knows it is happening.

- *Said a prayer, a request to the universe, or a request to my own inner strength to help me accept and tolerate the situation so I can have freedom from being controlled by it.*

- *Took a moment to see if I could find some meaning or value out of the situation that could help me accept and tolerate it. (This does not mean that I think it's OK that the thing happened.)*
  - Example 1: Someone who was anxious in social situations reported that although she wished she did not get so anxious, she believed that her difficulties caused her to be a kinder person who was more caring of others who might also feel shy and anxious. Thus,

she found meaning by working to talk to others who seemed to be feeling anxious and left out.

- Example 2: Someone whose ex had cheated on him said that he was now wiser about the type of person he chooses for a relationship.
- Note: Clients do not have to try to find meaning or value in situations if they do not want to do so.

Mindfulness Practice: Exercise from H-K1: Freeing Yourself . . . Acceptance

Once you have read and explained all the bullet points to the client, bring the focus back to the situation the client wrote earlier. Tell the client that you will lead him through some of the acceptance exercises now. Ask him to close his eyes as you read through each of the bullet points—leaving enough time for the client to mentally do each practice for a few moments between bullet points. Use the information you have gleaned from the client to tailor the relevant bullet points to fit the situation. Return to the "It is as it is" bullet point a few times between other bullet points. After the practice, discuss the client's experience and provide feedback.

- Remind the client that acceptance and tolerance do not mean that he will never be upset, angry, or sad. Instead, acceptance helps free the client from being controlled by a situation. One can be upset, angry, or sad about something without being tied up in knots or totally consumed by the situation.
- If the client said he did not feel any more accepting of the situation after doing the exercises, remind him that it takes time to build emotional muscles, and that acceptance exercises often take practice to become effective. In addition, the ability to accept will tend to wax and wane, so repeated practice is often needed to maintain acceptance and tolerance. Encourage the client to keep practicing several times in the upcoming week.

Assign Home Practice: H-K1: Freeing Yourself from Being Controlled: Acceptance

The home practice is to engage in the acceptance/tolerance exercises from *H-K1: Freeing Yourself from Being Controlled: Acceptance*. Instruct the client to do the exercises for the situation he wrote down in the session. Advise the client to try out all of the bullet points the first few times he practices, but then to feel free to focus on three or four favorites if he chooses. Different bullet points might also work more effectively for different situations. So each time the client does the acceptance practice, he has the choice of going through all the bullet points briefly—or instead spending time only on specific bullet points. Do not try to force the client to practice a bullet point if he clearly does not want to do so. For example, if the client does not want to find value out of the situation, respect him enough to let him choose.

Although the exercises are not assigned as daily practice, instruct the client to do the acceptance exercises at least three times in the upcoming week. The client only needs to complete the worksheet one of those times. The acceptance/tolerance exercises can replace one BEST B per day, although the client is free, of course, to do the exercises in addition to the BEST B. Also provide the client with an additional copy of H-K1 in case he wants to do the exercises for another situation as the week progresses.

Wrap Up and Plan for Upcoming Week (5 minutes)

Remind the client about the rest of the home practice: guided audio (five times), BEST B (at least once daily, with encouragement to do more BEST Bs during routine activities), Pleasant/ Fulfilling Activity (once daily), *H-K1: Freeing Yourself from Being Controlled: Acceptance* (at least three times during the week; can replace one BEST B per day), Daily Log.

Review the Home Practice the Week after Assigning *H-K1: Freeing Yourself from Being Controlled: Acceptance*

Home practice is reviewed in the week following the above session.

- Review the Daily Log, the Tracking Sheet, and the client's week as you normally would.
- If the client practiced the acceptance/tolerance exercises, provide affirmations and process what the experience was like for him. Encourage him to continue practicing.
- If he says the exercise didn't work, assess what he means by "didn't work."
  - Clients often think successful practice of acceptance/tolerance means that they are no longer at all upset by a situation. Remind the client that the purpose of acceptance and tolerance is not to become OK with everything that happens, like some sort of stereotypical Zen zombie. Instead, the purpose is to help lessen the amount of control the situation has over him. If the client had any moments when he felt less tied up in knots or less consumed by a situation, then the practice worked at least a little. If the client had times when he might have normally engaged in his target behavior in reaction to the situation but didn't, then the practice worked at least a little.
    - If he says he was not able to accept the situation at all, remind him that it takes time to build emotional muscles, and that these exercises often take practice to become effective.
    - Briefly walk the client through the bullet points to assess his experience. Gently provide feedback to increase effectiveness, if needed.
- Encourage the client to keep practicing acceptance/tolerance—even when not assigned. Be alert for relevant times to suggest acceptance/tolerance in the future.

Freeing Yourself from Being Controlled: Acceptance (Taking Back Your Power)

When you refuse to accept and tolerate something you can't immediately change (a situation, actions of another person, etc.), you give that thing power over you. You let that thing have at least a little control over your emotions and/or actions. That thing has the power to (1) lead you to do things that hurt *you* in the long run (ex: target behavior) and/or (2) get you so upset that you feel tied up in knots and ruminate about the thing. Either way, *you* are the one who suffers. This practice is about freeing yourself from being controlled and taking back your power by choosing to accept and tolerate the thing instead of letting it control your reactions.

Important: Accepting and tolerating does *not* mean that you approve. Accepting is a way to free yourself from being controlled and to ease your own distress. You are not necessarily saying that you accept that the thing will stay the same forever, but you're accepting and tolerating that it is that way *now*. You might even work to change the thing, but you accept that it's the way it is now.

Choose something that feels like it has power over your reactions. Be sure to pick something that you want to work to accept and tolerate. Write the facts, without opinions or judgments.

_____

_____

Take a few breaths and think about the thing you wrote above. Think about the facts; steer your mind away from judgments. Then do some combination of the following exercises for 3–5 minutes. Circle what you did.

- Was purposely aware of emotions, urges, sensations, and thoughts ["EST" of BEST B]. Did a quick mental body scan and breathed in to any tense areas. *Allowed tension to release with the breath.* Repeated until at least some tension was released.

- Reminded myself that I can have emotions, urges, sensations, and thoughts without them controlling me.

- Breathed and thought, "It is as it is" on each inbreath and each outbreath.

- Thought about the facts that had nothing to do with me that led to the current situation. Worked to understand how these facts combined to lead up to the situation. (This doesn't mean that it's OK that it happened or that I approve; it just means I want to free myself from feeling controlled by it.) This also helps remind me that things aren't always entirely about me, even when they affect me.

- [If involving another person] Thought about circumstances in the person's life that may have contributed to the thing I'm having trouble accepting. Worked to understand the situation based on the person's history and current circumstances. Did my best to steer clear of judgments and accept the thing about the person. (This doesn't mean I'm happy about the thing. It just means I want to accept it so I can free myself from feeling controlled by it.)

- [If involving another person] Thought about or imagined other things in the person's life that he/she might be concerned, sad, scared, and/or insecure about. (This does not mean I approve of the behavior or like the person—just that I can feel sympathy for her/him as a human being.) Allowed myself to feel pity for the person.

- Said a prayer, a request to the universe, or a request to my own inner strength to help me accept and tolerate the situation so I can have freedom from feeling controlled by it.

- Took a moment to see if I could find some meaning or value out of the situation that could help me accept and tolerate it. (This does not mean I think it's OK or good that the thing happened.)

You can go back and forth between skills in the same practice. Describe your experience on the back.

_____

Tracking Sheet

Please write the day and what you did each day in the appropriate column.

Day	Audio: Five Times	BEST B: At Least Once Daily Where? When?	Pleasant/Fulfilling Activity	Comments (Optional)

Home Practice Summary:
Freeing Yourself from Being Controlled (Acceptance/Tolerance)

1. **Do an audio practice at least 5 days this week.**

   Be sure to fill in the Tracking Sheet to record your practice.

2. **Do the BEST B at least once a day. (You're also encouraged to do a second BEST B each day while doing other activities.)**

   Be sure to fill in the Tracking Sheet to record your practice.

3. **Do one Pleasant/Fulfilling Activity or take one step toward a goal each day.**

   Be sure to fill in the Tracking Sheet to record your practice.

4. **Complete *H-K1: Freeing Yourself from Being Controlled: Acceptance.***

   Do some combination of the acceptance/tolerance exercises at least three times this week. (You can substitute this practice for one BEST B each day if you'd like.)

5. **Complete the Tracking Sheet and the Daily Log each day.**

   Fill out the Tracking Sheet and the Daily Log each day. This helps us both keep track of what works best for you, what gets in your way, and how you are feeling throughout the week.

Note: When you fill out the Tracking Sheet and the Daily Log, please do your best to be honest. You will not be judged about how much or little you have practiced, how strong or weak your urges are, or what behaviors you have or haven't engaged in during the week. The more honest you are on these forms, the more I can tailor your treatment to meet your needs. This will allow me to be more effective in helping you get closer to the kind of life you want to live. Also, please write any comments you have or anything that comes up during practice so we can talk about it at the next meeting.

MMT Session L
Freeing Yourself from Being Controlled and Taking Back Your Power, Part II: Acceptance and Tolerance of Self and Others

- Review the week (the client's experiences, home practice, target behavior; 15–20 minutes).
- Introduce new topic: accepting self and others (20–25 minutes)
  - Further discussion of the benefits of working to understand and accept (1) people whom the client may not like, and (2) people with whom the client is angry.
  - Discuss (again) how acceptance does not equal approval.
  - Discuss the benefits of working to understand and accept oneself (while also still working to change behavior that interferes with a life that feels fulfilling).
  - Identify an inter-/intrapersonal situation that the client is having difficulty accepting/tolerating. May suggest a slight variation of situation from previous week if needed.
  - Conduct mindfulness practice: *H-L1: Freeing Yourself from Being Controlled: Acceptance of Self and Others.*
  - Assign home practice exercise options from *H-L1: Freeing Yourself . . . Self and Others* (can replace one BEST B). Focus on others or self if possible.
- Wrap up and plan for upcoming week (5 minutes).
- Home practice: guided audio (five times), BEST B (at least once daily), Pleasant/Fulfilling Activity (once daily), acceptance/tolerance exercises from *H-L1: Freeing Yourself* (*at least three times; can replace one BEST B daily*), Daily Log.

Needed for session (all therapist sheets and handouts for this session are at the end of the Session L guidelines):

- Freeing Yourself . . . Self and Others (H-L1; two copies)
- Tracking Sheet (H-L2)
- Practice Summary (H-L3)
- Daily Log

SESSION L

This session provides clients with further opportunities to practice and generalize acceptance skills. Although the topic is quite similar to that of the previous week, the session is modified to focus explicitly on accepting/tolerating self and others.

Greet the Client and Review the Previous Week (15–20 Minutes)

See the instructions for home practice review at the end of the relevant session.

Introduce New Topic: Working to Accept Self and Others (20–25 Minutes)

Pilot research, clinical observation, and client feedback have shown that clients are more likely to integrate the acceptance (*Freeing Yourself*) exercises into daily life if they are covered in two sessions instead of just one (Wupperman et al., 2012, 2018). This session focuses on acceptance of self/others even if the client chose self or others as the focus in the previous week, as acceptance of self and others is a core facet of MMT.

Further Discuss the Benefits of Working to Understand and Accept (1) People Whom the Client May Not Like, and (2) People with Whom the Client Is Angry

Remind the client:

- *Working to accept and tolerate another person or the person's behavior does not mean that you like or approve of the person or the behavior.*
- *There is nothing wrong with feeling angry or upset with another person. However, when you refuse to accept and tolerate something you can't immediately change, you can give that person the power to control you (whether that person wants the power or not).*
- *That person's behavior can then (1) lead you to engage in behaviors that hurt you in the long run, and/or (2) get you so upset that you feel tied up in knots inside.*
- *Either way, you are the one who suffers.*
- *The purpose of working to accept and tolerate another person's behavior is so you can take back your power and free yourself from being controlled by other people.*
- *You can still feel angry or annoyed without feeling like the person's behavior controls you.*

Discuss the Benefits of Working to Understand and Accept Oneself, While Also Still Working to Change Behavior That Interferes with a Life That Feels as Fulfilling as It Could

Key points are similar to those listed in Session K. In addition:

- *Some people think that the only way they can improve themselves is by refusing to accept things about themselves they do not like.*
- *The truth is the opposite. By refusing to understand and accept yourself, you are likely to*

increase your feelings of hopelessness and self-hatred, and decrease your motivation. The result is that you (1) decrease your chances of improvement, and (2) allow the things you don't like about yourself to control your life.

- *Understanding and accepting yourself does not mean giving up. You can still work to change parts of yourself while accepting how you are at the moment. By working to understand and accept yourself, you increase your chances of being able to improve yourself in ways that move you toward a more fulfilling life.*

  - For example, one client was self-critical because she had reached her current age with no high school degree and only an entry-level job. Instead of continuing to tell herself that she was a failure, she worked to understand the basic reality that given some of her struggles, it was understandable that she had had difficulty finishing school and maintaining a good job. Instead of being controlled by self-judgment, she worked to accept the fact that she currently had a low-paying, physically demanding job—while also planning to look for other jobs once she established a more stable employment history.

- *Of course, we all have things about ourselves that cannot be changed. If you refuse to accept those things, they can become the primary focus of your life. But by working to understand and accept the things about yourself that can't be changed, you decrease the control that those things have over your life. You take back some of your power.*

  - One client's former husband divorced her at least partially because she had been so caught up in her target behavior. The client eventually attended treatment and moved past the target behavior, but it was too late to win back her ex-husband. Instead of continuing to ruminate about the lost relationship and berate herself for "ruining everything," the client worked to accept the reality that, based on her history, it made sense that the target behavior controlled her life for a while. She wasn't happy about it, but she worked to accept that her marriage was over. Accepting that fact helped ease her misery and free her to focus on her current life.

Work with the Client to Identify a Situation Involving Self or Others That the Client Is Having Difficulty Accepting and Tolerating

The client may choose a new situation or a slight variation on the situation chosen the previous week, depending on need. Situations often chosen by clients include working to accept:

- Difference in communication styles with partner, friend, child, or parent
- Behaviors by others with which the client feels irritated or angry
- Feeling rejected, criticized, or unsupported by a friend, romantic interest, family member, boss, etc.
- Relationship breakups
- Still having urges to engage in the target behavior
- Some of the negative consequences that have occurred because of the behavior
- Feeling socially anxious
- Not having the job, level of education, relationship, house, car, or other achievement/ security the person feels that she *should* have achieved
- Feeling treated unfairly by others

Work with the client to describe the facts of the situation without judgment, and then write the description of the situation on the *H-L1: Freeing Yourself* sheet.

Engage in Mindfulness Practice, Part II: Exercises from H-L1: Freeing Yourself from Being Controlled: Acceptance of Self and Others

Briefly talk through the bullet-pointed exercise options on *H-L1: Freeing Yourself,* customizing any to fit the client's current situation, if needed. Then ask the client to close her eyes (perhaps setting up the practice with the standard "three, two, one" induction) and lead the client through the exercises for approximately 5 minutes. You may read down the list or jump around. (Return to "It is as it is" between some of the other, more complex bullet points.) Afterward, process the client's reactions and answer any questions. Affirm, reflect, and validate.

Assign Home Practice: Acceptance/Tolerance Exercises from H-L1: Freeing Yourself from Being Controlled: Acceptance of Self and Others

Instruct the client to practice at least three times in the upcoming week. Although the client is instructed to do the exercises for the chosen situation, encourage her to also do the exercises for other situations in which she might benefit from working to understand and accept. The goal is for the client to begin automatically doing an acceptance exercise whenever she could benefit from doing so. (The acceptance exercises can replace one BEST B per day, although the client is free, of course, to do the acceptance exercises in addition to the BEST B. The client can record these practices under BEST B on the Tracking Sheet.)

Wrap Up and Plan for Upcoming Week (5 Minutes)

Remind the client about the rest of the home practice: guided audio (five times), BEST B (at least once daily, with encouragement to do more BEST Bs during routine activities), Pleasant/Fulfilling Activity (once daily), multiple practices from *H-L1: Freeing Yourself from Being Controlled: Acceptance of Self and Others* (three times; can replace one BEST B per day), Daily Log.

Review the Home Practice the Week after Assigning *H-L1: Freeing Yourself from Being Controlled: Acceptance of Self and Others*

Home practice is reviewed in the week following the above session.

- Review the Daily Log, the Tracking Sheet, and the client's week as you normally would.
- If the client practiced the acceptance/tolerance exercises, provide affirmations and process what the experience was like for her. Encourage her to continue practicing.
- If she says the exercises didn't work, assess what she means by "didn't work."
  - Clients often think that successful practice of acceptance/tolerance means that they are no longer at all upset by a situation. Remind the client that the purpose of the exercise is not be become OK with everything that happens. Instead, the purpose is to help free herself

from feeling *as* controlled by the situation. If the client had any moments when she felt less consumed by a situation, then the practice worked at least a little. If the client had times when she might have normally engaged in the target behavior in reaction to the situation but didn't, then the practice worked at least a little.

◆ If the client says that she was not able to accept the situation, remind her that it takes time to build emotional muscles, and that these exercises often take practice to become effective.

◆ Walk the client through the exercises to assess her experience. Gently provide feedback to increase effectiveness, if needed.

● Encourage the client to keep practicing acceptance/tolerance in the future—even when not assigned. Be alert for relevant times to suggest it in the future.

Freeing Yourself from Being Controlled:
Acceptance of Self and Others (Taking Back Your Power)

When you refuse to accept something about yourself or someone else that you can't immediately change (actions, characteristics, etc.), you give that thing power over you. You let that thing have at least some control over your emotions or actions. That thing has the power to: (1) lead you to do things that hurt *you* in the long run (ex: <u>target behavior</u>, avoid situations, say things you regret) and/or (2) get you so upset that you feel tied up in knots (and think about the thing so much that it gets in the way of your life). Either way, *you* are the one who suffers. This practice is about freeing yourself from being controlled and taking back your power by choosing to accept and tolerate the thing instead of letting it control your reactions.

Important: Accepting and tolerating does *not* mean you are giving up or that you approve. Accepting is a way to free yourself from being controlled and to ease your distress. You are not necessarily saying you accept that the thing will stay the same forever, but you're accepting and tolerating that it is the way it is *now*. You might even work to change the thing if that's possible, but you accept the way it is now.

Choose something that feels like it has power over your reactions. Be sure to pick something that you want to work to accept and tolerate. Write the facts, without opinions or judgments.

_____

_____

Take a few breaths and think about the thing you wrote above. Think about the facts; steer your mind away from judgments. Then do some combination of the following exercises for 3–5 minutes. Circle what you did.

- Was purposely aware of emotions, urges, sensations, and thoughts ("EST" of BEST B). Did a quick mental body scan and breathed in to any tense areas. *Allowed tension to release with the breath.* Repeated until at least some tension was released.

- Reminded myself that I can have emotions, urges, sensations, and thoughts without them controlling me.

- Breathed and thought, "It is as it is" on each inbreath and each outbreath.

- Thought about the facts that had nothing to do with me that led to the current situation. Worked to understand how these facts combined to lead up to the situation. (This doesn't mean that it's OK that it happened or that I approve; it just means I want to free myself from feeling controlled by it.) This also helps remind me that things aren't always entirely about me, even when they affect me.

- (If involving another person) Thought about circumstances in the person's life that may have contributed to the thing I'm having trouble accepting. Worked to understand the situation based on the person's history and current circumstances. Did my best to steer clear of judgments and accept the thing about the person. (This doesn't mean I'm happy about the thing. It just means I want to accept it so I can free myself from feeling controlled by it.)

- (If involving another person) Thought about or imagined other things in the person's life that he/she might be concerned, sad, scared, and/or insecure about. (This does not mean I approve of the behavior or like the person—just that I can feel sympathy for her/him as a human being.) Allowed myself to feel pity for the person.

- Said a prayer, a request to the universe, or a request to my own inner strength to help me accept and tolerate the situation so I can have freedom from feeling controlled by it.

- Took a moment to see if I could find some meaning or value out of the situation that could help me accept and tolerate it. (This does not mean I think that it's OK or good that the thing happened.)

You can go back and forth between skills in the same practice. Describe your experience on the back.

Tracking Sheet

Please write the day and what you did each day in the appropriate column.

Day	Audio: Five Times	BEST B: At Least Once Daily Where? When?	Pleasant/Fulfilling Activity	Comments (Optional)

Home Practice Summary: Freeing Yourself from Being Controlled (Acceptance/Tolerance of Self and Others)

1. **Do an audio practice at least 5 days this week.**

   Be sure to fill in the Tracking Sheet to record your practice.

2. **Do the BEST B at least once a day. (You're also encouraged to do a second BEST B each day while doing other activities.)**

   Be sure to fill in the Tracking Sheet to record your practice.

3. **Do one Pleasant/Fulfilling Activity or take one step toward a goal each day.**

   Be sure to fill in the Tracking Sheet to record your practice.

4. **Complete *H-L1: Freeing Yourself from Being Controlled: Self/Others.***

   Do some combination of the acceptance/tolerance exercises at least three times this week. (You can substitute the practice for one BEST B each day if you'd like.)

5. **Complete the Tracking Sheet and the Daily Log each day.**

   Fill out the Tracking Sheet and the Daily Log each day. This helps us both keep track of what works best for you, what gets in your way, and how you are feeling throughout the week.

Note: When you fill out the Tracking Sheet and the Daily Log, please do your best to be honest. You will not be judged about how much or little you have practiced, how strong or weak your urges are, or what behaviors you have or haven't engaged in during the week. The more honest you are on these forms, the more I can tailor your treatment to meet your needs. This will allow me to be more effective in helping you get closer to the kind of life you want to live. Also, please write any comments you have or anything that comes up during practice so we can talk about it at the next meeting.

MMT Session M
Experiencing and Expressing Understanding

- Review the week (the client's experiences, home practice, target behavior; 15–20 minutes).
- Engage in mindfulness practice: Sounds (5 minutes).
- Introduce new topic: experiencing and expressing understanding (15–20 minutes).
  - Explain how expressing understanding of others can help (1) improve relationships, (2) give one the power to make others feel good, and (3) help further free oneself from feeling controlled by one's reactions to others.
  - Explain and discuss *H-M1: Expressing Understanding*.
  - Introduce and discuss *H-M2: Examples of ETC (**E**xpressing Understanding, **T**hanking, **C**omplimenting)*.
  - Assign home practice: Track *ETC* skills (*H-M3*) throughout the week.
- Wrap up and plan for upcoming week (5 minutes).
- Home practice: guided audio (five times), BEST B (at least once daily), Pleasant/Fulfilling Activity (once daily), *H-M3: ETC*, Daily Log.

Needed for session (all therapist sheets and handouts for this session are at the end of the Session M guidelines):

- Mindfulness: Sounds (TS-M1)
- Expressing Understanding (H-M1)
- Examples of ETC (H-M2)
- ETC (H-M3)
- Tracking Sheet (H-M4)
- Practice Summary (H-M5)
- Daily Log

SESSION M

This session focuses on helping clients experience and express empathy, which can help clients (1) improve relationships and (2) gain freedom from feeling controlled by their reactions to others.

Greet the Client and Review the Previous Week (15–20 Minutes)

See the instructions for home practice review at the end of the relevant session.

Engage in Mindfulness Practice: *TS-M1: Sounds* (5 Minutes)

See the therapist sheet (TS-M1).

Introduce New Topic: Experiencing and Expressing Understanding (15–20 Minutes)

Clients may question how expressing understanding of others can help them work to stop their own dysregulated behavior. Some clients may also report that they are tired of being the one who has to "do the work" in relationships. They may also be concerned that the introduction of the topic implies that you assume they are not being as understanding as you feel they should. Thus, it's important to be explicit in explaining how the skill can help the client, while also explaining that even people who are already very understanding (including therapists!) can usually be helped by purposely working to increase their expression of that understanding.

Explain How Expressing Understanding of Others Can Benefit the Client

Explain that routinely expressing understanding can:

1. Improve relationships (which can increase positive emotions, decrease conflict, and increase social support);
2. Give the client the power to make other people feel good (which can help the client feel more powerful);
3. Further free the client from feeling controlled by his reactions to other people; and
4. Help the client gain and maintain freedom from his target behavior.

Explain and Discuss H-M1: Expressing Understanding

The handout provides instructions on basic ways of expressing understanding: (1) simple reflection, (2) reflection of potentially underlying emotions, (3) sharing understanding based on similar experiences, (4) expressing understanding even when one does not agree with the other person, and (5) expressing affirmation about appropriate details even when one does not fully agree with the other person.

As you read the sheet aloud, suggest examples of situations you think would be relevant to the client, and ask the client to share examples in his own life of how he might express understanding to people in various circumstances. Check to assess the client's understanding after each section. You're also encouraged to share any of your own experiences of having someone express understanding to you. Here's an actual example once shared by a therapist:

> *I was once sitting at my desk toward the end of a week in which everything seemed to go wrong. After I told the project manager about the most recent obstacle, she said, "This must be exhausting for you—especially since I know you care so much about this project." I did feel exhausted—and although the project manager's words did not make everything OK, I did feel a little comforted just hearing that someone else understood my reaction. I also felt gratitude for the person—which I still remember all this time later. So even though I teach the importance of expressing understanding, I still felt good when someone expressed understand toward me. It helped me feel just a little bit better. Even a small, passing comment can have the power to affect another person.*

The last two sections (expressing understanding and affirming even when one does not agree) tend to be the most difficult. Remind the client that the purpose of these and all sections of the handout are to help improve the client's relationships, help him have more power, and free him from feeling controlled by his reactions to other people. (In other words, the practices will ultimately help the client.) He is not *required* to practice all sections of the handout, but he is encouraged to at least try each section a few times—to test how he is affected.

Introduce and Explain H-M2: Examples of ETC

Explain the importance of compliments and expressions of gratitude:

> *As we get caught up in day-to-day life, it can be easy to notice things about a person that bother you or that you wish were different—but then take for granted things that you like and appreciate. But by working to notice and comment on the things you like or appreciate, you can gain the same benefits of expressing understanding. You can improve relationships, have the power to help someone feel a little better, and free yourself from being controlled—by your reactions to others, and by the target behavior. So what I'd like you to do this week is really work to find times when you can express understanding, thank people for doing things you appreciate, and compliment people for things you like about them. Let's look at some examples.*

Read through the ETC examples with the client. Point out that the ETC acronym is the same as the abbreviation for etcetera (etc.)—which might help the client remember it. Ask the client to think of possibilities for using the ETCs in his own life. Help him generate ideas if he has trouble in this area. (Be sure to instruct the client to only express gratitude or give compliments that he *really means*.) If the client has trouble generating ideas, assess whether his difficulty is related to trouble with understanding ETCs or with lack of social support. If the latter, gently suggest that the ETC week could be the perfect time to start (1) regaining/repairing contact with important others and/or (2) taking steps toward making new social connections. Validate the difficulty, as well as any anxiety, general reluctance, or feelings of shame or guilt that might exist in these areas.

Assign Home Practice: Use ETCs throughout the Week and Track with H-M3: ETC

Instruct the client to do his best to do at least one of the following each day: express understanding, thank someone, and/or compliment someone. Warn him that it can be difficult to find opportunities to offer ETCs unless he works hard to find chances to do so. Encourage him to work hard to find opportunities throughout the week in a variety of circumstances. Offering thanks and compliments can be simpler than expressing understanding, so encourage the client to focus particularly on expressing understanding. After each ETC, he is instructed to write down just a few words to remind himself of what he did, so he can discuss it with you the following session. In addition, ask the client to be mindful of how he feels each time he offers an ETC. Be sure to affirm the client if he seems eager to offer ETCs or reports that ETCs are natural for him. Affirming kindness and empathy can help the client become more fully aware of these qualities in himself and derive more value from focusing on these qualities in daily life.

Wrap Up and Plan for Upcoming Week (5 Minutes)

Remind the client about the rest of the home practice: guided audio (five times), BEST B (at least once daily, with encouragement to do more BEST Bs during routine activities), Pleasant/Fulfilling Activity (once daily), multiple ETC practices (*H-M1*), Daily Log.

Review the Home Practice the Week after Assigning
H-M1: Expressing Understanding

Home practice is reviewed in the week following the above session.

* Review the Daily Log, the Tracking Sheet, and the client's week as you normally would.
* If the client practiced ETCs, affirm and process what the experience was like for him.
  * Ask what he noticed about other people's reactions.
  * Ask what he felt like after offering ETCs.
    * Many clients report that they felt pleasure or even "warmth" when offering ETCs. If so, affirm. If not, validate and assure the client that just doing the ETCs are helpful in and of themselves.
  * If the client tended to focus on one activity (E, T, or C) to the exclusion of others, affirm the activities he did do, assess what got in the way of using the others, and encourage him to use more of the others in the following week
* If the client did not do any ETCs, assess the obstacles and respond accordingly.
  * Validate the difficulty and help the client generate ideas for offering ETCs in the upcoming week. Assign ETCs again—along with the new home practice.
* Encourage the client to keep practicing ETCs in the future—even when not assigned.

Mindfulness: Sounds—Therapist Script (5 Minutes)

Sit up, with your hands in your lap, feet on the floor. And allow your eyes to close. Three: Be aware of various sounds. (*Slight pause*) Two: Be aware of the feelings of your feet against the floor, body against the chair. (*Slight pause*) One: Be aware of your breathing—the physical sensations as you inhale and exhale. (*Pause*)

Now, gently shift your awareness away from physical sensations and back to the sounds. (*Slight pause*) Open your awareness to the sounds around you. (*Pause about 3 seconds*) Perhaps you may notice sounds in front of you (*pause*), on either side of you (*pause*), or behind you (*pause*). Some sounds may seem to be very close to you (*slight pause*); others may seem to be farther away. (*Pause about 5 seconds*) Some sounds may seem to take up most of your attention and overshadow other sounds. Allow yourself to be aware of those sounds (*slight pause*), and then see if you can also be aware of other sounds that might be softer and less distinct. (*Pause about 5 seconds*)

Open your attention to sounds that might be occurring between other sounds. (*Pause about 5 seconds*) Notice if you find yourself judging the sounds. Notice if you find yourself wishing that some sounds were softer or that some sounds would even go away. If this happens, gently bring your attention away from your *reactions* and instead focus on just being aware of the sounds themselves. (*Pause about 5 seconds*) Allow yourself to be curious about whether you can notice anything new about the sounds— any qualities about any of the sounds or combination of sounds you haven't noticed before. (*Pause about 5 seconds*) Notice how easy it is to get distracted by thoughts—how thoughts about your life can take you away from being fully aware of the sounds. When you notice yourself getting caught up in thoughts, give yourself credit for noticing, and then gently bring your awareness back to the sounds. (*Pause about 5 seconds*) See if you can find any rhythms or patterns in the sounds. (*Pause about 5 seconds*) Allow yourself to have a sense of curiosity about all the sounds that are happening around you—including sounds you may not even have noticed until this practice. (*Pause about 5 seconds*)

And now I'm going to be quiet for a while, and just allow yourself to be aware of the sounds. (*Pause 10–15 seconds*) When your attention wanders, just give yourself credit for noticing—bring your attention back to your breathing for a moment—and then gently guide your attention back to the sounds. (*Pause about 10 seconds*) As you go through the day, remember that if you start getting caught up in the events of life, you can take a moment to mentally step back and allow your mind to be still as you focus on sounds. (*Pause about 5 seconds*) And now, three: Gently bring your attention back to your breathing. (*Slight pause*) Two: Be aware of the sensations of your body against the chair and your feet against the floor. (*Slight pause*) One: Be aware of the sounds for one last moment. (*Slight pause*) And whenever you're ready, allow your eyes to open. (*Pause*) What was that like for you?

Expressing Understanding (Letting the Other Person Know You Can See Things from Her/His Perspective)

This will benefit <u>you</u> by improving your relationships, giving you the power to make others feel good, and helping free you from feeling controlled by others' actions.

There are different ways of expressing understanding:

1. **Really listen, and then reflect what the other person said.**
   Don't parrot every word, but instead reflect the general idea.
   > Sounds like you've had a busy day.
   > You did all that work and they didn't even act like they appreciated it!
   > So you've spent your entire day responding to other people's problems
   > You didn't get much sleep last night!

2. **Reflect what they might be feeling. (But let them correct you if you are wrong.)**
   > That must be really stressful.
   > That sounds sad.
   > You seem concerned.
   > How frustrating!
   > I bet you're excited!
   > Sounds like you had fun.
   > You must be tired after such a long day.

3. **If you can understand how they feel, then *tell them*.**
   > I can understand how you'd feel angry.
   > I'd be scared, too.
   > I'm sad to hear that you had to go through that.

   If you have been in a similar situation, tell them briefly—but don't turn the focus to yourself.

   Understanding example: "My friend used to say that same thing to me, so I know that it hurts."

   Self-focused example: "My friend used to say the same thing to me. One time, I got home late and I was trying to make a sandwich, and he called me and started saying . . ." (and so on).

4. **Show that you're doing your best to see it from the other person's perspective, even if you don't feel that way yourself; look for how the other person's feelings, thoughts, or actions make sense considering their history and current situation, even if you don't agree.**
   > I wish you wouldn't leave, but I can see that it's important to you.
   > I don't feel that way about it, but I can understand how you could.
   > I didn't mean to ignore you, but I can see that you thought I did—and so I can understand how you would feel upset about that.

5. **If you can find *anything* to compliment or affirm, do so—even if you don't agree with all of the person's actions. (This can be very difficult.)**
   > I admire you for caring so much about something, even though I wish you wouldn't go.
   > I didn't mean to ignore you, but I can see that you thought I did. I appreciate your trusting me enough to tell me. Can we talk about it?
   > I know it had to be difficult to tell me that. I appreciate your honesty.

ETC (Expressing Understanding, Thanking, or Complimenting) Example

Do *at least* one *E, T,* or *C* each day. Write down who you said it to and a short note about what you said. Focus especially on the *E—Expressing Understanding.*

	Expressed Understanding	**Thanked**	**Complimented**
Mon:	My roommate: Sounds like you had a rough day. I bet you're exhausted.		
Tue:	Relative: I know you're sad about your dog being sick. I'm sad that you have to go through that.	My friend: Thanks for listening. I really appreciate it.	My friend: Your food is always delicious. You're a great cook.
Wed:	My nephew: I can understand how you'd want to play after being at school, but you have to do your homework before you go to your friend's.	Thanked my landlord for keeping the lobby so clean.	
Thurs:	My friend: You've really worked hard on that.		Complimented cashier on being efficient at checking out customers quickly.
Fri:	My sibling: I understand how you'd be upset about that.		Complimented waitress on her earrings.
Sat:			Complimented colleague's musical taste.
Sun:	My friend: Sounds like you had a lot of fun.	Thanked my neighbor for getting my mail for me.	

ECT (Expressing Understanding, Thanking, or Complimenting)

Do *at least* one E, T, or C each day. Write down who you said it to and a short note about what you said. Focus especially on the *E*—Expressing Understanding.

	Expressed Understanding	Thanked	Complimented
Mon:			
Tue:			
Wed:			
Thurs:			
Fri:			
Sat:			
Sun:			

Tracking Sheet

Please write the day and what you did each day in the appropriate column.

Day	Audio: Five Times	BEST B: At Least Once Daily Where? When?	Pleasant/Fulfilling Activity	Comments (Optional)

Home Practice Summary: Expressing Understanding

1. **Do an audio practice at least 5 days this week.**

   Be sure to fill in the Tracking Sheet to record your practice.

2. **Do the BEST B at least once a day. (You're also encouraged to do a second BEST B each day while doing other activities.)**

   Be sure to fill in the Tracking Sheet to record your practice.

3. **Do one Pleasant/Fulfilling Activity or take one step toward a goal each day.**

   Be sure to fill in the Tracking Sheet to record your practice.

4. **Do your best to do at least one thing listed in *H-M3: ETC (Expressing Understanding, Thanking, or Complimenting)* each day.**

   Write down what you did.

5. **Complete the Tracking Sheet and the Daily Log each day.**

   Fill out the Tracking Sheet and the Daily Log each day. This helps us both keep track of what works best for you, what gets in your way, and how you are feeling throughout the week.

Note: When you fill out the Tracking Sheet and the Daily Log, please do your best to be honest. You will not be judged about how much or little you have practiced, how strong or weak your urges are, or what behaviors you have or haven't engaged in during the week. The more honest you are on these forms, the more I can tailor your treatment to meet your needs. This will allow me to be more effective in helping you get closer to the kind of life you want to live. Also, please write any comments you have or anything that comes up during practice so we can talk about it at the next meeting.

CHAPTER 12

Integrating and Generalizing
Planning for the Future

MMT Session N
Paving the Road: Building and Strengthening Connections

- Review the week and discuss termination (20 minutes).
- Engage in a mindfulness practice: Focus on Object (5 minutes).
- Introduce the new topic: paving the road: relationships (15 minutes).
  - Discuss the benefits of connections with other people and with one or more groups.
  - Work with the client to complete *H-N1: Paving the Road*.
    - Identify people in the client's life who have the potential to provide positive influence and/or support.
    - Identify a group or groups the client might like to join or increase involvement.
    - Discuss the first two steps needed to join or increase involvement with a group.
  - Assign home practice: Ask the client to commit to *at least one* connection-related activity during the next week. Discuss/normalize potential avoidance urges and anxiety.
- Wrap up and plan for upcoming week (5 minutes).
- Home practice: guided audio (five times), BEST B (at least once daily), Pleasant/Fulfilling Activity (once daily), one connection-related activity from *H-N1: Paving the Road*, Daily Log.

Needed for session (all therapist sheets and handouts for this session are at the end of the Session N guidelines):

- Mindfulness: Focus on Object (TS-N1)
- Paving the Road (H-N1)
- Tracking Sheet (H-N2)
- Practice Summary (H-N3)
- Daily Log

Session N

This session focuses on building social support, which is a protective factor against relapse.

Greet the Client and Review the Week; Mention Termination (20 minutes)

See the instructions for home practice review at the end of the relevant session. Along with the standard review, remind the client that you will only have two sessions left.[1] Briefly share that you will miss the client and be a little sad (if applicable), but also express confidence in the client (to the degree that you actually feel it). Normalize that the client may feel anxious and/or sad when she thinks about treatment ending. Reflect and validate before segueing to the mindfulness practice.

Note: Start to briefly mention termination at least 6–8 weeks before treatment ends, depending upon the length of time in treatment. Begin specifically discussing the client's potential reactions and your reactions at least 3 weeks before treatment ends.

Engage in a Mindfulness Practice: *TS-N1: Focus on Object* (5 minutes)

Choose a different object than the one you used in the earlier session. See *Mindfulness: Focus on Object (TS-N1)* at the end of this session.

Introduce New Topic: Paving the Road: Connections with Other People (15 minutes)

Remind clients of the importance of connecting with other people—both for remaining free from the target behavior, as well as for reaching and maintaining a life that feels fulfilling. Feel free to read the introductory paragraph from *H-N1: Paving the Road toward a More Fulfilling Life: Connections* or to paraphrase the entries in the following list. Connections with other people can:

- *Provide support (and we all need support at times),*
- *Help life feel more meaningful,*
- *Keep you [the client] from engaging in behavior you regret later, and*
- *Help keep you moving along the road toward the kind of person you want to be and the kind of life you want to live.*

While Discussing the Benefits of Connecting with Others, Be Sure to Validate Any Anxiety and/or Reluctance Expressed by the Client

The client may feel conflicting emotions about social connection, as she may have experienced rejection or mistreatment in previous interpersonal relationships. In these cases, validate the pain and hesitancy, while also gently urging the client to consider building connections with

---

[1] Insert other relevant number of remaining sessions, if needed.

people who treat her respectfully and possibly share more of her values. Normalize any anxiety and reluctance, while also sharing that many people have had (or attempted) relationships in which they were rejected and/or mistreated. Such instances do not mean that the client deserves such treatment or is different from other human beings. Such instances may instead mean that some of those people might not have had values consistent with the client's current values.

Work with the Client to Complete
H-N1: Paving the Road toward a More Fulfilling Life: Connections

As you work with the client to complete the form, be aware of her current level of social support and gently encourage her to take steps in the area(s) you think would be the most beneficial for her. Validate the difficulty, as well as any anxiety or reluctance.

The first section of the worksheet (A) asks the client to:

> Take a moment to think about people who provide positive influences in your life. These can be people you enjoy or feel comfortable around. They can be people who help you feel confident and/ or who provide support for you in general. They might also be people who inspire you. Please list as many as possible. You can list people you communicate with regularly, as well as people you haven't seen or spoken to in quite a while.

You may need to explain that the people the client chooses do not have to meet all of the criteria listed in the instructions. The client also does not have to feel 100% positive about the people she chooses. A person could be appropriate for the list as long as any of the following applies: The client (1) generally enjoys the person's company, (2) generally feels supported by the person, (3) tends to feel comfortable and "safe" around the person, (4) tends to feel confident around the person, or (5) any other criteria that seems generally positive. The only disqualifying criterion is encouraging the client to engage in her target behavior or to do anything else that might get in the way of being the kind of person she wants to be.

If the client lists three or fewer people (which is common), offer prompts that might help her think of additional possibilities: Family members? People the client may not have seen or spoken with in a while? People who live near the client? People from the client's current or former school/work/group? If the client continues having difficulty, focus on potentially strengthening relationships with people the client already knows (even if only casually) or on working to build new relationships. Work to generate ideas of people the client might like to become closer with and/or ways for the client to meet people with similar interests or values. During this time, be careful not to insinuate that the client is at all deficient or abnormal for only being able to think of zero to three people. Normalize and reflect—while also explaining that increasing social support can be helpful for most people—especially when working to maintain freedom from a target behavior. Instruct the client to continue to think of possible names to add to the list during the following week.

The second section of the worksheet (B1) instructs the client to think of groups or organizations she might like to get involved with or at least visit. Read the instructions aloud, and stress that she is just being asked to brainstorm ideas; nothing she writes on the list will be considered a commitment. Possibilities listed on the sheet include a support group, a meditation center, a community group, an opportunity to volunteer with an organization, a Meetup group, a class, a self-improvement group, a sports group, a spiritual/religious group, etc. After reading the list, suggest examples that fit some of the categories (or categories not on the list) that you think might be appropriate for the client.

If the client's target behavior has a relevant support group (12-step or otherwise) and she has not attended such a group, take a moment to process her reluctance while also gently encouraging her to give it a try. Many clients have previously formed social circles consisting primarily of people who engage in the target behavior as a routine part of socializing. In addition, some target behaviors (e.g., drinking alcohol) are part of standard socializing for most people, even those who do not have issues with the behavior. Thus, support groups can be invaluable for meeting people who (1) will not expect the client to engage in the target behavior, (2) will understand the client's struggles related to the behavior, and (3) will be available to provide support outside of the group. Of note is that some of these groups do not adhere to the same philosophy as MMT (because MMT does not endorse the 12-step disease model or think a lapse means that a person has lost all progress). You can educate the client that these particular items do not fit the way the target behavior is viewed in MMT (or most research), but let her know that she can still benefit from the social connections even if she doesn't agree 100% with everything discussed in the group. Remind her that most people are advised to attend four or five different meeting locations before choosing one (or before deciding they do not like support groups), as the style and tone of meetings vary greatly. For example, some 12-step meetings are small and friendly; others are large and lecture-style. Finally, some clients report not wanting to go to 12-step meetings because they do not identify as religious; however, the "higher power" mentioned in 12-step groups can be conceptualized as the universe or even the group itself. Some 12-step groups even identify as agnostic or atheist.

Another possibility—Meetup (*www.meetup.com*)—can be a particularly helpful resource, especially for clients who do not have relevant support groups for their target behavior (and/or who refuse to attend a support group). Meetup is not a dating site. Instead, it offers a way to meet other people with similar interests. Individuals can use keywords to search for groups in their area (e.g., book clubs, sports, politics, hiking, animal rights, vegetarian, single parents, sober). Individuals then "join" relevant groups (which costs no money and involves no commitment) and sign up to attend upcoming meetings. Many clients who have been through MMT have met friends through Meetup, but most have had to be encouraged by therapists to join the groups and attend meetings. Of course, the other listed groups may fit as well or better than Meetup; however, Meetup is the focus here because many therapists are not familiar with it.

For the next subsection (B2), ask the client to write down the name of the group she would be most likely to attend or increase involvement. Then work with the client to break down the steps she would need to take to eventually attend or increase involvement with the group. Break down the process into small steps (consistent with the *Goals* session), and write the steps on the back of the paper. Assure the client that writing the steps does not mean she has committed to *taking* any of the steps; instead the steps are there for her to use if she chooses to do so.

Assign Home Practice: Ask the Client to Commit to at Least One Connection-Related Activity for the Following Week

The final section (C) instructs the client to:

> Write down two connection-related activities you could take with a person and/or group this week. These activities can include the steps you wrote above, or they can include calling someone, meeting someone for coffee, visiting someone, inviting someone to visit you, sending a text or email, etc. Choose activities you don't do every week. Then circle one you *commit to doing this week*. Before you write anything and circle it, make sure you're willing to commit to following through *this week*. (You're free to do both activities or more, but you only need to *commit* to doing one.) Record the activities under *Pleasant/Fulfilling Activity* on your Tracking Sheet.

Read the instructions to the client and then discuss options. Stress that she should only record and circle what she *knows* she can do this week and is willing to commit to doing *no matter what*. Encourage the client to do more than one connection-related activity, but assure her that she is only committing to one. Remind her that any connection-related activity she does can be counted as one of her daily Pleasant/Fulfilling Activities on the Tracking Sheet. If the client chooses to text someone, check to make sure that the text will involve more than just saying "hi" to a casual friend with whom the client will likely not have any further contact. Nor should it be a text to someone the client already texts regularly. If the client chooses to take a step toward attending a group, tell the client that you would like for her either to attend the group or at least sign up to attend an upcoming meeting before the end of treatment if possible. Choose steps accordingly.

Finally, discuss when the client will be most likely to engage in the committed activity and make a plan for doing so. Troubleshoot potential obstacles. Normalize and discuss potential avoidance urges and anxiety that may arise prior to engaging in connection-related activities—as well as adaptive ways for the client to respond.

Wrap Up and Plan for Upcoming Week (5 Minutes)

Briefly mention the importance of continuing MMT practices after treatment ends, while also acknowledging that the client will likely not practice as often as she did when she knew she would be reporting her practice to you each week. Ask the client to begin thinking about what would constitute a feasible practice schedule after ending treatment. Tell her that you would rather have her commit to a light schedule that she keeps than to a stringent schedule that she does not keep. Common schedules include one or two audios per week and four to seven BEST Bs per week. Some people want to continue at least mentally tracking their pleasant activities, whereas others choose not to do so. Ask the client to start thinking about a feasible schedule, which you will discuss and implement after the following session. Home practice for this week includes guided audio (five times), BEST B (at least once daily), Pleasant/Fulfilling Activity (once daily), *H-N1: Paving the Road* sheet (at least one connection-related activity—which can count as a Pleasant/Fulfilling Activity), and Daily Log.

Review the Home Practice the Week after Assigning *H-N1: Paving the Road*

Home practice is reviewed in the week following the above session.

- Review the Daily Log, the Tracking Sheet, and the client's week as you normally would do.
- If the client engaged in at least one connection-related activity, affirm and process what the experience was like for her.
  - Ask if she was anxious beforehand and/or had urges to avoid. Validate, and then affirm the fact that she engaged in the activity despite the anxiety and urges.
  - Process the reaction of the client and others; reflect and validate.
  - If the client engaged in more than one connection-related activity, affirm strongly.
  - Briefly discuss additional connection-related activities (and or additional steps toward attending a group) the client can take in the upcoming week. Remind her that they can be recorded under Pleasant/Fulfilling Activities.
- If the client did not engage in the activity, assess obstacles and respond accordingly.
  - Validate the difficulty, and help the client generate ideas for doing such activities in the upcoming week. Remind her that they can be recorded under Pleasant/Fulfilling Activities.

Mindfulness: Focus on an Object

Choose a common object (e.g., leaf, rock, coin). Give the object to the client and begin:

Three: Be aware of sounds. (*Pause*) Two: Be aware of the feelings of your feet against the floor, body against the chair. (*Pause*) One: Be aware of your breath. (*Pause*) During this practice, I will provide some prompts and ask some questions. You do not need to answer the questions aloud.

The following is a template. After a few breaths, lead the client through variations on the following instructions. Pause for a few seconds between each instruction/question. Allow 4–5 minutes for the exercise.

- Focus on the sensations of holding the object in your hand. Be aware of any weight of the object. . . . Does it feel warm or cool? . . . Can you tell if it's rough or smooth?
- Open your eyes and study the object. Allow yourself to *really see* it. Notice the details you might normally miss. . . . Allow yourself to be curious. Notice the shape . . . the edges . . . the colors . . . the pattern. . . . Do your best to let go of judgments.
- Do your best to find some sort of beauty in the object.
- Now move the object around in your hands. Turn it over . . . rub the edges . . . bring it closer to your eyes or farther away.
- Notice how the light falls on the object. Does the color change at all?
- Is the object's surface rough or smooth? How does it feel to rub against your hand or fingers?
- Now I'm going to pause for a while to let you really look at the object. When you notice your mind wandering, just bring it back to your breath—and then back to the object. *[Give prompts to gently bring mind back to object every 10 seconds.]*

A point to make afterward: The client sees that object regularly—but probably rarely really *sees it. Sometimes we get so caught up in life that we forget to be curious about what's around us. We lose touch with the beauty. Encourage the client to look for the beauty in the upcoming week.*

Paving the Road toward a More Fulfilling Life: Connections

Connections with other people can provide support, help life feel more meaningful, keep you from engaging in behavior you regret later, and help keep you on the road toward the kind of person you want to be and the kind of life you want to live.

A. Take a moment to think about people who provide positive influences in your life. These can be people you enjoy or feel comfortable around. They can be people who help you feel confident and/or who provide support for you in general. They might also be people who inspire you. Please list as many as possible. You can list people you communicate with regularly, as well as people you haven't seen or spoken to in quite a while.

1. _____   5. _____

2. _____   6. _____

3. _____   7. _____

4. _____   8. _____

B1. Do your best to think of one or more groups or organizations you might like to get involved with or at least visit. *(This could be a support group, a meditation center, a community group, an opportunity to volunteer with an organization, a Meetup group, a class, a sports group, a spiritual/ religious group, etc.).* Write all possibilities in the following list. This is not a commitment. This exercise is to brainstorm options. Becoming involved can increase your sense of connectedness to others and provide opportunities to participate in fulfilling activities.

1. _____

2. _____

3. _____

4. _____

B2. Which of those groups would you be most likely to attend or become more involved with? Write the name of that group below. *Remember:* This is not a commitment. What steps would you need to take to attend (or become more involved with) that group? Write the steps on the back of this page. Be sure to break the process into small steps.

C. Write down two connection-related activities you could take with a person and/or group this week. These activities can include the steps you wrote above, or they can include calling someone, meeting someone for coffee, visiting someone, inviting someone to visit you, sending a text or email, etc. Choose activities you don't do every week. Then circle one you *commit to doing this week.* Before you write anything and circle it, make sure you're willing to commit to following through *this week.* (You're free to do both activities or more, but you only need to *commit* to doing one.) Record the activities under *Pleasant/Fulfilling Activity* on your Tracking Sheet.

1. _____

2. _____

Tracking Sheet

Please write the day and what you did each day in the appropriate column.

Day	Audio: Five Times	BEST B: At Least Once Daily Where? When?	Pleasant/Fulfilling Activity	Comments (Optional)

Home Practice Summary: Paving the Road

1. **Do an audio practice at least 5 days this week.**

   Be sure to fill in the Tracking Sheet to record your practice.

2. **Do the BEST B at least once a day. (You're also encouraged to do a second BEST B each day while doing other activities.)**

   Be sure to fill in the Tracking Sheet to record your practice.

3. **Do one Pleasant/Fulfilling Activity or take one step toward a goal each day.**

   Be sure to fill in the Tracking Sheet to record your practice.

4. **Complete at least one connection-related activity from *H-N1: Paving the Road*.**

   You can count each activity as one of your Pleasant/Fulfilling Activities.

5. **Complete the Tracking Sheet and the Daily Log each day.**

   Fill out the Tracking Sheet and the Daily Log each day. This helps us both keep track of what works best for you, what gets in your way, and how you are feeling throughout the week.

Note: When you fill out the Tracking Sheet and the Daily Log, please do your best to be honest. You will not be judged about how much or little you have practiced, how strong or weak your urges are, or what behaviors you have or haven't engaged in during the week. The more honest you are on these forms, the more I can tailor your treatment to meet your needs. This will allow me to be more effective in helping you get closer to the kind of life you want to live. Also, please write any comments you have or anything that comes up during practice so we can talk about it at the next meeting.

MMT Session O
Integrating and Generalizing

- Review the week (the client's experiences, home practice, target behavior; 15–20 minutes).
  - Further discuss termination. (Begin discussion several weeks before last session.)
  - Normalize sadness and anxiety, and share some of your own feelings.
- Engage in a mindfulness practice: Therapist's Choice (5 minutes).
- Introduce a new topic: integrating and generalizing (15–20 minutes).
  - Briefly review each MMT skill in *H-O1: Ways to Cope.*
  - Choose one skill to reassign: a skill the client needs to practice more and/or a skill the client might need to generalize to new situations.
  - Review *H-O2: Ways to Practice Mindfulness Every Day.*
  - Work with the client to create a practice schedule likely to be maintained once treatment ends. (Discussion may begin up to 3 weeks prior to session.)
  - Assign home practice: one MMT skill chosen in session, practice from *H-O2: Ways to Practice Mindfulness* at least two times, and other practices from the new schedule.
- Wrap up and plan for the upcoming week (5 minutes).
- Home practice: Audios, BEST Bs, Pleasant/Fulfilling Activities, and days of Daily Log will depend on modified schedule; *H-O2: Ways to Practice Mindfulness* two times, one MMT skill.

Needed for session (all therapist sheets and handouts for this session are at the end of the Session O guidelines):

- Mindfulness practice (therapist's choice)
- Ways to Cope (H-O1)
- Ways to Practice Mindfulness Every Day (H-O2)
- Tracking Sheet (H-O3)
- Practice Summary (H-O4)
- Daily Log
- Additional Sheet (for assignment this week; TBD, depending on client)

SESSION O

The purpose of this session is to review all skills and revisit the skills with which the client may need more practice.

Greet the Client and Review the Previous Week (15–20 Minutes)

Review the previous week as you normally would do. Briefly discuss and plan for termination. (As mentioned previously, therapists should begin mentioning termination 6–8 weeks before the final session.) The *integration and generalization* session may be offered one or more times, depending on whether you feel the client needs to revisit more than one skill. Regardless of the number of times it is offered, an *integration and generalization* session always occurs immediately prior to the termination session. Although discussion of termination should start several weeks before the last session, termination should receive in-depth focus in the session prior to the last session. Essential points to make include the following:

- Remind the client that you and he will be meeting only for one additional session.
- Share that you will miss the client and be a little sad (if applicable), regardless of whether or not the client endorses any negative feelings. *Note:* Do your best to be aware of the fact that you will no longer be seeing this human being whose life you have affected. It is very common for therapists to feel a little sad and/or miss the client after termination.
- Tell the client that if he is like most clients, he will feel at least some anxiety and sadness—as well as some increased urges in the days before and after the final session.
  - If the client denies these feelings, validate and normalize, but also tell him that they might start within the next few days or even right after the last session.
  - Remind the client that the next few weeks may be a higher-risk time due to the transition. Express confidence in the client's ability to continue moving down the road while also preparing him for coping with potential risks.

Engage in a Mindfulness Practice: Therapist's Choice (5 Minutes)

Choose which mindfulness practice you would like to lead. (If you are conducting a version of MMT that is shorter than 20 weeks, you are encouraged to choose one of mindfulness exercises you missed when combining or skipping sessions.)

Introduce New Topic: Integration and Generalization (15–20 minutes)

Most clients would benefit from additional practice of at least some of the MMT skills. This session may be repeated if the client needs additional practice of multiple skills. If the session is conducted more than once for clients in treatment for a fixed number of weeks, it would count as one of the flex sessions.

Briefly Review Each MMT Skill in H-01: Ways to Cope

H-O1: Ways to Cope provides a quick reference of all the primary MMT skills. Encourage the client to keep the list handy and practice skills even after treatment ends, so the skills continue to "sink in" and eventually become automatic ways of coping. The list can also be used by the client as a reminder of ways to respond to urges—which might be especially crucial in the few weeks following treatment.

- Review the list with the client, and provide a brief explanation of each skill.
    - If you are new to MMT, take a moment before the session to revisit instructions for some of the skills with which you do not feel as familiar.
    - Briefly check the client's memory and understanding of each skill, and provide a succinct review of each.
- Ask whether the client needs any additional copies of any skill (in other words, whether the client has lost any of the handouts). If so, provide the client with those handouts either that day or the following week.
    - It can be helpful to have all the primary MMT handouts already printed. You will need access to the handout for whichever skill you and the client choose to review in depth, plus you will then be ready for any replacement sheets the client might need.
        - It can also be helpful to *always* have all handouts printed and easily available. Sometimes a client's life will warrant revisiting a previously learned skill, even if that skill wasn't the intended focus of the session.
    - See *H-O1: Ways to Cope* for a list of handout names and numbers.
- Choose one skill to assign again. After going through each of the items, work together to pick one skill that will be assigned again during the upcoming week. Or, if you already know of a skill you believe the client needs but has not mastered, you may choose that skill before the session. Choose a skill with which the client needs more work and/or that the client needs to generalize to a new situation. Do not choose one of the skills that the client has already had the option of practicing each week (e.g., an audio, Pleasant/Fulfilling Activities, or BEST B), and do not choose an item that is more of an "extra" (e.g., thinking about the destination). Briefly review the chosen skill with the client, and assign the skill for the upcoming week.

Review H-02: Ways to Practice Mindfulness Every Day

Explain that mindfulness practice is somewhat like physical exercise in that continued exercise is needed to keep the muscles strong. Then review *H-O2: Ways to Practice Mindfulness Every Day*. Read through each item and ask for the client's reactions. Then ask the client to circle the number by any exercise he would be open to practicing at some point. (Circling a number is not a commitment.) Ask the client to choose one exercise (other than the BEST B or the audios) to practice at least twice in the upcoming week. Talk about what time of day the client might practice and how he will remember to do so. (It can often be helpful to set a phone alarm for each day at the approximate time—or to tape a reminder in the general area the client will be practicing the exercise.) The exercise needs to be something the client will likely have a chance to do *at least* twice in the upcoming week. The goal is to have the client eventually engage in the practice routinely when he engages in the relevant activity. Tell the client that he is welcome to practice more than one exercise, but that it is important to practice the exercise he has chosen at least twice.

Continue to Work with the Client to Create a Practice Schedule Likely to Be Maintained after Treatment Ends

As a continuation on the above theme, talk with the client about the importance of continuing MMT practices after treatment ends, while also acknowledging that the client will probably not practice as often as he did when he knew he would be reporting his practice to you. Discuss what would constitute a feasible practice schedule after ending treatment. Remind him that you would rather have him commit to a light schedule that he keeps than to a stringent schedule that he does not keep. You may suggest a schedule to the client, which may partially be based on your knowledge of his current level of practice.

Standard posttreatment schedules include one or two audio practices per week (which works best when at least one is scheduled for a certain day of the week, such as every Sunday) and a BEST B four or five times per week, with encouragement for the client to revisit other practices regularly. The client may or may not decide to continue a schedule of Pleasant/Fulfilling Activities. Once you agree upon a tentative schedule, assign that schedule for the upcoming week. The client can then practice that schedule this week as a test run.

Remind the Client of Home Practice

Briefly review the assignment of one MMT skill chosen in session and one practice from *H-O2: Ways to Practice Mindfulness Every Day* (at least two times).

Wrap Up and Plan for Upcoming Week (5 Minutes)

Review the new schedule for audios, BEST B, Daily Log, and (perhaps) Pleasant/Fulfilling Activities. Remind the client that he will likely feel sad and/or anxious at some points this week. Validate his emotions while also expressing your confidence in him. Help plan for potentially difficult moments.

Ways to Cope

The following list offers suggestions of ways to ride out urges, to cope with potential problems, and/or to keep moving toward a life that feels more like the life you want.

1. *BEST B (H-B2)*

2. *Coping Toolbox* (*H-A2*; Do as many of the activities as needed.)

3. Do a *Pleasant and/or Fulfilling Activity.* (See *H-E1* for suggestions.)

4. *Awareness of Thoughts*—and awareness that you can choose whether or not to act on thoughts, which can lead you to move toward or away from your destination (See *H-G1* and *H-G3*.)

5. Putting up *Urge Roadblocks (H-F1)*

6. *Break Down a Goal* into small steps and then take a step. (See *H-H1* and *H-H2*.)

7. *OFFER:* To say "No" (*H-I1* and *H-I2*) or to ask for something (*H-J1* and *H-J2*)
   - **O**ther (express what the other person might be feeling),
   - **F**acts (tell the facts),
   - **F**eelings (tell your feelings or consequences for you),
   - **E**xplain (explain what you want or why you're saying "no"),
   - **R**eward (tell the other person how she/he can benefit).

8. *Freeing Yourself from Being Controlled:* gaining back your power by practicing acceptance/tolerance exercises (*H-K1* and *H-L1*)

9. *"May You Be"* meditation for others and self

10. *Expressing Understanding of Others* and *Expressing Understanding, Thanking, or Complimenting; ETC.* (*H-M1* and *H-M3*)

11. *Paving the Road:* building connections with others (*H-N1*)

12. *Ways to Practice Mindfulness Every Day (H-O2)*

13. Create a list of positive and negative consequences of engaging in the target behavior.

14. Imagine the Mirror Exercise.

15. Do one of the audios. (Ex: Color Body Scan, Body Movement, etc.).

16. Remind yourself of the progress you have made. Do you want to go back?

17. Think of the destination (*your* destination).

18. _____

19. _____

20. _____

Ways to Practice Mindfulness Every Day

1. Continue to engage in the BEST B.

2. Continue to do the audio practices.

3. At one meal each day, *take a moment to look at your food and really notice the appearance* of the food. As you bring the food toward your mouth, allow yourself to be aware of the smell (if applicable). Then focus your attention on the taste, texture, and temperature as you chew and swallow your first three bites (or more) of the food.

4. *Take a few moments to notice shapes and colors when you walk somewhere* (whether it's across a parking lot, down a street, or down a hallway). Allow yourself to look for interesting shapes and/or color combinations. Choose a color or shape you will notice. ("I will notice things that are green" Or "I will notice things that are somewhat circular.")

5. *Choose one physical activity you perform daily,* and bring your attention to the physical sensations for approximately 30 seconds. The activity may be brushing your teeth, washing your face, brushing your hair, walking down/upstairs, etc. (You are encouraged to stick with one activity for at least a week, and preferably longer.)

6. *Before getting out of bed each day,* gently bring your attention to your breathing, and be aware of physical sensations for three inbreaths and three outbreaths.
   - You can also choose a different cue; for example, (a) when you first sit in your car (before starting the engine), (b) whenever you sit down for your coffee (before starting to drink it), (c) right before you leave your home in the morning, and so on.

7. *Before going to sleep each night,* gently be aware of the physical sensations for three inbreaths and three outbreaths.
   - Other potential cues for awareness of three breaths include (a) right before you get out of your car, (b) when you first arrive home after being out, etc.

8. *Whenever you wait in line at a store or wait for mass transit,* allow yourself to notice your reactions. Are you feeling anxious? Irritated? Pressured? Bored? Allow yourself to feel your emotions—and then gently practice acceptance.

9. Every day *take a moment to think of someone in your life* (family member, friend, neighbor, etc.). Do your best to imagine what it might be like to be that person. Think about some difficulties, struggles, and pain that person might experience: lonely at times, not fitting in, money worries, scared, shy, sad, bored, problems at work, health problems, etc. Really try to imagine what it must be like to be that person. Send up thoughts of comfort or a prayer of comfort for the person.

10. *Create your own cue for a short mindfulness practice:*

_____

_____

Tracking Sheet

Please write the day and what you did each day in the appropriate column.

Day	Audio: Five Times	BEST B: At Least Once Daily Where? When?	Pleasant/Fulfilling Activity	Comments (Optional)

Home Practice Summary: Integrating

1. Do the audio practice according to the schedule you chose in session.

2. Do the BEST B according to the schedule you chose in session.

3. Do Pleasant/Fulfilling Activities or take steps toward a goal according to the schedule you chose in session.

4. Complete the MMT skill chosen in session. What was the skill? _____

5. Practice one exercise from *H-O2: Ways to Practice Mindfulness Every Day* at least twice during the week.

6. Complete the Tracking Sheet and the Daily Log according to the schedule you chose in session.

MMT Session P
Termination: Planning for Continued Progress toward a Valued Life

- Review the week. Ask for feedback on the practice schedule chosen last week; encourage the client to do her best to continue that schedule or a modified version (15–20 minutes).
- Engage in a mindfulness practice: BEST B (5–6 minutes).
- Introduce the new topic: planning for the future and goodbye (20–25 minutes).
  - Validate the client's work in treatment.
  - Ask for feedback about the client's experiences in treatment, and provide your own view of the client's progress. Discuss plans for the future, potential obstacles, and areas for continued focus.
  - Work with client to complete *H-P1: Reminders*.
  - Give the client the *H-P3: Remember* sheet.
  - Discuss the client's reaction to termination. Normalize anxiety and sadness. You are encouraged to share that you will miss the client and think of the client each week at session time. (Only share this if it is true.)
  - Give the client a card or other concrete reminder of the treatment experience.
  - Ask about the rest of the day; work with the client to set a plan.
  - Wrap up and say goodbye.

Needed for session (all therapist sheets and handouts for this session are at the end of the Session P guidelines):

- Reminders (H-P1)
- Ways to Cope (H-P2)
- Remember (H-P3)
- Tracking Sheet (H-O3; optional)
- Daily Log (optional)
- Any additional sheets you choose

Session P

This session will serve as a chance to review treatment progress, process emotions, review plans for the future, and say goodbye.

Greet the Client, Review the Week, and Review the Home Practice (15–20 Minutes)

- Briefly review the Daily Log and validate reported emotions and urges.
- Review the Tracking Sheet by asking the client what she thought about the practice schedule she chose for the previous week. Modify it, if necessary, and encourage the client to do her best to continue practicing according to that schedule. (Tell her that she is free to practice more than the minimum, of course, but stress the importance of practicing the minimum.) Again briefly discuss potential days and times to do the practice. You are encouraged to ask the client to set alarms for the chosen days—which can be helpful for the first few weeks.
- *Warn the client that many people have urges to stop the home practice for a while when they no longer have anyone who will hold them accountable.* Many say they consider it a break. *However, once clients stop the home practice, they tend to have difficulty starting it again.* Thus, emphasize the importance of working to continue the new schedule of home practice *without* taking a break.
- Briefly review the MMT skill you assigned the previous week.
- Briefly ask about *H-O2: Ways to Practice Mindfulness Every Day* (one exercise practiced at least twice). Affirm the client for engaging in the practice, if applicable, and encourage her to continue this and/or other listed practices. Additional practices may be added as regular practices or completed periodically, as needed.
- If the client lapsed into her target behavior this past week (which is rare but of course not impossible), validate the difficulty of ending treatment while stressing that a lapse is not a relapse. (Use the destination metaphor.) Do not conduct a functional analysis; instead, work with the client on a plan to get through the next few days without additional lapses. Potentially offer referrals to further treatment.

Engage in a Mindfulness Practice: BEST B (5–6 Minutes)

Tell the client you will lead her in one last in-session BEST B. Although you will turn your body around and ask her to sit up and close her eyes, you will not begin the practice by counting from three to one. Instead, you will conduct a BEST B more consistent with how the client will likely practice on her own. Just begin by mentioning the breath, and conduct a BEST B that lasts approximately 3 minutes. You do not need to read a script; just do your best to relate the gist of the BEST B customized to fit the last session. Example:

- *And now, focus your attention on your breath for a few breaths. Allow yourself to be aware of the sensations in your chest and stomach as you breathe in and breathe out.* (Pause)
- *Gently bring your attention to your emotions and urges, as well as to any related physical sensations. You may be feeling sadness. Maybe anxiety. Maybe urges. Maybe something else.*

Label the emotions and urges. (Pause) *Remind yourself that emotions and urges won't make your head explode, and they don't predict the future. You can have emotions and urges and choose whether or not you act on them.* (Pause approximately 10–15 seconds)

- *Gently shift your attention to focus primarily on physical sensations. Do a brief scan of your body, and if any area feels tight or tense, imagine that your breath goes to that area and seeps through it. When you exhale, some of the tightness may or may not leave with the breath. There is no right or wrong way to feel.* (Pause approximately 10 seconds)

- *Allow yourself to be aware of your thoughts. Label the first few thoughts that come into your head as "just thoughts." Just say to yourself, "That's a thought." "That's a thought."* (Pause) *Your brain spews out thoughts based on what it was taught to believe in the past. Remember: Thoughts don't necessarily equal facts. You can have a thought and choose whether or not to act on it.* (Pause approximately 15 seconds)

- *Now, gently bring your attention back to your breath. Allow yourself to be aware of the sensations in your chest and stomach as you breathe in and breathe out.* (Slight pause) *Now, take this moment to commit to yourself to act in a way that fits the kind of person you want to be. Here's my suggestion: I'd like you to commit to continuing to do the practices and moving toward the life that fits your values. At times, you'll probably have urges to stop doing the practices and using the skills, but I'd like you to make a commitment to do your best to keep doing whatever it takes to continue to move forward.* (Pause about 10 seconds) *Really make that commitment to yourself. And be aware of what that feels like.* (Pause about 10 seconds) *Whenever you're ready, allow your eyes to open.*

Introduce New Topic: Planning for the Future and Saying Goodbye (20–25 minutes)

Be sure to leave at least 20 minutes for the following activities.

Review the Client's Progress and Overall Therapy Experience

- Validate and affirm the client's work and effort over the course of treatment.
- Ask for feedback about the client's experiences in treatment. Ask about progress as well as difficulties in treatment and future concerns.
- Share your own views about the client's progress, including areas that still need focus.
- Discuss plans for addressing future known and potential obstacles.

Start by briefly validating and affirming the client's progress. Mention the amount of difficulty the client has already overcome and validate the amount of effort the client has made. Elicit feedback about the client's experience in treatment, and reflect and affirm each answer to draw out further information. Potential questions include:

- *How do you feel about your life and yourself now compared to right before you started this treatment?*
- *How do you feel different now than when you started? Tell me more about that.*
- *What did you find most helpful about treatment? What did you find most difficult?*

- *What challenges do you see ahead?*
- *What do you want to continue working toward?*

Example of the beginning of such a conversation follows.

THERAPIST: [After validating and affirming effort] Before we talk more about my view of the progress you've made, I'd like to hear your experience. Take a moment to think about your life right around the time you started coming here. How do you feel about your life and yourself now—compared to your life then?

CLIENT: (*Pause*) Definitely different. I was so discouraged then.

THERAPIST: I remember how discouraged you were. You seem a little sad when you talk about it now.

CLIENT: It's a little sad just thinking about how long I felt that way. I thought that that was just how life was always going to be.

THERAPIST: That *is* sad. (*Slight pause*) And you feel different now.

CLIENT: Of course. For one thing, the [target behavior] is different.

THERAPIST: To say the least! Would you have believed when you first came here that in just 6 months, you would have gone more than 4 months without any [target behavior]?

CLIENT: No. I didn't think it was possible.

THERAPIST: You really did a lot of work. I know it felt impossible at first—but you did it anyway.

CLIENT: Yeah, it was not fun at first, but it feels good now.

THERAPIST: I'm glad. You deserve to feel good about it. So the [target behavior] has decreased. What else feels different?

CLIENT: Well, I feel calmer.

THERAPIST. Tell me more about that.

CLIENT: (*Pause*) Sometimes it's like I don't get as anxious. But sometimes it's like I might get as anxious at first, but then I don't lose control. Before I came here, I could get in an argument with Chris, and I could lose a whole weekend just feeling anxious about whether we'd stay together and how much I'd messed up. Or I'd do the [target behavior] just to shut down. And now it's like I still get anxious about those things, but now I can live my life without feeling controlled.

THERAPIST: So, sometimes the anxiety is less intense, and other times you might still feel the anxiety as strongly—but you don't feel controlled by it. You're able to live a life that you value.

CLIENT: Yeah, that's it.

THERAPIST: The anxiety might not be pleasant, but it doesn't get in the way as much anymore.

CLIENT: I don't listen to that self-critical voice as much.

THERAPIST: That's a big deal! I know that was one of the hardest things for you—not getting caught up in those critical thoughts.

After processing the client's view of his progress, take a moment to share your own perspective. You likely will already have shared some of your views when reflecting and affirming the client's feedback, but the client can also benefit from hearing your views independently of your reaction to his comments.

I want spend a little time talking about my take on your progress. A lot will be similar to what we just talked about—but I think it's important enough that it's OK if you hear some of it twice.

When giving feedback, place an especially strong focus on skills the client has mastered, difficulties she has overcome, and values and goals to which she has moved closer. Also share your experience of working with her. At the same time, gently communicate areas in which she still needs to work. For example, if the client has become abstinent from the target behavior and obtained a job, but has not yet built much of a social support network, you would affirm her abstinence, job, and overall therapeutic work—while also pointing out that she still needs to work on building a social network. You could then briefly talk about potential plans for doing so and ways to potentially cope with obstacles that might interfere with the plan (e.g., social anxiety).

If the client is still struggling with the target behavior (but is in a program that has to end), affirm the progress the client has made (which may include gaining skills to be more effective in other areas of life, or decreasing the frequency of the target behavior). Encourage the client to continue treatment at whatever facility to which you have referred her. Stress that some people might take longer than others to get past the behavior; the fact that she needs to be referred to another program does not mean she cannot eventually get past the behavior. The fact that the client has continued to attend treatment is a good indicator of her eventual success.

If the client has chosen to work to continue the target behavior in moderation (or if the client's target behavior is one that requires some form of moderation), review the moderation plan as well as red flags you and the client have identified as signs the client may be at risk for slipping back to the old behavior. (See *moderation* in Chapter 6, pp. 87–90.) Discuss potential courses of action to take if red flags occur.

If the client has moved passed the dysregulated behavior and is being referred for other treatment (PTSD, personality symptoms, couple therapy, etc.), briefly discuss the status of that referral, while also reinforcing the client's desire to continue working to move forward.

Finally, for all clients, discuss the probability of increased urges, sadness, and anxiety over the course of the next few weeks. These first weeks after leaving treatment hold a higher risk for lapse, so prepare the client for the potential of increased urges, and assure her that the increase will not be permanent. Discuss ways in which the client can cope with any urges that might occur.

Work with the Client to Complete H-P1: Reminders

As a continuation of the discussion about urges, introduce *H-P1: Reminders*. The worksheet takes up half a page. The page should be cut in half, so it is easier to fold and keep in a wallet. You can use the remaining half as a scratch pad for writing and refining the client's list before completing the actual handout.

The first portion instructs the client to list *reasons to continue moving toward the destination and remain free from target behavior*. The reasons can be reasons why the client does not want to revert to the target behavior (i.e., negative consequences of the behavior), as well as reasons why the client wants to continue moving forward (liking self better; improved relationships, etc.). Advise the client to choose reminders that bring up emotional reactions; in other words, you want the client to choose negative consequences that would be distressing and reasons to move forward that are meaningful (or potentially meaningful) in the client's life. Potential negative consequences tend to be more effective for many clients, so instruct the client to have at least a couple of negative consequences.

Once the list of *reasons* is complete, ask the client to list *a few reminders of ways to cope to ride out urges*. The client is instructed to write four things she commits to doing when experiencing urges. The first method of coping—BEST B—is already listed. Work with the client to decide which skills might be the most effective for her to use during high-risk times. Consult *H-P2: Ways to Cope* for ideas. The client is free to choose skills from MMT, and she can also write anything else that she thinks would be helpful.

Once the client has completed *H-P1: Reminders,* review it and discuss how she will get herself to use the coping skills when she has urges. Encourage her to keep the sheet somewhere she can access easily, such as a wallet or a pocket of a purse. Ask her to read through the list whenever she notices herself experiencing urges—or even if she is tempted to engage in the behavior without noticing urges. You might also want to encourage her to read through the list every day for the next week or two, regardless of whether she is experiencing urges.

Also give the client *H-P3: Remember,* which contains key MMT phrases.

Discuss Reaction to Termination

After completing *H-P1: Reminders,* tell the client how many minutes are left in session, and bring the conversation back to the fact that the client is completing treatment.

- You are strongly encouraged to express that you are feeling at least a little sad, you will miss seeing the client, and you will think of the client and hope she is doing well. You can also say that you will think of her particularly strongly at her standard session time each week. At the same time, also share how glad and/or proud you are that she was able to complete treatment.
  - As always, do not be fake. Only say it if it is true. But work to remember that this is a human being who has worked with you through pain and intense struggles.
- Tell the client that if she is like most people, she will feel at least some anxiety and sadness—as well as some increased urges.
  - This discussion can be very difficult to have. It can feel like you are saying, "I know I am very valuable to you and therefore you will miss me"—which can feel awkward and uncomfortably vulnerable. Since you just mentioned feeling sad about the client ending treatment, you open yourself up to feelings of being rejected if the client denies sadness. (Yes, even though you are a professional, you are also still human.) Do your best to risk (and perhaps tolerate) those potential feelings of rejection.
    - In follow-up research, many clients reported extremely positive reactions to hearing that they were important enough for a therapist to actually miss (Wupperman et al.,

2018). Some clients reported that the knowledge helped them cope with their own sadness in the days after treatment ended—even when they did not realize they were feeling sad until after the termination session.

■ Some clients *will* deny feeling sad or anxious (which may feel uncomfortable for you—and that's OK). In these cases, tell the client that whatever she does or doesn't feel is fine, and that urges or sadness/anxiety may (or may not) start within the next few days. Some clients truly may not feel any negative emotions about leaving. However, many clients who deny such emotions may have trouble admitting vulnerable emotions (to themselves and/or others), especially when related to caring about a person they will no longer be able to see. These reactions do not lessen the importance of the client knowing that *you* care about her ending treatment.

■ Spend a few moments processing and validating the client's anxiety and/or sadness. Also express your belief in the client's ability to continue moving down the road toward the life that she wants, even while reminding her that the course will not always be easy and that she will still have times of urges.

Give the Client a Card and/or Some Other Concrete Reminder of Her/His Work with You

● One possibility is a greeting card (the kind that are blank on the inside) with just a few sentences sharing your thoughts and wishing the client well. (Just sign your full name if possible—without a title in front of it.) Give clients the opportunity to read the card in session or after they leave. (Clients often choose to wait until after they leave.)

● At various times, MMT therapists have also chosen to give clients interesting rocks, seashells, Silly Putty in an egg (that description will make sense if you know what Silly Putty is), and small notebooks. The object is less important than the fact that you are giving it.

● Encourage the client to take a moment to think about her progress in treatment whenever she sees the card and/or object in the future.

● Some clients also say they would like clean copies of the Tracking Sheet and Daily Log. Be prepared to provide copies of those, as well as *H-P2: Ways to Cope* and any sheet requested the week before. (Providing the Tracking Sheet will give you another chance to mention the importance of continuing the home practice without taking a break.)

Ask What the Client Will Be Doing the Rest of the Day

If she does not have any plans, encourage her to plan something. Briefly talk through what she will/might do.

Wrap Up and Say Goodbye

Wish the client well. Tell her you will think of her (if it is true). If at all possible, take a few moments after the session to reflect on your experience with the client.

Reminders

Reasons to Continue Moving toward the Destination and Remain Free from <u>Target Behavior:</u>

1. _____

2. _____

3. _____

4. _____

5. _____

A Few Reminders of Ways I Can Cope to Ride Out Urges

I will do AT LEAST ONE (even when I don't feel like doing it) when I experience increased urges:

1. Do a BEST B.

2. _____

3. _____

4. _____

5. _____

- -

H-P2

Ways to Cope

The following list offers suggestions of ways to ride out urges, to cope with potential problems, and/ or to keep moving toward a life that feels more like the life you want.

1. *BEST B (H-B2)*

2. *Coping Toolbox* (*H-A2*; Do as many of the activities as needed.)

3. Do a *Pleasant and/or Fulfilling Activity.* (See *H-E1* for suggestions.)

4. *Awareness of Thoughts*—and awareness that you can choose whether or not to act on thoughts, which can lead you to move toward or away from your destination (See *H-G1* and *H-G3*.)

5. Putting up *Urge Roadblocks (H-F1)*

6. *Break Down a Goal* into small steps and then take a step. (See *H-H1* and *H-H2*.)

7. *OFFER:* To say "No" (*H-I1* and *H-I2*) or to ask for something (*H-J1* and *H-J2*)
   - **O**ther (express what the other person might be feeling),
   - **F**acts (tell the facts),
   - **F**eelings (tell your feelings or consequences for you),
   - **E**xplain (explain what you want or why you're saying "no"),
   - **R**eward (tell the other person how she/he can benefit).

8. *Freeing Yourself from Being Controlled:* gaining back your power by practicing acceptance/ tolerance exercises (*H-K1* and *H-L1*)

9. *"May You Be"* meditation for others and self

10. *Expressing Understanding of Others and Expressing Understanding, Thanking, or Complimenting; ETC.* (*H-M1* and *H-M3*)

11. *Paving the Road:* building connections with others (*H-N1*)

12. *Ways to Practice Mindfulness Every Day (H-O2)*

13. Create a list of positive and negative consequences of engaging in the target behavior.

14. Imagine the Mirror Exercise.

15. Do one of the audios. (Ex: Color Body Scan, Body Movement, etc.).

16. Remind yourself of the progress you have made. Do you want to go back?

17. Think of the destination (*your* destination).

18. _____

19. _____

20. _____

Remember . . .

- Emotions and urges will not make your head explode. You can survive emotions and urges without trying to turn them off.

- Urges do not predict the future. You can have an urge without acting on it. You can ride out the urge.

- Thoughts do not necessarily equal facts. Thoughts do not predict the future. You can have a thought without acting on it.

An emotion is just an emotion.

An urge is just an urge.

A sensation is just a sensation.

A thought is just a thought.

You can have emotions, urges, and thoughts *without* acting on them.

You can have emotions, urges, sensations, and thoughts—and still continue making progress toward your destination.

MMT Flex Sessions
Clinician Chooses Topic and Timing of the Session

- Review the week (the client's experiences, home practice, target behavior; 15–? minutes).
- Focus on the topic that you believe needs additional work. Possibilities include:
  - Issues with motivation, commitment, and/or rapport.
  - In-depth work on problems with home practice, attendance, and/or decreasing the target behavior.
  - Further (repeated) explanation on how the practice "works."
  - Topics relevant to the client's specific target behavior.
  - Other topics you and the client agree need to be addressed.
- Remind the client of home practice, and wrap up the session (5 minutes).
- Review home practice: basic activities listed on the Tracking Sheet (consistent with where the client is in treatment), Daily Log, and any additional practice the therapist chooses to assign.

Needed for session:

- Tracking Sheet (version depending on when the flex session is conducted)
- Daily Log
- Any additional sheets you choose

FLEX SESSIONS

Flex sessions allow the therapist to choose the session topic(s) based on client needs. Most flex sessions focus on one or more of the following: (1) addressing issues with motivation and/or commitment, (2) additional work on skills with which the client has difficulty and/or needs help generalizing, (3) additional work on shaping to decrease the target behavior, (4) additional focus on diversity-related issues, (5) necessary case management activities, and/or (6) other topics you and the client agree need to be addressed.

Flex sessions may also be used to incorporate treatment techniques specifically designed for the client's particular dysregulated behavior. The caveat would be that the incorporated techniques should be consistent with MMT's conceptualization of clients and core principles of treatment.

Although the therapist chooses the primary topic(s) of the session, all flex sessions maintain the template of beginning by reviewing the previous week and ending by reminding the client about home practice (and providing the client with the Tracking Sheet and Daily Log).

The 16-week version of MMT includes one flex session and one semi-flex session. The 20-week version includes three flex sessions and one semi-flex session. Therapists may use these flex sessions any time during the treatment. If the treatment is not time-limited, the therapist may use as many flex sessions as deemed necessary; however, it is recommended that the therapist not use multiple flex sessions in a row, as that could risk the client's becoming bored by home practice that never changes and losing motivation after not being exposed to new material.

CHAPTER 13

Conclusion

Training Opportunities and Online Resources

Clients in treatment for dysregulated behavior are suffering. They suffer due to the consequences of the dysregulated behavior, and they often suffer even more (in the short term) when they work to stop the dysregulated behavior. The strategies and procedures in this book were developed to help clients move past their suffering and move closer to lives that feel fulfilling and meaningful. However, making such progress can be excruciatingly painful, and clients who work to stop such behavior deserve credit for their courage, their strength, and their tremendous effort in working toward change even in the face of their pain.

Caring therapists are not immune to the suffering of clients. In general, human beings try *not* to experience pain, but therapists choose a profession that *guarantees* they will interact with suffering on a regular basis. As a result, although working with clients can be rewarding, it can also feel stressful, emotionally draining, and even painful. Yet therapists choose to do such work anyway. The importance of this fact should not be minimized.

I hope you will take time to regularly remind yourself of your own courage, kindness, and strength of character in choosing the field you chose and doing the work you do. I hope you allow yourself to experience reverence at the honor of having human beings trust you enough to show vulnerabilities they may share with few (if any) other people. And I hope you allow yourself to have some awe for the fact that your daily job gives you the chance to help decrease suffering and help human beings literally change their lives.

MMT TRAINING

As with all therapies, the explanations in a book can provide only the most basic guidelines for conducting MMT. Thus, in order to provide MMT effectively for your clients, you are strongly encouraged to attend an MMT training if at all possible. A partial list of MMT introductory workshops can be found on the MMT website (*http://mindfulnessandmodificationtherapy.com*). In addition, we are also available to conduct trainings around the country, with options that include public workshops, customized trainings for specific groups or clinics, and individualized supervision. For more information about potentially scheduling an MMT training, please contact us through the MMT website.

ONLINE RESOURCES

In addition, please use this book as a reference and tool for sharpening your skills as you conduct sessions and encounter new issues with clients. Chapters 2–5 are intended to be especially amenable to repeated reading. As a reminder, therapist sheets, scripts, handouts, and guided audios are also available online (see the box at the end of the table of contents).

Finally, updates on MMT research and other information can be found on the MMT website.

Thank you for reading this book. And thank you for doing the work that you do.

References

Allen, K. L., Byrne, S. M., Oddy, W. H., & Crosby, R. D. (2013). Early onset binge eating and purging eating disorders: Course and outcome in a population-based study of adolescents. *Journal of Abnormal Child Psychology, 41*(7), 1083–1096.

Baker, T. B., Piper, M. E., McCarthy, D. E., Majeskie, M. R., & Fiore, M. C. (2004). Addiction motivation reformulated: An affective processing model of negative reinforcement. *Psychological Review, 111*(1), 33–51.

Bateman, A. W., & Fonagy, P. (2004). Mentalization-based treatment of BPD. *Journal of Personality Disorders, 18*(1), 36–51.

Berking, M., & Whitley, B. (2014). *Affect regulation training: A practitioner's manual.* New York: Springer Science + Business Media.

Borders, A., Earleywine, M., & Jajodia, A. (2010). Could mindfulness decrease anger, hostility, and aggression by decreasing rumination? *Aggressive Behavior, 36*(1), 28–44.

Bowen, S., Chawla, N., & Marlatt, G. A. (2010). *Mindfulness-based relapse prevention for addictive behaviors: A clinician's guide.* New York: Guilford Press.

Bowen, S., Witkiewitz, K., Clifasefi, S. L., Grow, J., Chawla, N., Hsu, S. H., et al. (2014). Relative efficacy of mindfulness-based relapse prevention, standard relapse prevention, and treatment as usual for substance use disorders: A randomized clinical trial. *JAMA Psychiatry, 71*(5), 547–556.

Bulik, C. M., Sullivan, P. F., Carter, F. A., & Joyce, P. R. (1997). Lifetime comorbidity of alcohol dependence in women with bulimia nervosa. *Addictive Behaviors, 22*(4), 437–446.

Castonguay, L. G., & Hill, C. E. (2012). The corrective experience: A core principle for therapeutic change. In L. G. Castonguay & C. E. Hill (Eds.), *Transformation in psychotherapy: Corrective experiences across cognitive behavioral, humanistic, and psychodynamic approaches* (pp. 3–10). Washington, DC: American Psychological Association.

Cheetham, A., Allen, N. B., Yücel, M., & Lubman, D. I. (2010). The role of affective dysregulation in drug addiction. *Clinical Psychology Review, 30*(6), 621–634.

Cooper, M. L., Frone, M. R., Russell, M., & Mudar, P. (1995). Drinking to regulate positive and negative emotions: A motivational model of alcohol use. *Journal of Personality and Social Psychology, 69*(5), 990–1005.

Day, N. L., Helsel, A., Sonon, K., & Goldschmidt, L. (2013). The association between prenatal alcohol exposure and behavior at 22 years of age. *Alcoholism: Clinical and Experimental Research, 37*(7), 1171–1178.

de Souza, I. C. W., de Barros, V. V., Gomide, H. P., Mendes Miranda, T. C., de Paula Menezes, V., Kozasa, E. H., et al. (2015). Mindfulness-based interventions for the treatment of smoking: A systematic literature review. *Journal of Alternative and Complementary Medicine, 21*(3), 129–140.

Díaz-Morales, J. F., Ferrari, J. R., & Cohen, J. R. (2008). Indecision and avoidant procrastination: The role of morningness–eveningness and time perspective in chronic delay lifestyles. *Journal of General Psychology, 135*(3), 228–240.

Dimeff, L. A., & Koerner, K. (2007). *Dialectical behavior therapy in clinical practice: Applications across disorders and settings.* New York: Guilford Press.

Eisenberg, N., & Morris, A. S. (2002). Children's emotion-related regulation. In R. V. Kail (Ed.), *Advances in child development and behavior* (Vol. 30, pp. 189–229). San Diego, CA: Academic Press.

Eysenck, S. B., & Eysenck, H. J. (1978). Impulsiveness and venturesomeness: Their position in a dimensional system of personality description. *Psychological Reports, 43*(3, Pt. 2), 1247–1255.

Fix, R. L., & Fix, S. T. (2013). The effects of mindfulness-based treatments for aggression: A critical review. *Aggression and Violent Behavior, 18*(2), 219–227.

Godfrey, K. M., Gallo, L. C., & Afari, N. (2015). Mindfulness-based interventions for binge eating: A systematic review and meta-analysis. *Journal of Behavioral Medicine, 38*(2), 348–362.

Goldman, D., Oroszi, G., & Ducci, F. (2005). The genetics of addictions: Uncovering the genes. *Nature Reviews Genetics, 6*(7), 521–532.

Goodman, A. (2008). Neurobiology of addiction: An integrative review. *Biochemical Pharmacology, 75*(1), 266–322.

Gratz, K. L. (2006). Risk factors for deliberate self-harm among female college students: The role and interaction of childhood maltreatment, emotional inexpressivity, and affect intensity/reactivity. *American Journal of Orthopsychiatry, 76*, 238–250.

Greenberg, L. S. (2004). Emotion-focused therapy. *Clinical Psychology and Psychotherapy, 11*(1), 3–16.

Griffiths, M. (2005). A "components" model of addiction within a biopsychosocial framework. *Journal of Substance Use, 10*(4), 191–197.

Hayes, A. M., Beevers, C. G., Feldman, G. C., Laurenceau, J., & Perlman, C. (2005). Avoidance and processing as predictors of symptom change and positive growth in an integrative therapy for depression. *International Journal of Behavioral Medicine, 12*(2), 111–122.

Hayes, S., Strosahl, K., & Wilson, K. (2011). *Acceptance and commitment therapy: The process and practice of mindful change* (2nd ed.). New York: Guilford Press.

Holzel, B. K., Carmody, J., Vangel, M., Congleton, C., Yerramsetti, S. M., Gard, T., et al. (2011). Mindfulness practice leads to increases in regional brain gray matter density. *Psychiatry Research: Neuroimaging, 191*(1), 36–43.

Kabat-Zinn, J. (1982). An outpatient program in behavioral medicine for chronic pain patients based on the practice of mindfulness meditation: Theoretical considerations and preliminary results. *General Hospital Psychiatry, 4*(1), 33–47.

Kabat-Zinn, J. (2002). *Guided mindfulness meditation* [CD recordings]. Lexington, MA: Sounds True.

Kabat-Zinn, J. (2005). *Full catastrophe living: Using the wisdom of your body and mind to face stress, pain, and illness* (15th anniversary ed.). New York: Delta/Bantam Dell.

Kelly, A. C., & Tasca, G. A. (2016). Within-persons predictors of change during eating disorders treatment: An examination of self-compassion, self-criticism, shame, and eating disorder symptoms. *International Journal of Eating Disorders, 49*(7), 716–722.

Klonsky, E. D. (2007). The functions of deliberate self-injury: A review of the evidence. *Clinical Psychology Review, 27*(2), 226–239.

Klonsky, E. D., & Muehlenkamp, J. J. (2007). Self-injury: A research review for the practitioner. *Journal of Clinical Psychology, 63*(11), 1045–1056.

Koch, A. J., D'Mello, S. D., & Sackett, P. R. (2015). A meta-analysis of gender stereotypes and bias in experimental simulations of employment decision making. *Journal of Applied Psychology, 100*(1), 128–161.

Koekkoek, B., Hutschemaekers, G., van Meijel, B., & Schene, A. (2011). How do patients come to be seen as "difficult"?: A mixed-methods study in community mental health care. *Social Science and Medicine, 72*(4), 504–512.

Koekkoek, B., van Meijel, B., & Hutschemaekers, G. (2006). "Difficult patients" in mental health care: A review. *Psychiatric Services, 57*(6), 795–802.

Krause, E. D., Mendelson, T., & Lynch, T. R. (2003). Childhood emotional invalidation and adult psychological distress: The mediating role of emotional inhibition. *Child Abuse and Neglect, 27*(2), 199–213.

Kristeller, J. L. (2015). Mindfulness, eating disorders, and food intake regulation. In B. D. Ostafin, M. D. Robinson, & B. P. Meier (Eds.), *Handbook of mindfulness and self-regulation* (pp. 199–215). New York: Springer Science + Business Media.

Krug, I., Treasure, J., Anderluh, M., Bellodi, L., Cellini, E., di Bernardo, M., et al. (2008). Present and lifetime comorbidity of tobacco, alcohol and drug use in eating disorders: A European multicenter study. *Drug and Alcohol Dependence, 97*(1–2), 169–179.

Lavender, J. M., Jardin, B. F., & Anderson, D. A. (2009). Bulimic symptoms in undergraduate men and women: Contributions of mindfulness and thought suppression. *Eating Behaviors, 10*(4), 228–231.

Leung, A. K., Liou, S., Qui, L., Kwan, L. Y., Chiu, C., & Yong, J. C. (2014). The role of instrumental emotion regulation in the emotions–creativity link. *Emotion, 14*(5), 846–856.

Linehan, M. M. (1993a). *Cognitive-behavioral treatment of borderline personality disorder.* New York: Guilford Press.

Linehan, M. M. (1993b). *Skills training manual for treating borderline personality disorder.* New York: Guilford Press.

Lisman, J., & Sternberg, E. J. (2013). Habit and nonhabit systems for unconscious and conscious behavior: Implications for multitasking. *Journal of Cognitive Neuroscience, 25*(2), 273–283.

Lundh, L., Karim, J., & Quilisch, E. (2007). Deliberate self-harm in 15-year-old adolescents: A pilot study with a modified version of the deliberate self-harm inventory. *Scandinavian Journal of Psychology, 48*(1), 33–41.

Manley, R. S., & Boland, F. J. (1983). Side-effects and weight gain following a smoking cessation program. *Addictive Behaviors, 8*(4), 375–380.

McFarlane, T., Olmsted, M. P., & Trottier, K. (2008). Timing and prediction of relapse in a transdiagnostic eating disorder sample. *International Journal of Eating Disorders, 41*(7), 587–593.

McLellan, A. T., Lewis, D. C., O'Brian, C. P., & Kleber, H. D. (2000). Drug dependence, a chronic medical illness: Implications for treatment, insurance, and outcomes evaluation. *Journal of the American Medical Association, 284*(13), 1689–1695.

Merriam-Webster Online. (n.d.). [Definition of *manipulate*]. Retrieved February 9, 2017, from *www.merriam-webster.com/dictionary/manipulate.*

Mezzich, A. C., Tarter, R. E., Giancola, P. R., Lu, S., Kirisci, L., & Parks, S. (1997). Substance use and risky sexual behavior in female adolescents. *Drug and Alcohol Dependence, 44*(2–3), 157–166.

Milkman, K. L., Akinola, M., & Chugh, D. (2015). What happens before?: A field experiment exploring how pay and representation differentially shape bias on the pathway into organizations. *Journal of Applied Psychology, 100*(6), 1678–1712.

Miller, W. R., Benefield, R. G., & Tonigan, J. S. (1993). Enhancing motivation for change in problem drinking: A controlled comparison of two therapist styles. *Journal of Consulting and Clinical Psychology, 61*(3), 455–461.

Miller, W. R., & Rollnick, S. (2012). *Motivational interviewing: Helping people change.* (3rd ed.). New York: Guilford Press.

Miller, W. R., Walters, S. T., & Bennett, M. E. (2001). How effective is alcoholism treatment in the United States? *Journal of Studies on Alcohol, 62*(2), 211–220.

Moulton, S. J., Newman, E., Power, K., Swanson, V., & Day, K. (2015). Childhood trauma and eating psychopathology: A mediating role for dissociation and emotion dysregulation? *Child Abuse and Neglect, 39,* 167–174.

Moyers, T. B., & Miller, W. R. (2013). Is low therapist empathy toxic? *Psychology of Addictive Behaviors, 27*(3), 878–884.

Moyers, T. B., Miller, W. R., & Hendrickson, S. M. L. (2005). How does motivational interviewing work?: Therapist interpersonal skill predicts client involvement within motivational interviewing sessions. *Journal of Consulting and Clinical Psychology, 73*(4), 590–598.

Neff, K. D., Kirkpatrick, K. L., & Rude, S. S. (2007). Self-compassion and adaptive psychological functioning. *Journal of Research in Personality, 41*(1), 139–154.

Nixon, M. K., Cloutier, P. F., & Aggarwal, S. (2002). Affect regulation and addictive aspects of repetitive self-injury in hospitalized adolescents. *Journal of the American Academy of Child and Adolescent Psychiatry, 41*(11), 1333–1341.

Petry, N. M., Stinson, F. S., & Grant, B. F. (2005). Comorbidity of DSM-IV pathological gambling and other psychiatric disorders: Results from the National Epidemiologic Survey on Alcohol and Related Conditions. *Journal of Clinical Psychiatry, 66*(5), 564–574.

Post, F. (1994). Creativity and psychopathology: A study of 291 world-famous men. *British Journal of Psychiatry, 165*(2), 22–34.

Project MATCH Research Group. (1998). Matching patients with alcohol disorders to treatments: Clinical implications from Project MATCH. *Journal of Mental Health, 7*(6), 589–602.

Racine, E., Bell, E., Zizzo, N., & Green, C. (2015). Public discourse on the biology of alcohol addiction: Implications for stigma, self-control, essentialism, and coercive policies in pregnancy. *Neuroethics, 8*(2), 177–186.

Raymond, N. C., Neumeyer, B., Thuras, P., Weller, C. L., Eckert, E. D., Crow, S. J., et al. (1999). Compulsive and impulsive traits in individuals with obese binge eating disorder and bulimia nervosa. *Eating Disorders: Journal of Treatment and Prevention, 7*(4), 299–317.

Saucier, D. A., Miller, C. T., & Doucet, N. (2005). Differences in helping whites and blacks: A meta-analysis. *Personality and Social Psychology Review, 9*(1), 2–16.

Segal, Z. V., Williams, J. M. G., & Teasdale, J. D. (2002). *Mindfulness-based cognitive therapy for depression*. New York: Guilford Press.

Selby, E. A., Bulik, C. M., Thornton, L., Brandt, H. A., Crawford, S., Fichter, M. M., et al. (2010). Refining behavioral dysregulation in borderline personality disorder using a sample of women with anorexia nervosa. *Personality Disorders: Theory, Research, and Treatment, 1*(4), 250–257.

Sirois, F. M., & Kitner, R. (2015). Less adaptive or more maladaptive?: A meta-analytic investigation of procrastination and coping. *European Journal of Personality, 29*(4), 433–444.

Spinella, M., Martino, S., & Ferri, C. (2013). Mindfulness and addictive behaviors. *Journal of Behavioral Health, 2*(1), 1–7.

Tenenbaum, H. R., & Ruck, M. D. (2007). Are teachers' expectations different for racial minority than for European American students?: A meta-analysis. *Journal of Educational Psychology, 99*(2), 253–273.

Vansteelandt, K., Claes, L., Muehlenkamp, J., De Cuyper, K., Lemmens, J., Probst, M., et al. (2013). Variability in affective activation predicts non-suicidal self-injury in eating disorders. *European Eating Disorders Review, 21*(2), 143–147.

White, W. L., & Miller, W. R. (2007). The use of confrontation in addiction treatment: History, science and time for change. *Counselor, 8*(4), 12–30.

Williams, J. M. G., Fennell, M., Barnhofer, T., Crane, R., & Silverton, S. (2015). *Mindfulness and the transformation of despair: Working with people at risk of suicide*. New York: Guilford Press.

Witkiewitz, K. A., & Bowen, S. (2010). Depression, craving, and substance use following a randomized trial of mindfulness-based relapse prevention. *Journal of Consulting and Clinical Psychology, 78*(3), 362–374.

Witkiewitz, K. A., Lustyk, M. K., & Bowen, S. (2013). Retraining the addicted brain: A review of hypothesized neurobiological mechanisms of mindfulness-based relapse prevention. *Psychology of Addictive Behaviors, 27*(2), 351–365.

Witkiewitz, K. A., & Marlatt, G. A. (2007). *Therapist's guide to evidence-based relapse prevention.* San Diego, CA: Elsevier Academic Press.

Wolfe, S., Kay-Lambkin, F., Bowman, J., & Childs, S. (2013). To enforce or engage: The relationship between coercion, treatment motivation and therapeutic alliance within community-based drug and alcohol clients. *Addictive Behaviors, 38*(5), 2187–2195.

Wupperman, P., Burns, N., Edwards, E. E., Pugach, C., & Spada, A. (2019a). *Mindfulness and modification therapy for behavioral dysregulation: Results from a pilot trial targeting binge eating.* Manuscript in preparation.

Wupperman, P., Burns, N., Pugach, C., & Edwards, E. (2019b). *Treatment for individuals with severe mental illness who use drugs while maintained on methadone: Mindfulness and modification therapy.* Manuscript under review.

Wupperman, P., Burns, N., Spada, A., Pugach, C., & Shapiro, R. (2018). *Case studies of mindfulness and modification therapy for a variety of dysregulated behaviors.* Unpublished data.

Wupperman, P., Cohen, M. G., Haller, D. L., Flom, P., Litt, L. C., & Rounsaville, B. J. (2015). Mindfulness and modification therapy for behavioral dysregulation: A comparison trial focused on substance use and aggression. *Journal of Clinical Psychology, 71*(10), 964–978.

Wupperman, P., Fickling, M., Klemanski, D. H., Berking, M., & Whitman, J. B. (2013). Borderline personality features and harmful dysregulated behavior: The mediational effect of mindfulness. *Journal of Clinical Psychology, 69*(9), 903–911.

Wupperman, P., Marlatt, G. A., Cunningham, A., Bowen, S., Berking, M., Mulvihill-Rivera, N., et al. (2012). Mindfulness and modification therapy for behavioral dysregulation: Results from a pilot study targeting alcohol use and aggression in women. *Journal of Clinical Psychology, 68*(1), 50–66.

Wupperman, P., Neumann, C. S., & Axelrod, S. R. (2008). Do deficits in mindfulness underlie borderline personality features and core difficulties? *Journal of Personality Disorders, 22*(5), 466–482.

Index

Note. *f* following a page number indicates a figure.

List of Audio Files

Track	Title	Run Time	URL
1.	*Color Body Scan*	12:41	www.guilford.com/MMT-scan
2.	*Body Movement*	14:10	www.guilford.com/MMT-movement
3.	*Mirror*	13:54	www.guilford.com/MMT-mirror
4.	*Mighty Tree*	8:52	www.guilford.com/MMT-tree
5.	*May You Be*	10:43	www.guilford.com/MMT-may
6.	*Thoughts*	8:01	www.guilford.com/MMT-thoughts
7.	*Sounds*	6:26	www.guilford.com/MMT-sounds